Yellow Flags: Quarantine volume 5
October 2020-November 2020

Guy Breshears

<Published by Guy Breshears>

First Printing: <2022>

ISBN: 978-988-75614-4-6

Other books by the author:

Loyal till Death: A Diary of the 13th New York Artillery

Major Granville Haller: Dismissed with Malice

To Seize Their Lands: Manifest Destiny in Washington State

Visit http://www.heritagebooks.com for more information of these books

Of Papers and Protests: Hong Kong responds to Occupy Central, volumes 1, 2, 3, 4, 5

Tales of a Traveler

Block Rosary: Hong Kong

Catholic answers: towards government and education

Visit http://www.lulu.com/spotlight/gbreshears for more information about these books

For more information about this book contact the publisher:

Guy Breshears
PO Box 88409
Sham Shui Po Post Office
Kowloon
Hong Kong

Published in Hong Kong

Dedication

To my wife who has stood by me ever since I have arrived in Hong Kong. I could not have survived without her continuing support.

Also, to Our Lady of China: Pray for all that live here so that those who govern will do so with equal justice for all. Finally, pray for the faithful who live here and have recourse to thee

Introduction

Why the title of "yellow flags"? In the past a yellow flag flying from a ship meant, according to the International Code of Signal (ICS) flags, that it was under quarantine due to an infectious illness. It has nothing to do, as some may claim, with protests that have been part of Hong Kong since 2014.

Today, a ship flying a solid yellow flag means that it is free from any illness and it requests boarding by government officials and given clearance to dock as well as being certified of having no infectious illness onboard.

But with the advent of radio and other means of communication there is currently no quarantine flag officially listed in the ICS. If you see a single yellow flag on a ship coming into a harbor it means that the ship's captain is declaring that the ship is healthy. Double yellow flags flying means that the ship requests a health inspection before docking.

On 31 December 2019, while most of Hong Kong was getting ready to celebrate the coming of the New Year the Centre for Health Protection issued a statement that they were closely monitoring a cluster of pneumonia cases in Wuhan. No one knew what exactly the problems were nor could they foresee events that these "pneumonia cases" would cause for both Hong Kong and the rest of the world.

The Hong Kong government was slow to react and didn't seem to take it very seriously when more news came from China about this new type of infection. They insisted to keep borders open and everyone treat it like a common flu season.

Many of the older generation of Hong Kongers took a different approach since many of them had lived through SARS and didn't want to see that happen again. So they started wearing masks and taking other precautions. If the government didn't want to do much, then the people would do something.

Finally, after lots of dragging their feet and making excuses, the government acted. On advice from China they slowly shut down many of the boarder crossing check points and started to issue social distancing rules. They also closed schools and many people, including the government, were told to work from home.

People started to panic and started to stockpile handmasks, sanitizers, rice, and toilet paper, to name a few. Prices also went up as people saw limited supplies as a way to make money.

The government tried to calm the people about hoarding supplies but it didn't work well. It was only after the various stores limit the amount of items you could purchase that the supplies of items began to increase.

In terms of facemask supplies, many private organizations were able to go around the world and purchase larges quantities of masks. The government kept on promising that they had bought a large supply of masks but it was mostly empty promises. A few eventually showed up.

With China facing it's own health crisis it was nearly impossible to get masks from there. So the government made a program to help local Hong Kong businesses to start making masks. Some have done well and others have gone away.

In late May 2020 schools were re-opened on a limited basis as well as loosening of social distance rules. It was hoped that since the number of cases were lower than normal then it would just be a matter of time before Hong Kong got back to re-building lost revenue and get back to normal.

In July 2020 with most people going about their business a new wave hit Hong Kong with total number of people being reported infected surpassing the number that were infected during SARS. The government was puzzled of where it came from and who they might have infected. Social distancing rules were put back into effect, schools were closed for the summer, and many people were ordered to work from home. People started to worry again as toilet paper and rice disappeared off store shelves and stores were forced to limit quantities so that more people would be able to get some of the basic things they needed to survive.

At the end of government announcements of the Centre for Health Protection they write:

To prevent pneumonia and respiratory tract infection, members of the public should always maintain good personal and environmental hygiene. They are advised to:

• Wear a surgical mask when taking public transport or staying in crowded places. It is important to wear a mask properly, including performing hand hygiene before wearing and after removing a mask;

• Perform hand hygiene frequently, especially before touching the mouth, nose or eyes, after touching public installations such as handrails or doorknobs, or when hands are contaminated by respiratory secretions after coughing or sneezing;
• Maintain drainage pipes properly and regularly (about once a week) pour about half a litre of water into each drain outlet (U-trap) to ensure environmental hygiene;
• Cover all floor drain outlets when they are not in use;
• After using the toilet, put the toilet lid down before flushing to avoid spreading germs;
• Wash hands with liquid soap and water, and rub for at least 20 seconds. Then rinse with water and dry with a disposable paper towel. If hand washing facilities are not available, or when hands are not visibly soiled, performing hand hygiene with 70 to 80 per cent alcohol-based handrub is an effective alternative;
• Cover your mouth and nose with tissue paper when sneezing or coughing. Dispose of soiled tissues into a lidded rubbish bin, then wash hands thoroughly; and
• When having respiratory symptoms, wear a surgical mask, refrain from work or attending class at school, avoid going to crowded places and seek medical advice promptly.

While this is good advice it is not included in this edition for their daily announcements. Also, any attachments or annexes, or other references made are also not include in this book.

The prophets that have been before me, and before thee from the beginning, and have prophesied concerning many countries, and concerning great kingdoms, of war, and of affliction, and of famine.[1]

[1] Jeremias 28:8 (Douay-Rheims version)

Table of Contents

October 1[1]

FEHD steps up inspections at food premises relating to anti-epidemic measures

****

The Food and Environmental Hygiene Department (FEHD) conducted a joint operation with the Police yesterday (September 30) to step up inspections at catering business premises including bars in the Central and Western District, and remind food business operators and food handlers to strictly comply with the relevant requirements under the Prevention and Control of Disease (Requirements and Directions) (Business and Premises) Regulation (Cap. 599F) (the Regulation).

A spokesman for the FEHD said, "The latest directions issued by the Secretary for Food and Health in relation to catering business premises under the Regulation remain effective, under which food business operators and food handlers have to comply with a series of requirements and restrictions. Among these, the number of customers at any bar or pub must not exceed half of the normal seating capacity of the premises and no more than two persons may be seated together at one table; live performance and dancing must not be allowed in any catering business premises; a mask must be worn at all times within the premises, except when the person is consuming food or drink; and body temperature screening must be conducted before the person is allowed to enter the catering premises and hand sanitisers must be provided."

"During the operation in Lan Kwai Fong of the Central and Western District last night, the FEHD inspected 17 catering business premises (including bars) and initiated legal proceedings of prosecution against the operators of seven premises. These are mainly about violating the requirements on the distance between tables and wearing a mask at all times within the premises except when consuming food or drink," the spokesman said.

The spokesman said that the FEHD will continue to step up inspections at food premises across the territory and conduct joint operations with the Police in the long holidays to ensure that food business operators and food handlers strictly comply with the directions under the Regulation, and will take enforcement actions against offenders so as to minimise the risk of transmission of COVID-19 in food premises.

Under the Regulation, licensees and operators of food premises must strictly comply with the series of requirements and restrictions. Contravening the requirements and restrictions is a criminal offence. Offenders are subject to a maximum fine of $50,000 and imprisonment for six months.

The spokesman appealed to food business operators and food handlers to comply with the relevant regulation on prevention and control of disease in a concerted and persistent manner, with a view to keeping workers, customers and the public safe. The FEHD will continue to step up inspections and take stringent enforcement actions against offenders in defiance of relevant

[1] https://www.info.gov.hk/gia/general/202010/01.htm

legislations on prevention and control of disease as well as environmental hygiene and food safety issues.

Issued at HKT 0:36

CE's speech at National Day reception

****

Following is the speech (English translation) by the Chief Executive, Mrs Carrie Lam, at the National Day Reception in Celebration of the 71st Anniversary of the Founding of the People's Republic of China today (October 1):

Distinguished guests, fellow citizens,

I am very pleased to celebrate National Day with you, which this year coincides with the Mid-Autumn Festival. With the easing of the third wave of the epidemic that has plagued our city since early July, members of the public have gradually resumed work and students have returned to school. We can all celebrate these special occasions with relatives and friends while strictly observing social distancing and other precautionary measures.

The year 2020 has presented mankind with an unprecedented public health crisis. As of today, the number of confirmed COVID-19 cases worldwide has exceeded 33 million while the death toll has sadly reached one million. With the exception of China, the epidemic situation around the globe shows no signs of abating and is even rapidly worsening in some places, dealing a heavy blow to various sectors and industries and resulting in rising unemployment. It seems we have some time to go before we can emerge from the economic doldrums.

On the other hand, by vigorously suppressing and strictly controlling the epidemic, our country has already regained its economic momentum. In the first half of this year, there was a "V-shaped" rebound in China's Gross Domestic Product (GDP) in the second quarter with a growth rate of 3.2 per cent after a sharp drop of 6.8 per cent in the first quarter. This has made China a rare bright spot among major economies and has shown once again the shift of the global economic focus from the West to the East.

The success of our country's anti-epidemic work did not come easy. As we saw from TV reports, in order to curb the spread of the virus, our compatriots in the Mainland stayed at home and strictly followed all the rules; cities were locked down; medical and healthcare staff worked round-the-clock to treat patients; supply and support teams acted as one to fight the virus. As President Xi Jinping said at a ceremony commending role models in China's fight against

COVID-19 on September 8, the fight against the epidemic was a race against time and a battle that required resolute courage and unwavering determination.

Over the past nine months, the Central Government has been paying great attention to the epidemic situation in Hong Kong and has responded positively to requests from the Hong Kong Special Administrative Region (HKSAR) Government, including supplying personal protective equipment, exporting mask production machines, assisting Hong Kong residents stranded in the Mainland and overseas to return home, and supporting three major projects to help Hong Kong suppress the third wave of the epidemic and enhance our capability to treat more patients in future. With the full assistance of the Central Government, the large-scale Universal Community Testing Programme was successfully completed in mid-September, while construction of a temporary hospital and a community treatment facility has also commenced.

The Central Government's assistance to Hong Kong in fighting the epidemic demonstrates, once again, that it has always given Hong Kong its full support in overcoming various difficulties and challenges since our return to the Motherland. Other examples include support rendered to ride out and overcome the serious threats to Hong Kong's financial stability posed by the 1997 Asian financial crisis, the life and health risks and economic recession caused by the 2003 SARS outbreak, and the negative impact of the 2008 global financial tsunami.

Apart from creating a safe haven for us in times of turmoil, and giving us a shot in the arm when needed, the Central Government has also leveraged Hong Kong's role in planning and taking forward the country's overall development and has actively promoted exchanges and co-operation between Hong Kong and the Mainland. The work of the current-term Government is an example. In the past three years, thanks to the support of Central Government leaders and the co-ordination of relevant ministries, the HKSAR Government has signed over 90 co-operation agreements with the Mainland. Strategically important ones include the "Framework Agreement on Deepening Guangdong-Hong Kong-Macao Cooperation in the Development of the Greater Bay Area" signed with the National Development and Reform Commission (NDRC) and the governments of Guangdong and Macao in July 2017; the "Arrangement between the NDRC and the Government of the HKSAR for Advancing Hong Kong's Full Participation in and Contribution to the Belt and Road Initiative" signed with the NDRC in December 2017; the "Arrangement on Enhancing Innovation and Technology Cooperation between the Mainland and Hong Kong" signed with the Ministry of Science and Technology in September 2018; the "Arrangement on Reciprocal Recognition and Enforcement of Judgments in Civil and Commercial Matters by the Courts of the Mainland and of the HKSAR" signed with the Supreme People's Court in January 2019; and the "Agreement Concerning Amendment to the CEPA Agreement on Trade in Services" signed with the Ministry of Commerce in November 2019. All this shows that the Central Government always gives us strong backing and helps maintain Hong Kong's prosperity and stability, whether Hong Kong is facing good times or bad, difficulties or opportunities.

To help extract Hong Kong from our economic predicament, we must create new engines of economic growth with the continued support of the Central Government. We have to help Hong Kong's professional services sector and enterprises target business opportunities in the Mainland market and capitalise on Hong Kong's unique role as a connector to the world under the development model of "domestic and international dual circulation" propelled by our country. The HKSAR Government will participate more actively in the drafting of the outline of our country's 14th Five-Year Plan, and will seek the Central Government's support to strengthen and enhance Hong Kong's status as an international financial centre and a global aviation hub. We will also take forward the development of the Guangdong-Hong Kong-Macao Greater Bay Area at full steam and deepen our work with Shenzhen in developing an international innovation and technology hub.

Having gone through the social unrest arising from the legislative amendment exercise of the Fugitive Offenders Ordinance in mid-2019, and having implemented the National Security Law in mid-2020, we should see very clearly that if we are to keep Hong Kong moving forward, overcome economic challenges, and meet pubic aspirations for improved livelihoods and democracy, we must have a safe and stable social environment, adhere to the "One Country" principle, safeguard national sovereignty and security, correctly understand the relationship between "One Country" and "Two Systems", and act in accordance with the Constitution and the Basic Law. Over the past three months, the plain truth is and it is obvious to see that stability has been restored to society while national security has been safeguarded, and our people can continue to enjoy their basic rights and freedoms in accordance with the law. So, no matter how severe some foreign governments, holding "double-standards", are going to level unjustified accusations against the authorities in charge of implementing the National Security Law, or aggressively imposing further sanctions against HKSAR officials responsible for safeguarding national security, I and my relevant colleagues will continue to discharge our duty to safeguard national security in accordance with the law without fear or anxiety.

I believe that as long as we uphold the "One Country, Two Systems" principle and the Basic Law wholeheartedly, work together to seize the opportunities presented by our country's new development model, communicate in a sensible way and find common ground among differences, we can certainly make Hong Kong, our home, an even better place.

May I wish our country continued prosperity and progress, Hong Kong social harmony and stability, and everyone a happy National Day and Mid-Autumn Festival.

Thank you very much.

Issued at HKT 10:02

CHP investigates 10 additional confirmed cases of COVID-19

****

The Centre for Health Protection (CHP) of the Department of Health has announced that as of 0.00am, October 1, the CHP was investigating 10 additional confirmed cases of coronavirus

disease 2019 (COVID-19), taking the number of cases to 5 098 in Hong Kong so far (comprising 5 097 confirmed cases and one probable case).

Among the newly reported cases announced, nine had a travel history during the incubation period.

The CHP's epidemiological investigations and relevant contact tracing on the confirmed cases are ongoing. For case details and contact tracing information, please see the Annex or the list of buildings with confirmed cases of COVID-19 in the past 14 days and the latest local situation of COVID-19 available on the website "COVID-19 Thematic Website" (www.coronavirus.gov.hk).

In view of the severe epidemic situation, the CHP called on members of the public to avoid going out, having social contact and dining out. They should put on a surgical mask and maintain stringent hand hygiene when they need to go out. The CHP strongly urged the elderly to stay home as far as possible and avoid going out. They should consider asking their family and friends to help with everyday tasks such as shopping for basic necessities.

A spokesman for the CHP said, "Given that the situation of COVID-19 infection remains severe and that there is a continuous increase in the number of cases reported around the world, members of the public are strongly urged to avoid all non-essential travel outside Hong Kon

"The CHP also strongly urges the public to maintain at all times strict personal and environmental hygiene, which is key to personal protection against infection and prevention of the spread of the disease in the community. On a personal level, members of the public should wear a surgical mask when having respiratory symptoms, taking public transport or staying in crowded places. They should also perform hand hygiene frequently, especially before touching the mouth, nose or eyes.

"As for household environmental hygiene, members of the public are advised to maintain drainage pipes properly, regularly pour water into drain outlets (U-traps) and cover all floor drain outlets when they are not in use. After using the toilet, they should put the toilet lid down before flushing to avoid spreading germs."

Moreover, the Government has launched the website "COVID-19 Thematic Website" (www.coronavirus.gov.hk) for announcing the latest updates on various news on COVID-19 infection and health advice to help the public understand the latest updates. Members of the public may also gain access to information via the COVID-19 WhatsApp Helpline launched by the Office of the Government Chief Information Officer. Simply by saving 9617 1823 in their phone contacts or clicking the link wa.me/85296171823?text=hi, they will be able to obtain information on COVID-19 as well as the "StayHomeSafe" mobile app and wristband via WhatsApp.

Issued at HKT 17:05

Public hospitals daily update on COVID-19 cases

****

The following is issued on behalf of the Hospital Authority:

As at 9am today (October 1), 10 COVID-19 confirmed patients were discharged from hospital in the last 24 hours. So far, a total of 4 837 patients with confirmed or probable infection have been discharged.

At present, there are 639 negative pressure rooms in public hospitals with 1 155 negative pressure beds activated. A total of 118 confirmed patients are currently hospitalised in 16 public hospitals, among which 10 patients are in critical condition, eight are in serious condition and the remaining 100 patients are in stable condition.

The Hospital Authority will maintain close contact with the Centre for Health Protection to monitor the latest developments and to inform the public and healthcare workers on the latest information in a timely manner.

Details of the above-mentioned patients are as follows:

Patient condition	Case numbers
Discharged	1316, 1498, 2479, 3215, 4921, 4987, 4988, 5063, 5073, 5084
Critical	1401, 1989, 2912, 3496, 3764, 4641, 4706, 4833, 4937, 4990
Serious	1650, 3904, 4100, 4101, 4433, 4746, 4788, 4969

Issued at HKT 18:05

QEH announces a nurse tested preliminarily positive for COVID-19

****

The following is issued on behalf of the Hospital Authority:

Queen Elizabeth Hospital (QEH) made an announcement today (October 1) regarding a nurse tested preliminarily positive for COVID-19:

A nurse of a general medical ward at QEH has onset of cough on September 28, and attended Accident and Emergency Department on September 30 due to fever. The hospital arranged a COVID-19 deep throat saliva test for him. The test result was preliminarily positive this morning (October 1). The patient is currently receiving isolation treatment at the hospital and is in stable condition.

The hospital reported the case to the Centre for Health Protection (CHP) upon the preliminary test result of the nurse and conducted epidemiological tracing. The nurse concerned performed routine clinical duties in the ward and was equipped with appropriate personal protective equipment during his work. He did not have any contact with COVID-19 confirmed patients in the past two weeks. So far, no patient in the ward is classified as a close contact.

In addition, six staff members who had meals respectively with the nurse at different time are classified as close contacts. They are all asymptomatic and need to be quarantined. The hospital will follow up with the CHP for their condition.

According to the guideline, the hospital adopted admission screening for all in-patients. All existing patients in the ward were tested negative on admission. The preliminary investigation shows that there is no evidence suggesting the staff member acquired the disease in the hospital. The hospital has conducted tests for the patients and the staff members in the ward. So far, 29 staff members and 44 patients are tested negative.

As a precautionary measure, admission of patients to the ward concerned has been suspended. The hospital has arranged thorough cleansing and disinfection for the ward concerned. QEH will continue to closely monitor the health of our staff members and patients and communicate with the CHP about the latest situation.

Issued at HKT 20:25

October 2[2]

Grave sweepers urged to stagger grave-sweeping activities over wider period before and after Chung Yeung Festival

****

To prevent the spread of COVID-19, the Food and Environmental Hygiene Department (FEHD) today (October 2) appealed to members of the public to stagger grave-sweeping

---

[2] https://www.info.gov.hk/gia/general/202010/02.htm

activities over a wider period before and after the Chung Yeung Festival (October 25), to avoid grave sweeping during the peak period on the day of the Chung Yeung Festival so as to avoid overcrowding, which might increase the risk of disease transmission.

A spokesman for the FEHD urged people visiting cemeteries and columbaria paying respect to ancestors during the festival to avoid meal gatherings at worship sites or in crowded places. They are also urged to maintain appropriate social distancing with other people as far as possible, comply with relevant regulations on prevention and control of disease, maintain good personal hygiene and keep the environment clean when sweeping graves.

The spokesman said, "The opening hours of public columbaria under the FEHD will be extended to 7am to 7pm two weeks before and after the Chung Yeung Festival (the period between October 10 to November 8) to lessen crowd conditions. The FEHD will provide special cleaning services such as disinfection of handrails and lift buttons inside public cemeteries and columbaria during the festival period, and deploy more staff to clear undergrowth and remove rubbish, and empty bottles and containers left behind by grave sweepers. We will also remove water in containers and incense burners, and level the ground surface to prevent accumulation of water. Furthermore, additional litter bins and toilet facilities will be provided."

The spokesman urged the public to co-operate by clearing stagnant water and rubbish before leaving to prevent mosquito breeding. Containers such as lunch boxes, drink cans, plastic bags and buckets for burning incense should also be removed. As a precaution against mosquitoes, grave sweepers are advised to wear light-coloured long-sleeved tops and trousers, and apply insect repellent to exposed parts of their body.

The FEHD has also advised managers of private cemeteries to take similar precautions against mosquitoes.

To protect the environment and to prevent hill fires, members of the public are encouraged to replace incense burning with flowers when paying tribute to their ancestors. Grave sweepers should take extra care when burning incense, which should only be carried out inside a designated joss paper furnace or iron bucket. They should make sure that all fires have gone out before leaving. Grave sweepers are also reminded to keep flammable items (such as alcohol antiseptic sprays and alcohol-based instant hand sanitisers) away from fires.

The Government has been promoting green burials, and the FEHD has set up the Internet Memorial Service webpage (www.memorial.gov.hk) and its mobile application for members of the public to pay tribute to their deceased beloved ones anywhere and anytime.

The spokesman also urged the public to pay attention to special traffic and transport arrangements which will be implemented during the Chung Yeung Festival. Access to cemeteries and columbaria of the FEHD will be closed to all vehicles while the special traffic and transport arrangements are in operation, except for those with permission. The spokesman reminded the public that on Saturdays, Sundays and the public holiday of the two weeks before and after Chung Yeung Festival, Nim Wan Road to Tsang Tsui Columbarium will be closed. Grave sweepers are not allowed to walk, drive or take a taxi to Tsang Tsui Columbarium, and they have to take the KMB special route 56S plying between MTR Tuen Mun Station and Tsang Tsui Columbarium.

For details of the special traffic and transport arrangements in the vicinity of cemeteries and crematoria during the Chung Yeung Festival, please visit the Transport Department website (www.td.gov.hk).

Issued at HKT 16:00

Public may collect CuMask+™ at over 300 locations starting October 5

****

The Innovation and Technology Bureau announced today (October 2) that citizens who have not obtained the CuMask+™ may collect them at post offices across the territory from October 5 to 31. Residents of public rental housing estates under the Hong Kong Housing Authority (HA) and rental estates under the Hong Kong Housing Society (HS) may also collect the CuMask+™ from their respective estate management offices.

Procedures for collecting CuMask+™

Citizens should present to the staff at post offices or estate management offices the original of their own Hong Kong identity card (HKID) (copies will not be accepted). The staff will input the citizen's HKID number into a computer or a handheld device immediately and provide two adult-sized CuMask+™ if the citizen has not obtained a mask, or one adult-sized CuMask+™ if the citizen has already obtained a mask. The computers and handheld devices used by post offices or estate management offices will not store any personal data of the citizens.

Collection points

(1) Post offices

Citizens can visit any of the 121 post offices (except mobile post offices) during the respective office hours to collect the CuMask+™. Taking into account the sizes of individual post offices and the availability of other collection point(s) in the area, the number of masks available for collection at each post office each day will vary. Citizens can check the relevant information at the following website:
www.hongkongpost.hk/en/about_us/network/cuMaskOffices/index.html.

(2) Public Rental Housing Estate Management Offices under the HA

Residents of the 186 public rental housing estates under the HA can visit their respective estate management offices to collect the CuMask+™ during the time slots listed below (excluding estate management offices in Tenants Purchase Scheme estates and Buy or Rent Option courts):

October 5 to 9 (Monday to Friday)

2pm to 5pm

October 12 to 30 (Mondays to Fridays, except public holidays)

9.30am to 12.30pm and 2pm to 5pm

(3) Rental Estate Management Offices under the HS

Residents of the 20 rental estates under the HS can visit their respective estate management offices to collect the CuMask+™ during the timeslots listed below:

Mondays to Fridays (except public holidays)

8.30am to 12.30pm and 1.30pm to 5.30pm

Office hours of Sha Tau Kok Chuen Estate Management Office:

Mondays to Fridays

8.45am to 12.45pm and 1.30pm to 4.30pm

Office hours of Tui Min Hoi Chuen Estate Management Office:

Mondays and Thursdays

8.30am to 12.30pm

Tuesdays

8.30am to 12.30pm and 1.30pm to 5.30pm

Authorised collection arrangements

Those who are unable to collect the mask(s) in person may authorise others to collect the CuMask+™ on their behalf at post offices or estate management offices. Each authorisee can collect the mask(s) on behalf of a maximum of two authorisers on each occasion. Detailed arrangements are as follows:

(1) Collection of masks at post offices on behalf of others

The authorisee should present to the staff at post offices a copy (photocopy or electronic copy) of the authoriser's HKID and the original or a copy (photocopy or electronic copy) of the authorisation letter signed by the authoriser. The authorisation letter should include the name and HKID number of the authoriser and the name and HKID number of the authorisee, and specify that the authorisation is for collection of the adult-sized CuMask+™. A template of the authorisation letter has been uploaded onto the CuMask+™ website (qmask.gov.hk) for reference. The authorisee should also present to the staff the original of his/her HKID to prove his/her identity.

(2) Collection of masks at estate management offices on behalf of tenants of public rental housing estates of the HA and rental estates of the HS

The authorisee should present to the staff at estate management offices the original of the tenancy agreement of the unit in which the authoriser resides and a copy (photocopy or electronic copy) of the authoriser's HKID. The name of the authoriser must appear on the tenancy agreement. There is no need to present a separate authorisation letter, but the authorisee should present to the staff the original of his/her HKID to prove his/her identity.

The staff at post offices or estate management offices will input the HKID number of the authoriser into a computer or a handheld device immediately to verify the eligibility of the authoriser. The staff will also input the name and HKID number of the authorisee into the computer or the handheld device. The information will be immediately transmitted to the central system, solely for record-keeping purposes in relation to mask distribution. The computers and handheld devices used by post offices or estate management offices will not store any personal data of the citizens.

Enquiries

For details about the CuMask+™ or other enquiries, including the addresses of public rental housing estate management offices under the HA and rental estate management offices under the HS, please visit the CuMask+™ website (qmask.gov.hk). Citizens may also call the hotline at 3142 2313 or check via the WhatsApp Helpline 9617 1823.

Issued at HKT 16:00

CHP investigates seven additional confirmed cases of COVID-19

****

The Centre for Health Protection (CHP) of the Department of Health has announced that as of 0.00am, October 2, the CHP was investigating seven additional confirmed cases of coronavirus disease 2019 (COVID-19), taking the number of cases to 5 105 in Hong Kong so far (comprising 5 104 confirmed cases and one probable case).

Among the newly reported cases announced, four had a travel history during the incubation period.

The CHP's epidemiological investigations and relevant contact tracing on the confirmed cases are ongoing. For case details and contact tracing information, please see the Annex or the list of buildings with confirmed cases of COVID-19 in the past 14 days and the latest local situation of COVID-19 available on the website "COVID-19 Thematic Website" (www.coronavirus.gov.hk).

In view of the severe epidemic situation, the CHP called on members of the public to avoid going out, having social contact and dining out. They should put on a surgical mask and maintain stringent hand hygiene when they need to go out. The CHP strongly urged the elderly to stay home as far as possible and avoid going out. They should consider asking their family and friends to help with everyday tasks such as shopping for basic necessities.

A spokesman for the CHP said, "Given that the situation of COVID-19 infection remains severe and that there is a continuous increase in the number of cases reported around the world, members of the public are strongly urged to avoid all non-essential travel outside Hong Kong.

"The CHP also strongly urges the public to maintain at all times strict personal and environmental hygiene, which is key to personal protection against infection and prevention of the spread of the disease in the community. On a personal level, members of the public should wear a surgical mask when having respiratory symptoms, taking public transport or staying in crowded places. They should also perform hand hygiene frequently, especially before touching the mouth, nose or eyes.

"As for household environmental hygiene, members of the public are advised to maintain drainage pipes properly, regularly pour water into drain outlets (U-traps) and cover all floor drain outlets when they are not in use. After using the toilet, they should put the toilet lid down before flushing to avoid spreading germs."

Moreover, the Government has launched the website "COVID-19 Thematic Website" (www.coronavirus.gov.hk) for announcing the latest updates on various news on COVID-19 infection and health advice to help the public understand the latest updates. Members of the public may also gain access to information via the COVID-19 WhatsApp Helpline launched by the Office of the Government Chief Information Officer. Simply by saving 9617 1823 in their phone contacts or clicking the link wa.me/85296171823?text=hi, they will be able to obtain information on COVID-19 as well as the "StayHomeSafe" mobile app and wristband via WhatsApp.

Issued at HKT 17:10

Public hospitals daily update on COVID-19 cases

****

The following is issued on behalf of the Hospital Authority:

As at 9am today (October 2), six COVID-19 confirmed patients were discharged from hospital in the last 24 hours. So far, a total of 4 843 patients with confirmed or probable infection have been discharged.

At present, there are 639 negative pressure rooms in public hospitals with 1 155 negative pressure beds activated. A total of 122 confirmed patients are currently hospitalised in 17 public hospitals, among which 10 patients are in critical condition, eight are in serious condition and the remaining 104 patients are in stable condition.

The Hospital Authority will maintain close contact with the Centre for Health Protection to monitor the latest developments and to inform the public and healthcare workers on the latest information in a timely manner.

Details of the above-mentioned patients are as follows:

Patient condition	Case numbers
Discharged	4934, 4962, 4979, 5009, 5015, 5035
Critical	1401, 1989, 2912, 3496, 3764, 4641, 4706, 4833, 4937, 4990
Serious	1650, 3904, 4100, 4101, 4433, 4746, 4788, 4969

Issued at HKT 18:43

FEHD reminds catering business operators and public to strictly comply with anti-epidemic regulations

****

The Food and Environmental Hygiene Department (FEHD) today (October 2) reminded catering business operators and food handlers again to strictly comply with the directions under the Prevention and Control of Disease (Requirements and Directions) (Business and Premises) Regulation (Cap. 599F), and the public should also comply with relevant anti-epidemic regulations when patronising restaurants. The FEHD will continue to step up inspections at food premises in various districts and take enforcement actions against offenders so as to minimise the risk of transmission of COVID-19 in food premises.

A spokesman for the FEHD said, "The latest directions issued by the Secretary for Food and Health in relation to catering business premises under the Regulation and the related legislative amendments have already come into effect, under which food business operators and food handlers have to continue to comply with a series of requirements and restrictions. Members of the public also have to comply with the related regulation on group gatherings at catering premises."

"The FEHD inspected over 1 250 catering business premises yesterday (October 1) and today. No violation of related regulation on group gatherings at catering premises is observed, but legal proceedings of prosecution were initiated against the operators of more than ten premises. These are mainly about violating the requirements on the distance between tables and wearing a mask at all times within the premises except when consuming food or drink," the spokesman said.

"The FEHD will continue to strengthen manpower deployment to step up inspections at food premises in various districts across the territory, and conduct joint operations with the Police to ensure that the relevant requirements and restrictions under the Regulations are complied with."

The FEHD spokesman appealed to food business operators and food handlers to comply with the relevant Regulation on prevention and control of disease in a concerted and persistent manner, with a view to keeping workers, customers and the public safe. Under the Regulation, licensees and operators of food premises must strictly comply with the series of requirements and restrictions. Contravening the requirements and restrictions is a criminal offence. Offenders are subject to a maximum fine of $50,000 and imprisonment for six months.

The spokesman also appealed to the public to comply with the relevant restriction on group gatherings and cooperate to facilitate compliance with the relevant anti-epidemic measures when patronising restaurants. In the premises, members of the public must wear a mask except when eating or drinking, maintain social distancing at all times, and avoid sharing of tables as far as possible. In addition, they must not consume food or drink in areas adjacent to the premises.

Issued at HKT 19:17

October 3[3]

[3] https://www.info.gov.hk/gia/general/202010/03.htm

Public hospitals daily update on COVID-19 cases

****

The following is issued on behalf of the Hospital Authority:

As at 9am today (October 3), six COVID-19 confirmed patients were discharged from hospital in the last 24 hours. So far, a total of 4 849 patients with confirmed or probable infection have been discharged.

At present, there are 639 negative pressure rooms in public hospitals with 1 155 negative pressure beds activated. A total of 123 confirmed patients are currently hospitalised in 17 public hospitals, among which 10 patients are in critical condition, eight are in serious condition and the remaining 105 patients are in stable condition.

The Hospital Authority will maintain close contact with the Centre for Health Protection to monitor the latest developments and to inform the public and healthcare workers on the latest information in a timely manner.

Details of the above-mentioned patients are as follows:

Patient condition	Case numbers
Discharged	4911, 4928, 4929, 5041, 5054, 5062
Critical	1401, 1989, 2912, 3496, 3764, 4641, 4706, 4833, 4937, 4990
Serious	1650, 3904, 4100, 4101, 4433, 4746, 4788, 4969

Issued at HKT 17:12

CHP investigates four additional confirmed cases of COVID-19

****

The Centre for Health Protection (CHP) of the Department of Health has announced that as of 0.00am, October 3, the CHP was investigating four additional confirmed cases of coronavirus

disease 2019 (COVID-19), taking the number of cases to 5 109 in Hong Kong so far (comprising 5 108 confirmed cases and one probable case).

Among the newly reported cases announced, three had a travel history during the incubation period.

The CHP's epidemiological investigations and relevant contact tracing on the confirmed cases are ongoing. For case details and contact tracing information, please see the Annex or the list of buildings with confirmed cases of COVID-19 in the past 14 days and the latest local situation of COVID-19 available on the website "COVID-19 Thematic Website" (www.coronavirus.gov.hk).

In view of the severe epidemic situation, the CHP called on members of the public to avoid going out, having social contact and dining out. They should put on a surgical mask and maintain stringent hand hygiene when they need to go out. The CHP strongly urged the elderly to stay home as far as possible and avoid going out. They should consider asking their family and friends to help with everyday tasks such as shopping for basic necessities.

A spokesman for the CHP said, "Given that the situation of COVID-19 infection remains severe and that there is a continuous increase in the number of cases reported around the world, members of the public are strongly urged to avoid all non-essential travel outside Hong Kong.

"The CHP also strongly urges the public to maintain at all times strict personal and environmental hygiene, which is key to personal protection against infection and prevention of the spread of the disease in the community. On a personal level, members of the public should wear a surgical mask when having respiratory symptoms, taking public transport or staying in crowded places. They should also perform hand hygiene frequently, especially before touching the mouth, nose or eyes.

"As for household environmental hygiene, members of the public are advised to maintain drainage pipes properly, regularly pour water into drain outlets (U-traps) and cover all floor drain outlets when they are not in use. After using the toilet, they should put the toilet lid down before flushing to avoid spreading germs."

Moreover, the Government has launched the website "COVID-19 Thematic Website" (www.coronavirus.gov.hk) for announcing the latest updates on various news on COVID-19 infection and health advice to help the public understand the latest updates. Members of the public may also gain access to information via the COVID-19 WhatsApp Helpline launched by the Office of the Government Chief Information Officer. Simply by saving 9617 1823 in their phone contacts or clicking the link wa.me/85296171823?text=hi, they will be able to obtain information on COVID-19 as well as the "StayHomeSafe" mobile app and wristband via WhatsApp.

Issued at HKT 17:45

FEHD continues to step up inspections at food premises relating to anti-epidemic measures

****

The Food and Environmental Hygiene Department (FEHD) conducted joint operations with the Police today (October 3) to step up inspections at catering business premises (including "Dai Pai Dongs") in Sai Kung and Sham Shui Po districts and remind food business operators and food handlers to strictly comply with the relevant requirements under the Prevention and Control of Disease (Requirements and Directions) (Business and Premises) Regulation (Cap. 599F), and the public should also comply with the restriction in relation to group gatherings under the anti-epidemic regulation when patronising restaurants.

A spokesman for the FEHD said, "According to the directions issued by the Secretary for Food and Health in relation to catering business premises under the Regulation, food business operators and food handlers have to strictly comply with a series of requirements and restrictions. Among these, the number of customers at any premises must not exceed half of its normal seating capacity, no more than four persons may be seated together at one table at catering premises; a mask must be worn at all times within the premises, except when the person is consuming food or drink; and body temperature screening must be conducted before the person is allowed to enter the catering premises and hand sanitisers must be provided. According to the latest amendments of the anti-epidemic regulation and directions, members of the public also have to comply with the related restriction on group gatherings that no more than four persons may be seated at one table at catering premises."

Under the Regulation, licensees and operators of food premises must strictly comply with the series of requirements and restrictions. Contravening the requirements and restrictions is a criminal offence. Offenders are subject to a maximum fine of $50,000 and imprisonment for six months. Persons who violate the group gathering restriction of Prevention and Control of Disease (Prohibition in Group Gathering) Regulation (Cap. 599G) are subject to a fixed penalty of $2,000.

"During the operations in Sai Kung and Sham Shui Po districts today, the FEHD inspected some 40 catering business premises and initiated legal proceedings of prosecution against the operators of seven premises. Apart from violating the requirements on the distance between tables, enforcement for violating other legislations on causing public obstruction is also included," the spokesman said.

The spokesman said that the FEHD will continue to step up inspections at food premises across the territory and conduct joint operations with the Police to ensure that food business operators, food handlers and the public strictly comply with the directions under the regulation and will take enforcement actions against offenders so as to minimise the risk of transmission of COVID-19 in food premises.

The FEHD spokesman appealed to food business operators and food handlers to comply with the relevant Regulation on prevention and control of disease in a concerted and persistent manner, with a view to keeping workers, customers and the public safe.

Issued at HKT 23:10

October 4[4]

CHP investigates five additional confirmed cases of COVID-19

****

The Centre for Health Protection (CHP) of the Department of Health has announced that as of 0.00am, October 4, the CHP was investigating five additional confirmed cases of coronavirus disease 2019 (COVID-19), taking the number of cases to 5 114 in Hong Kong so far (comprising 5 113 confirmed cases and one probable case).

Among the newly reported cases announced, three had a travel history during the incubation period.

The CHP's epidemiological investigations and relevant contact tracing on the confirmed cases are ongoing. For case details and contact tracing information, please see the Annex or the list of buildings with confirmed cases of COVID-19 in the past 14 days and the latest local situation of COVID-19 available on the website "COVID-19 Thematic Website" (www.coronavirus.gov.hk).

In view of the severe epidemic situation, the CHP called on members of the public to avoid going out, having social contact and dining out. They should put on a surgical mask and maintain stringent hand hygiene when they need to go out. The CHP strongly urged the elderly to stay home as far as possible and avoid going out. They should consider asking their family and friends to help with everyday tasks such as shopping for basic necessities.

A spokesman for the CHP said, "Given that the situation of COVID-19 infection remains severe and that there is a continuous increase in the number of cases reported around the world, members of the public are strongly urged to avoid all non-essential travel outside Hong Kong.

"The CHP also strongly urges the public to maintain at all times strict personal and environmental hygiene, which is key to personal protection against infection and prevention of the spread of the disease in the community. On a personal level, members of the public should wear a surgical mask when having respiratory symptoms, taking public transport or staying in crowded places. They should also perform hand hygiene frequently, especially before touching the mouth, nose or eyes.

"As for household environmental hygiene, members of the public are advised to maintain drainage pipes properly, regularly pour water into drain outlets (U-traps) and cover all floor drain outlets when they are not in use. After using the toilet, they should put the toilet lid down before flushing to avoid spreading germs."

[4] https://www.info.gov.hk/gia/general/202010/04.htm

Moreover, the Government has launched the website "COVID-19 Thematic Website" (www.coronavirus.gov.hk) for announcing the latest updates on various news on COVID-19 infection and health advice to help the public understand the latest updates. Members of the public may also gain access to information via the COVID-19 WhatsApp Helpline launched by the Office of the Government Chief Information Officer. Simply by saving 9617 1823 in their phone contacts or clicking the link wa.me/85296171823?text=hi, they will be able to obtain information on COVID-19 as well as the "StayHomeSafe" mobile app and wristband via WhatsApp.

Issued at HKT 17:36

Public hospitals daily update on COVID-19 cases

****

The following is issued on behalf of the Hospital Authority:

As at 9am today (October 4), 12 COVID-19 confirmed patients were discharged from hospital in the last 24 hours. So far, a total of 4 861 patients with confirmed or probable infection have been discharged.

At present, there are 639 negative pressure rooms in public hospitals with 1 155 negative pressure beds activated. A total of 115 confirmed patients are currently hospitalised in 17 public hospitals, among which 10 patients are in critical condition, eight are in serious condition and the remaining 97 patients are in stable condition.

The Hospital Authority will maintain close contact with the Centre for Health Protection to monitor the latest developments and to inform the public and healthcare workers on the latest information in a timely manner.

Details of the above-mentioned patients are as follows:

Patient condition	Case numbers
Discharged	2079, 4969, 4971, 5012, 5013, 5044, 5046, 5049, 5056, 5060, 5101, 5109
Critical	1401, 1989, 2912, 3496, 3764, 4641, 4706, 4833, 4937, 4990

Serious	1650, 3904, 4100, 4101, 4433, 4746, 4788, 5088

Issued at HKT 17:53

October 5[5]

Public hospitals daily update on COVID-19 cases

****

The following is issued on behalf of the Hospital Authority:

As at 9am today (October 5), three COVID-19 confirmed patients were discharged from hospital in the last 24 hours. So far, a total of 4 864 patients with confirmed or probable infection have been discharged.

At present, there are 633 negative pressure rooms in public hospitals with 1 131 negative pressure beds activated. A total of 117 confirmed patients are currently hospitalised in 17 public hospitals, among which 11 patients are in critical condition, eight are in serious condition and the remaining 98 patients are in stable condition.

The Hospital Authority will maintain close contact with the Centre for Health Protection to monitor the latest developments and to inform the public and healthcare workers on the latest information in a timely manner.

Details of the above-mentioned patients are as follows:

Patient condition	Case numbers
Discharged	5031, 5032, 5045
Critical	1401, 1989, 2912, 3496, 3764, 4641, 4706, 4833, 4937, 4990, 5110
Serious	1650, 3904, 4100, 4101, 4433, 4746, 4788, 5088

[5] https://www.info.gov.hk/gia/general/202010/05.htm

Issued at HKT 17:28

CHP investigates 11 additional confirmed cases of COVID-19

****

The Centre for Health Protection (CHP) of the Department of Health has announced that as of 0.00am, October 5, the CHP was investigating 11 additional confirmed cases of coronavirus disease 2019 (COVID-19), taking the number of cases to 5 125 in Hong Kong so far (comprising 5 124 confirmed cases and one probable case).

Among the newly reported cases announced, seven had a travel history during the incubation period.

The CHP's epidemiological investigations and relevant contact tracing on the confirmed cases are ongoing. For case details and contact tracing information, please see the Annex or the list of buildings with confirmed cases of COVID-19 in the past 14 days and the latest local situation of COVID-19 available on the website "COVID-19 Thematic Website" (www.coronavirus.gov.hk).

In view of the severe epidemic situation, the CHP called on members of the public to avoid going out, having social contact and dining out. They should put on a surgical mask and maintain stringent hand hygiene when they need to go out. The CHP strongly urged the elderly to stay home as far as possible and avoid going out. They should consider asking their family and friends to help with everyday tasks such as shopping for basic necessities.

A spokesman for the CHP said, "Given that the situation of COVID-19 infection remains severe and that there is a continuous increase in the number of cases reported around the world, members of the public are strongly urged to avoid all non-essential travel outside Hong Kong.

"The CHP also strongly urges the public to maintain at all times strict personal and environmental hygiene, which is key to personal protection against infection and prevention of the spread of the disease in the community. On a personal level, members of the public should wear a surgical mask when having respiratory symptoms, taking public transport or staying in crowded places. They should also perform hand hygiene frequently, especially before touching the mouth, nose or eyes.

"As for household environmental hygiene, members of the public are advised to maintain drainage pipes properly, regularly pour water into drain outlets (U-traps) and cover all floor drain outlets when they are not in use. After using the toilet, they should put the toilet lid down before flushing to avoid spreading germs."

Moreover, the Government has launched the website "COVID-19 Thematic Website" (www.coronavirus.gov.hk) for announcing the latest updates on various news on COVID-19 infection and health advice to help the public understand the latest updates. Members of the public may also gain access to information via the COVID-19 WhatsApp Helpline launched by the Office of the Government Chief Information Officer. Simply by saving 9617 1823 in their phone contacts or clicking the link wa.me/85296171823?text=hi, they will be able to obtain information on COVID-19 as well as the "StayHomeSafe" mobile app and wristband via WhatsApp.

Issued at HKT 18:35

EDB to provide one-off relief grant to kindergartens and private schools

****

The Education Bureau (EDB) today (October 5) issued letters or circular memorandum to all kindergartens (KGs), private primary and secondary day schools as well as private schools offering non-formal curriculum (PSNFCs) (generally referred to as "tutorial schools") informing them the details of a one-off relief grant under the third round of the Anti-epidemic Fund.

A spokesman for the EDB said that following the approval of the third round of the Anti-epidemic Fund by the Finance Committee of the Legislative Council last Monday (September 28), the EDB has made immediate arrangements for progressively disbursing subsidies related to the areas of education. To alleviate the financial hardship arising from the suspension of face-to-face teaching due to the coronavirus disease 2019, the Anti-epidemic Fund will provide the above-mentioned schools with a one-off grant. The grant ranging from $30,000 to $80,000 will be provided to each KG and private primary and secondary day school. The additional expenditure is estimated to be $67.5 million, benefitting some 1 000 KGs and about 180 private primary and secondary day schools. Details are as follows:

- Schools joining the kindergarten education scheme (Scheme-KGs) will receive a grant ranging from $30,000 to $80,000, depending on their types (i.e. half-day, whole-day and long whole-day) and sizes;

- For non-Scheme KGs, each KG will receive a grant of $40,000;

- Private primary and secondary day schools (including English Schools Foundation schools, international schools, Private Independent Schools and other private primary and secondary day schools offering formal curriculum) will each receive $40,000.

Regarding PSNFCs, a one-off relief grant of $20,000 will be given to each PSNFC registered under the Education Ordinance on or before the resumption of face-to-face classes by phases on September 23 and that is in operation on the date of issuance of the circular memorandum. The additional expenditure is estimated to be $60 million, benefitting some 3 000 PSNFCs.

Depending on the disbursement arrangements for respective grants, the EDB will disburse the subsidy to schools about one month after obtaining the funding from the Anti-epidemic Fund or in about one month upon receipt of fully completed application forms or payees' information.

Issued at HKT 20:06

October 6[6]

Public hospitals daily update on COVID-19 cases
****

The following is issued on behalf of the Hospital Authority:

As at 9am today (October 6), 11 COVID-19 confirmed patients were discharged from hospital in the last 24 hours. So far, a total of 4 875 patients with confirmed or probable infection have been discharged.

At present, there are 626 negative pressure rooms in public hospitals with 1 119 negative pressure beds activated. A total of 117 confirmed patients are currently hospitalised in 17 public hospitals, among which 10 patients are in critical condition, nine are in serious condition and the remaining 98 patients are in stable condition.

The Hospital Authority will maintain close contact with the Centre for Health Protection to monitor the latest developments and to inform the public and healthcare workers on the latest information in a timely manner.

Details of the above-mentioned patients are as follows:

Patient condition	Case numbers
Discharged	4737, 4933, 4935, 5025, 5053, 5065, 5075, 5082, 5092, 5119, 5120
Critical	1401, 1989, 2912, 3496, 3764, 4706, 4833, 4937, 4990, 5110
Serious	1650, 3904, 4100, 4101, 4433, 4641, 4746, 4788, 5088

[6] https://www.info.gov.hk/gia/general/202010/06.htm

Issued at HKT 18:00

CHP investigates eight additional confirmed cases of COVID-19

****

The Centre for Health Protection (CHP) of the Department of Health has announced that as of 0.00am, October 6, the CHP was investigating eight additional confirmed cases of coronavirus disease 2019 (COVID-19), taking the number of cases to 5 133 in Hong Kong so far (comprising 5 132 confirmed cases and one probable case).

Among the newly reported cases announced, three had a travel history during the incubation period.

The CHP's epidemiological investigations and relevant contact tracing on the confirmed cases are ongoing. For case details and contact tracing information, please see the Annex or the list of buildings with confirmed cases of COVID-19 in the past 14 days and the latest local situation of COVID-19 available on the website "COVID-19 Thematic Website" (www.coronavirus.gov.hk).

A spokesman for the CHP said, "During the CHP's epidemiological investigations and relevant contact tracing on the confirmed cases, we will compile and upload (www.chp.gov.hk/files/pdf/building_list_eng.pdf) a list of buildings that confirmed patients had visited from two days before the onset of symptoms. Given that cases of local infection continue to occur from time to time, members of the public are urged to seek medical attention immediately if they believe that they had visited the same place at an identical time with a confirmed patient and feel unwell subsequently. If they remain asymptomatic but are concerned that they have been infected, they can also visit the Hospital Authority's designated general out-patient clinics (www.ha.org.hk/haho/ho/covid-19/GOPC_extend_EN.pdf) to obtain specimen collection packs and collect deep throat saliva specimens for free COVID-19 testing."

In view of the severe epidemic situation, the CHP called on members of the public to avoid going out, having social contact and dining out. They should put on a surgical mask and maintain stringent hand hygiene when they need to go out. The CHP strongly urged the elderly to stay home as far as possible and avoid going out. They should consider asking their family and friends to help with everyday tasks such as shopping for basic necessities.

The spokesman said, "Given that the situation of COVID-19 infection remains severe and that there is a continuous increase in the number of cases reported around the world, members of the public are strongly urged to avoid all non-essential travel outside Hong Kong.

"The CHP also strongly urges the public to maintain at all times strict personal and environmental hygiene, which is key to personal protection against infection and prevention of the spread of the disease in the community. On a personal level, members of the public should wear a surgical mask when having respiratory symptoms, taking public transport or staying in

crowded places. They should also perform hand hygiene frequently, especially before touching the mouth, nose or eyes.

"As for household environmental hygiene, members of the public are advised to maintain drainage pipes properly, regularly pour water into drain outlets (U-traps) and cover all floor drain outlets when they are not in use. After using the toilet, they should put the toilet lid down before flushing to avoid spreading germs."

Moreover, the Government has launched the website "COVID-19 Thematic Website" (www.coronavirus.gov.hk) for announcing the latest updates on various news on COVID-19 infection and health advice to help the public understand the latest updates. Members of the public may also gain access to information via the COVID-19 WhatsApp Helpline launched by the Office of the Government Chief Information Officer. Simply by saving 9617 1823 in their phone contacts or clicking the link wa.me/85296171823?text=hi, they will be able to obtain information on COVID-19 as well as the "StayHomeSafe" mobile app and wristband via WhatsApp.

Issued at HKT 20:05

Government extends social distancing measures under Prevention and Control of Disease Ordinance

****

The Government will gazette directions and specifications under the Prevention and Control of Disease (Requirements and Directions) (Business and Premises) Regulation (Cap. 599F), the Prevention and Control of Disease (Prohibition on Group Gathering) Regulation (Cap. 599G) and the Prevention and Control of Disease (Wearing of Mask) Regulation (Cap. 599I) today (October 6) to largely maintain the social distancing measures currently in place. These measures will take effect at 0.00am on October 9 for a period of seven days till October 15.

A spokesman for the Food and Health Bureau said, "It is worrying that local confirmed cases with unknown sources of infection continued to be reported in recent days, indicating the existence of silent transmission chains in the community. While there has yet to be a significant rebound of the epidemic situation, it is noted that the seven-day average number of locally confirmed cases has not dropped further in the past week, and even showed signs of rebound in the past few days. Moreover, the seven-day average number of cases of unknown sources continued to increase after reaching a low level early last week. The epidemic situation certainly allows no room for optimism."

"We understand that members of the public are experiencing anti-epidemic fatigue to different extents and have become less alert in combating the epidemic, after many months of fighting against the disease. However, if each of us as a member of society does not comply strictly with the various epidemic control and social distancing measures and does not remain vigilant in maintaining personal and environmental hygiene, the risk of a rebound of the epidemic would be extremely high and we may well be on the verge of a large-scale community outbreak. As the latest virus strain has higher transmissibility, the epidemic may worsen rapidly in a very short period of time, possibly causing the fourth wave of the local epidemic to arrive early."

Since late August, the Government, having regard to the fact that the epidemic has subsided from its peak in late July, has relaxed or adjusted the various social distancing measures under a refined and sophisticated approach in a gradual and orderly manner, so as to allow social and economic activities to resume as far as possible under the new normal. The measures include relaxing the restriction on the number of persons allowed in group gatherings in public places, extending the hours when dine-in services are allowed in catering premises and relaxing the number of persons allowed to be seated together at one table therein, reopening all catering business and scheduled premises, and allowing team sports at sports premises.

Taking into account the latest public health risk assessment, starting this Friday (October 9), apart from refinements to the measures to allow team sports at public skating rinks, the Government will maintain all other requirements and restrictions applicable to catering business and scheduled premises.

The spokesman added, "As we have stressed time and again, co-operation and self-discipline of members of the public are the keys to the effectiveness of social distancing measures in preventing the spread of the disease in the community. Only with the co-operation of society as a whole can the Government continue to allow resumption of social and economic activities in a gradual and orderly manner. Therefore, the public's concerted efforts in fighting the epidemic and compliance with requirements and restrictions applicable to individual premises are of utmost importance. Otherwise, when there is another large-scale outbreak in the community, the Government will have no choice but to significantly tighten social distancing measures in order to safeguard public health."

The Government calls on the public to continue maintaining the awareness of epidemic prevention when resuming social and economic activities, and to continue to stay vigilant in maintaining personal and environmental hygiene with a view to making concerted efforts to prevent another outbreak in the community and to prevent the hard work the entire community has put in for almost three months from going in vain. The Government will continue to closely monitor the development of the epidemic situation and review and adjust the various measures in place from time to time while striking a balance among disease prevention and control, economic needs and level of acceptance of the society, and will announce the latest social distancing measures in a timely manner.

The requirements and restrictions under the latest directions and specifications (details of the arrangements for premises under Cap. 599F at Annex 1) are as follows:

(I) Catering premises and scheduled premises

The requirements and restrictions applicable to catering business and scheduled premises will be maintained to a large extent (see Annex 1 for details) during the seven-day period from October 9 to 15, 2020. Amongst others, activities and facilities involving higher health risks such as dancing activities, steam and sauna facilities and ball pits will continue to be suspended or prohibited from opening. To provide more opportunities for the general public to exercise to maintain physical and mental health so that the public will be fit to continue to combat the epidemic, the latest directions will allow team sports at public skating rinks with the maximum number of persons allowed at more than four persons based on the particular team sports activities.

Persons responsible for carrying on catering businesses and managers of scheduled premises that contravene the statutory requirements under Cap. 599F would have committed a criminal offence. Offenders are subject to a maximum fine of $50,000 and imprisonment for six months.

(II) Group gatherings

Unless exempted, the prohibition on group gatherings of more than four persons in public places will continue during the seven-day period from October 9 to 15, 2020

Any person who participates in a prohibited group gathering; organises a prohibited group gathering; owns, controls or operates the place of such gathering and knowingly allows the taking place of such gathering, commits an offence under Cap. 599G. Offenders are liable to a maximum fine of $25,000 and imprisonment for six months. Persons who participate in a prohibited group gathering may discharge liability for the offence by paying a fixed penalty of $2,000.

(III) Mask-wearing requirement

The mandatory mask-wearing requirement under Cap. 599I will be extended for a period of seven days from October 9 to 15, 2020. During the aforementioned period, a person must wear a mask all the time when the person is boarding or onboard a public transport carrier, is entering or present in an MTR paid area, or is entering or present in a specified public place (i.e. all public places, save for outdoor public places in country parks and special areas as defined in section 2 of the Country Parks Ordinance (Cap. 208)).

Under Cap. 599I, if a person does not wear a mask in accordance with the requirement, an authorised person may deny that person from boarding a public transport carrier or entering the area concerned, as well as require that person to wear a mask and disembark from the carrier or leave the said area. A person in contravention of the relevant provision commits an offence and the maximum penalty is a fine at level 2 ($5,000). In addition, authorised public officers may issue fixed penalty notices to persons who do not wear a mask in accordance with the requirement and such persons may discharge liability for the offence by paying a fixed penalty of $2,000.

Issued at HKT 21:40

October 7[7]

8th Hong Kong Games postponed

****

The 8th Hong Kong Games (HKG) has been postponed for a year due to the COVID-19 epidemic situation. Athlete selection in the 18 districts, originally scheduled to start this year, will be held from April 2021 to January 2022 instead, while inter-district sports competitions will begin in March 2022.

District athlete selection for the 8th HKG was scheduled to begin in September this year. However, as the epidemic situation has been fluctuating, the Leisure and Cultural Services Department has been obliged to implement corresponding disease prevention and control measures by temporarily closing some recreation and sports facilities and suspending recreation and sports programmes and competitions. As a result, athlete selection has not started yet. The process cannot be held within a short period, as athletes require sufficient time to undergo training in the recently reopened sports facilities before taking part in the selection.

To safeguard public health and to ensure a high standard for the Games, the 8th HKG Organising Committee decided to postpone the event for a year to 2021 and 2022. The arrangement will allow sufficient time for the 18 District Councils and other co-organisers to better prepare for district athlete selection, inter-district sports competitions and community participation programmes. Spectators will be allowed to watch the competitions on-site if circumstances permit.

Publicity and promotional activities for the 8th HKG will be launched soon. For the latest news of the Games, please visit the dedicated website at www.hongkonggames.hk.

Issued at HKT 10:00

Public hospitals daily update on COVID-19 cases

****

The following is issued on behalf of the Hospital Authority:

---

[7] https://www.info.gov.hk/gia/general/202010/07.htm

As at 9am today (October 7), 10 COVID-19 confirmed patients were discharged from hospital in the last 24 hours. So far, a total of 4 885 patients with confirmed or probable infection have been discharged.

At present, there are 627 negative pressure rooms in public hospitals with 1 119 negative pressure beds activated. A total of 115 confirmed patients are currently hospitalised in 17 public hospitals, among which 10 patients are in critical condition, eight are in serious condition and the remaining 97 patients are in stable condition.

The Hospital Authority will maintain close contact with the Centre for Health Protection to monitor the latest developments and to inform the public and healthcare workers on the latest information in a timely manner.

Details of the above-mentioned patients are as follows:

Patient condition	Case numbers
Discharged	4999, 5011, 5017, 5019, 5020, 5026, 5064, 5070, 5079, 5094
Critical	1401, 1989, 2912, 3496, 3764, 4706, 4833, 4937, 4990, 5110
Serious	1650, 3904, 4100, 4101, 4433, 4746, 4788, 5088

Issued at HKT 18:00

CHP investigates 11 additional confirmed cases of COVID-19

****

The Centre for Health Protection (CHP) of the Department of Health has announced that as of 0.00am, October 7, the CHP was investigating 11 additional confirmed cases of coronavirus disease 2019 (COVID-19), taking the number of cases to 5 144 in Hong Kong so far (comprising 5 143 confirmed cases and one probable case).

Among the newly reported cases announced, two had a travel history during the incubation period.

The CHP's epidemiological investigations and relevant contact tracing on the confirmed cases are ongoing. For case details and contact tracing information, please see the Annex or the list of buildings with confirmed cases of COVID-19 in the past 14 days and the latest local situation of COVID-19 available on the website "COVID-19 Thematic Website" (www.coronavirus.gov.hk).

A spokesman for the CHP said, "During the CHP's epidemiological investigations and relevant contact tracing on the confirmed cases, we will compile and upload (www.chp.gov.hk/files/pdf/building_list_eng.pdf) a list of buildings that confirmed patients had visited from two days before the onset of symptoms. Given that cases of local infection continue to occur from time to time, members of the public are urged to seek medical attention immediately if they believe that they had visited the same place at an identical time with a confirmed patient and feel unwell subsequently. If they remain asymptomatic but are concerned that they have been infected, they can also visit the Hospital Authority's designated general out-patient clinics (www.ha.org.hk/haho/ho/covid-19/GOPC_extend_EN.pdf) to obtain specimen collection packs and collect deep throat saliva specimens for free COVID-19 testing."

In view of the severe epidemic situation, the CHP called on members of the public to avoid going out, having social contact and dining out. They should put on a surgical mask and maintain stringent hand hygiene when they need to go out. The CHP strongly urged the elderly to stay home as far as possible and avoid going out. They should consider asking their family and friends to help with everyday tasks such as shopping for basic necessities.

A spokesman for the CHP said, "Given that the situation of COVID-19 infection remains severe and that there is a continuous increase in the number of cases reported around the world, members of the public are strongly urged to avoid all non-essential travel outside Hong Kong.

"The CHP also strongly urges the public to maintain at all times strict personal and environmental hygiene, which is key to personal protection against infection and prevention of the spread of the disease in the community. On a personal level, members of the public should wear a surgical mask when having respiratory symptoms, taking public transport or staying in crowded places. They should also perform hand hygiene frequently, especially before touching the mouth, nose or eyes.

"As for household environmental hygiene, members of the public are advised to maintain drainage pipes properly, regularly pour water into drain outlets (U-traps) and cover all floor drain outlets when they are not in use. After using the toilet, they should put the toilet lid down before flushing to avoid spreading germs."

Moreover, the Government has launched the website "COVID-19 Thematic Website" (www.coronavirus.gov.hk) for announcing the latest updates on various news on COVID-19 infection and health advice to help the public understand the latest updates. Members of the public may also gain access to information via the COVID-19 WhatsApp Helpline launched by the Office of the Government Chief Information Officer. Simply by saving 9617 1823 in their phone contacts or clicking the link wa.me/85296171823?text=hi, they will be able to obtain information on COVID-19 as well as the "StayHomeSafe" mobile app and wristband via WhatsApp.

Issued at HKT 18:56

October 8[8]

Public hospitals daily update on COVID-19 cases

****

The following is issued on behalf of the Hospital Authority:

As at 9am today (October 8), five COVID-19 confirmed patients were discharged from hospital in the last 24 hours. So far, a total of 4 890 patients with confirmed or probable infection have been discharged.

At present, there are 627 negative pressure rooms in public hospitals with 1 119 negative pressure beds activated. A total of 121 confirmed patients are currently hospitalised in 17 public hospitals, among which 10 patients are in critical condition, eight are in serious condition and the remaining 103 patients are in stable condition.

The Hospital Authority will maintain close contact with the Centre for Health Protection to monitor the latest developments and to inform the public and healthcare workers on the latest information in a timely manner.

Details of the above-mentioned patients are as follows:

Patient condition	Case numbers
Discharged	5050, 5078, 5093, 5102, 5114
Critical	1401, 1989, 2912, 3496, 3764, 4706, 4833, 4937, 4990, 5110
Serious	1650, 3904, 4100, 4101, 4433, 4746, 4788, 5088

Issued at HKT 18:35

[8] https://www.info.gov.hk/gia/general/202010/08.htm

CHP investigates 18 additional confirmed cases of COVID-19

****

The Centre for Health Protection (CHP) of the Department of Health has announced that as of 0.00am, October 8, the CHP was investigating 18 additional confirmed cases of coronavirus disease 2019 (COVID-19), taking the number of cases to 5 162 in Hong Kong so far (comprising 5 161 confirmed cases and one probable case).

Among the newly reported cases announced, four had a travel history during the incubation period.

The CHP's epidemiological investigations and relevant contact tracing on the confirmed cases are ongoing. For case details and contact tracing information, please see the Annex or the list of buildings with confirmed cases of COVID-19 in the past 14 days and the latest local situation of COVID-19 available on the website "COVID-19 Thematic Website" (www.coronavirus.gov.hk).

A spokesman for the CHP said, "During the CHP's epidemiological investigations and relevant contact tracing on the confirmed cases, we will compile and upload (www.chp.gov.hk/files/pdf/building_list_eng.pdf) a list of buildings that confirmed patients had visited from two days before the onset of symptoms. Given that cases of local infection continue to occur from time to time, members of the public are urged to seek medical attention immediately if they believe that they had visited the same place at an identical time with a confirmed patient and feel unwell subsequently. If they remain asymptomatic but are concerned that they have been infected, they can also visit the Hospital Authority's designated general out-patient clinics (www.ha.org.hk/haho/ho/covid-19/GOPC_extend_EN.pdf) to obtain specimen collection packs and collect deep throat saliva specimens for free COVID-19 testing."

In view of the severe epidemic situation, the CHP called on members of the public to avoid going out, having social contact and dining out. They should put on a surgical mask and maintain stringent hand hygiene when they need to go out. The CHP strongly urged the elderly to stay home as far as possible and avoid going out. They should consider asking their family and friends to help with everyday tasks such as shopping for basic necessities.

The spokesman said, "Given that the situation of COVID-19 infection remains severe and that there is a continuous increase in the number of cases reported around the world, members of the public are strongly urged to avoid all non-essential travel outside Hong Kong.

"The CHP also strongly urges the public to maintain at all times strict personal and environmental hygiene, which is key to personal protection against infection and prevention of the spread of the disease in the community. On a personal level, members of the public should wear a surgical mask when having respiratory symptoms, taking public transport or staying in crowded places. They should also perform hand hygiene frequently, especially before touching the mouth, nose or eyes.

"As for household environmental hygiene, members of the public are advised to maintain drainage pipes properly, regularly pour water into drain outlets (U-traps) and cover all floor drain outlets when they are not in use. After using the toilet, they should put the toilet lid down before flushing to avoid spreading germs."

Moreover, the Government has launched the website "COVID-19 Thematic Website" (www.coronavirus.gov.hk) for announcing the latest updates on various news on COVID-19 infection and health advice to help the public understand the latest updates. Members of the public may also gain access to information via the COVID-19 WhatsApp Helpline launched by the Office of the Government Chief Information Officer. Simply by saving 9617 1823 in their phone contacts or clicking the link wa.me/85296171823?text=hi, they will be able to obtain information on COVID-19 as well as the "StayHomeSafe" mobile app and wristband via WhatsApp.

Issued at HKT 18:40

EDB to provide one-off relief grant to suppliers of catering services for schools and post-secondary education institutions and providers of interest classes and school bus services for schools

****

The Education Bureau (EDB) is issuing circular memoranda today and tomorrow (October 8 and 9) to all primary, secondary and special schools and kindergartens to inform them of the details about the provision of relief grants under the third round of the Anti-epidemic Fund for suppliers of catering services for schools and providers of interest classes and school bus services for schools. The EDB has also distributed application forms through the post-secondary education institutions to the catering outlets operating on their campuses.

A spokesman for the EDB said that one-off relief grants under the third round of the Anti-epidemic Fund will be provided to the suppliers and service providers concerned as their services and income were affected during periods of suspension of classes and cessation of on-campus activities. The additional expenditure is estimated to be $248.9 million. Details are as follows:

(1) Operators of catering outlets (namely tuck shops, canteens and restaurants) at primary schools, secondary schools and post-secondary education institutions: a one-off relief grant of $40,000 to each outlet;

(2) Lunchbox providers of primary and secondary schools: a one-off relief grant of $5,000 per school each provider is serving;

(3) School bus drivers, school private light bus drivers and escorts (commonly called "nannies"): a one-off relief grant of $6,700 for each driver and $6,700 per vehicle for escorts (the subsidy of $6,700 will be shared among nannies based on their proportion of service time if more than one nanny serve in the same vehicle);

(4) Instructors, coaches, trainers and operators of interest classes engaged by schools: a one-off relief grant of $5,000 to each operator/service provider.

Depending on the disbursement arrangements for respective grants, the EDB will generally effect payment in about a month upon receipt of duly completed and certified application forms.

Issued at HKT 18:57

General outpatient clinics enhance distribution hours of specimen collection packs

****

The following is issued on behalf of the Hospital Authority:

To tie in with the Government's epidemic control strategy, the Hospital Authority (HA) today (October 8) announced that starting from tomorrow (October 9) the specimen collection packs' distribution time will be enhanced at general outpatient clinics (GOPCs), thereby assisting individuals, who feel they have a higher risk of exposure and are experiencing mild discomfort, to obtain a specimen collection pack for a COVID-19 test.

The HA spokesperson said, "To facilitate more members of the public to receive COVID-19 tests, specimen collection packs can now be obtained at the 46 GOPCs (see attached list) during the daytime service hours (9am to 1pm and 2pm to 5pm) starting from tomorrow.

"Since July 27, HA GOPCs have distributed nearly 60,000 specimen collection packs. Over 36,000 specimens were tested by the laboratory, and over 60 were positive for COVID-19.

"The specimens collected by this programme are handled by an accredited local private laboratory. For specimens testing positive for COVID-19, the cases will be reported to the Centre for Health Protection (CHP) for confirmation in accordance with the prevailing mechanism. The participants concerned will be notified by the CHP for admission to public hospitals for isolation as soon as possible. Participants should assume a negative test result if they do not receive a notification in three working days after the specimen submission."

Distribution points of specimen collection packs will be set up near the entrance of the 46 GOPCs to appropriately segregate the persons obtaining the specimen collection packs from the patients attending medical consultations. Members of the public can obtain the specimen collection packs (with contents including a specimen collection bottle, packaging plastic bags, guidelines for collection of deep throat saliva samples, etc) between 9am to 1pm and 2pm to 5pm from Monday to Friday (except public holidays) at the distribution points of specimen collection packs of the aforementioned clinics. Only one pack should be taken by each person while stocks last.

The HA spokesperson reminded participants that they are required to submit the deep throat saliva specimen within three working days, together with the necessary information, for laboratory tests. The collection points near the entrance of the 46 clinics will be open between 10am and 11am from Monday to Saturday (except public holidays).

The HA spokesperson also reminded the public to wear their own masks and maintain social distancing while collecting packs or submitting the specimens.

Issued at HKT 19:15

FEHD steps up inspections at food premises and takes stringent enforcement actions relating to anti-epidemic measures

****

The Food and Environmental Hygiene Department (FEHD) today (October 8) stepped up inspections at catering business premises in Tuen Mun District and Central and Western District. The FEHD conducted joint operations with the Police to step up inspections at catering business premises in Tuen Mun District and remind food business operators and food handlers to strictly comply with the relevant requirements under the Prevention and Control of Disease (Requirements and Directions) (Business and Premises) Regulation (Cap. 599F) (the Regulation), and the public to comply with the restriction in relation to group gatherings under the anti-epidemic regulations and directions when patronising restaurants.

During the operations in Tuen Mun District and Central and Western Districts today, the FEHD inspected some 30 catering business premises. During the joint operation with the Police in Tuen Mun District, the FEHD issued fixed penalty tickets to 19 persons found seated at two tables inside a VIP room of the catering business premises for violating the requirement of no more than four persons should be seated together at one table. The FEHD also initiated the procedure on prosecuting that catering business premises in Tuen Mun District and six catering business premises in a large shopping complex in Admiralty for violating the directions in relation to catering business. These are mainly about violating the requirements on the distance between tables, wearing a mask at all times within the premises except when consuming food or drink and the number of persons at one table.

A spokesman for the FEHD said, "According to the directions issued by the Secretary for Food and Health in relation to catering business premises under the Regulation, food business operators and food handlers have to strictly comply with a series of requirements and restrictions. Among these, the number of customers at any premises must not exceed half of its normal seating capacity, no more than four persons may be seated together at one table at catering premises; a mask must be worn at all times within the premises, except when the person is consuming food or drink; body temperature screening must be conducted before the person is allowed to enter the catering premises and hand sanitisers must be provided. According to the relevant anti-epidemic regulations and directions, members of the public also have to comply with the related restriction on group gatherings at catering business premises, that is no more than four persons may be seated at one table."

Under the Regulation, licensees and operators of food premises must strictly comply with the series of requirements and restrictions. Contravening the requirements and restrictions is a criminal offence. Offenders are subject to a maximum fine of $50,000 and imprisonment for six months. Persons who violate the group gathering restriction of Prevention and Control of Disease (Prohibition in Group Gathering) Regulation (Cap. 599G) are subject to a fixed penalty of $2,000.

The spokesman said that the FEHD will continue to step up inspections at food premises across the territory and conduct joint operations with the Police to ensure that food business operators, food handlers and the public strictly comply with the directions under the regulation and will take enforcement actions against offenders so as to minimise the risk of transmission of COVID-19 in food premises.

The FEHD spokesman appealed to food business operators and food handlers to comply with the relevant Regulation on prevention and control of disease in a concerted and persistent manner, with a view to keeping workers, customers and the public safe, and to members of the public to comply with the related regulations and directions relating to group gatherings at catering business premises.

Issued at HKT 23:14

October 9[9]

Cinemas Subsidy Scheme under AEF 3.0 opens for applications

****

The Cinemas Subsidy Scheme under the third-round Anti-epidemic Fund is open for applications from today (October 9) to October 20.

The Scheme will provide a one-off subsidy of $50,000 per screen to each existing cinema licensed as a place of public entertainment with commercial operation in July 2020. The maximum subsidy for a cinema circuit is $1.5 million.

The application details of the Scheme are available at Create Hong Kong's website (www.createhk.gov.hk).

---

[9] https://www.info.gov.hk/gia/general/202010/09.htm

Issued at HKT 11:00

One-off grant to registered sports coaches under third round of Anti-epidemic Fund open for application

****

A spokesman for the Leisure and Cultural Services Department (LCSD) said today (October 9) that the One-off Grant to Registered Sports Coaches scheme, relaunched under the third round of the Anti-epidemic Fund, is now open for application. The scheme will provide a one-off grant of $5,000 for each eligible registered sports coach.

Due to the deteriorating COVID-19 epidemic situation in mid-July, the Government further tightened up the social distancing measures. Most of the LCSD facilities were temporarily closed again from July 15, only to be gradually reopened in mid-September. As a result, many sports training activities that heavily relied on the provision of LCSD facilities were suspended again, in particular those handled by private coaches during the peak season of the summer vacation. The one-off grant scheme aims to further provide timely financial relief to eligible registered sports coaches.

Sports coaches registered under National Sports Associations or recognised sports organisations who had provided coaching services from April 1, 2019, to September 30, 2020, are eligible to apply. They can submit applications to the Sports Funding Office of the LCSD by November 30. The grant will be disbursed in batches around two months after receipt of the completed application form and relevant documents.

The application form and the guidelines of the scheme are available from the website (www.lcsd.gov.hk/en/programmes/programmeslist/sss/subsidyscheme.html) or the 18 District Leisure Services Offices of the LCSD. Please contact the Sports Funding Office at 2601 7411 for enquiries.

Issued at HKT 11:00

Places of Amusement Licence Holders Subsidy Scheme under third round of Anti-epidemic Fund open for application

****

A spokesman for the Leisure and Cultural Services Department (LCSD) said today (October 9) that the Places of Amusement Licence Holders Subsidy Scheme (the Scheme), re-launched under the third round of the Anti-epidemic Fund, is now open for application. The Scheme provides a one-off subsidy of $50,000 to billiard establishments, public bowling alleys and public skating rinks operating with a licence issued under the Places of Amusement Regulation (Cap 132BA). It aims to provide subsidies to the eligible licence holders whose businesses have been directly affected by the COVID-19 and anti-epidemic and social distancing measures imposed by the Government.

Holders of a valid Places of Amusement Licence issued by the Director of Leisure and Cultural Services under the Places of Amusement Regulation (Cap 132BA) on October 9, 2020, are eligible for application. Eligible licence holders should submit their applications to the Licensing and Prosecution Unit under the LCSD. The deadline for application is November 8. Upon submission of the completed application form and supporting documents, the disbursement of subsidies could generally be made in batches around two weeks after the deadline of the application.

Application forms and guidelines will be sent to each licence holder by mail or can be obtained from the website (www.lcsd.gov.hk/en/licensing/subsidyscheme.html). For enquiries, please contact the Licensing and Prosecution Unit at 2601 8799.

Issued at HKT 15:00

Successful completion of community treatment facility expansion at AsiaWorld-Expo

****

With the support of the Central Government, the community treatment facility (CTF) expansion at AsiaWorld-Expo (AWE) was successfully completed. A ceremony was conducted today (October 9) during which the facility was officially handed over to the Hospital Authority (HA).

The Secretary for Development, Mr Michael Wong, expressed his gratitude to the Central Government, the Guangdong Provincial Government and the Shenzhen Municipal Government for implementing the project.

Mr Wong said that relevant construction works commenced on September 19 and were swiftly completed within three weeks, providing an addition of nearly 1 000 beds in Halls 8 to 11 of AWE, with some equipped with negative pressure facilities.

The Chief Executive of the HA, Dr Tony Ko, said that 900 beds of the CTF were installed at Halls 1 and 2 of AWE earlier. Coupled with the newly completed CTF in Halls 8 to 11, Hong Kong's ability to cope with another potential wave of the epidemic in the future will be greatly enhanced, reducing the pressure on public hospitals.

Before the ceremony, Mr Wong, together with the Under Secretary for Food and Health, Dr Chui Tak-yi; Dr Ko; the Director of Architectural Services, Mrs Sylvia Lam; and representatives from the Shenzhen Municipal Government, inspected the newly completed CTF, including modular units of beds, negative pressure facilities, medical stations as well as the air-conditioning and air filtration system.

Mr Wong thanked the concerted efforts of the project team for collaborating with the Hong Kong SAR and Shenzhen Governments as well as the staff members of the HA to overcome different challenges at various stages of the project such that the works could be completed earlier under the tight schedule.

At the temporary hospital project adjacent to AWE, which is also supported by the Central Government, relevant construction works also commenced on September 19. The contractor is carrying out foundation works at the site. At the same time, fabrication of modular units in Mainland factories is also underway. The construction works are expected to be completed within four months. Upon completion, the temporary hospital will provide negative pressure wards that can accommodate over 800 beds and associated medical facilities.

Issued at HKT 15:40

CHP investigates eight additional confirmed cases of COVID-19

****

The Centre for Health Protection (CHP) of the Department of Health has announced that as of 0.00am, October 9, the CHP was investigating eight additional confirmed cases of coronavirus disease 2019 (COVID-19), taking the number of cases to 5 170 in Hong Kong so far (comprising 5 169 confirmed cases and one probable case).

Among the newly reported cases announced, one had a travel history during the incubation period.

The CHP's epidemiological investigations and relevant contact tracing on the confirmed cases are ongoing. For case details and contact tracing information, please see the Annex or the list of buildings with confirmed cases of COVID-19 in the past 14 days and the latest local situation of COVID-19 available on the website "COVID-19 Thematic Website" (www.coronavirus.gov.hk).

A spokesman for the CHP said, "During the CHP's epidemiological investigations and relevant contact tracing on the confirmed cases, we will compile and upload (www.chp.gov.hk/files/pdf/building_list_eng.pdf) a list of buildings that confirmed patients had visited from two days before the onset of symptoms. Given that cases of local infection continue to occur from time to time, members of the public are urged to seek medical attention immediately if they believe that they had visited the same place at an identical time with a confirmed patient and feel unwell subsequently. If they remain asymptomatic but are concerned that they have been infected, they can also visit the Hospital Authority's designated general out-patient clinics (www.ha.org.hk/haho/ho/covid-19/GOPC_extend_EN.pdf) to obtain specimen collection packs and collect deep throat saliva specimens for free COVID-19 testing."

In view of the severe epidemic situation, the CHP called on members of the public to avoid going out, having social contact and dining out. They should put on a surgical mask and maintain stringent hand hygiene when they need to go out. The CHP strongly urged the elderly to stay home as far as possible and avoid going out. They should consider asking their family and friends to help with everyday tasks such as shopping for basic necessities.

A spokesman for the CHP said, "Given that the situation of COVID-19 infection remains severe and that there is a continuous increase in the number of cases reported around the world, members of the public are strongly urged to avoid all non-essential travel outside Hong Kong.

"The CHP also strongly urges the public to maintain at all times strict personal and environmental hygiene, which is key to personal protection against infection and prevention of the spread of the disease in the community. On a personal level, members of the public should wear a surgical mask when having respiratory symptoms, taking public transport or staying in crowded places. They should also perform hand hygiene frequently, especially before touching the mouth, nose or eyes.

"As for household environmental hygiene, members of the public are advised to maintain drainage pipes properly, regularly pour water into drain outlets (U-traps) and cover all floor drain outlets when they are not in use. After using the toilet, they should put the toilet lid down before flushing to avoid spreading germs."

Moreover, the Government has launched the website "COVID-19 Thematic Website" (www.coronavirus.gov.hk) for announcing the latest updates on various news on COVID-19 infection and health advice to help the public understand the latest updates. Members of the public may also gain access to information via the COVID-19 WhatsApp Helpline launched by the Office of the Government Chief Information Officer. Simply by saving 9617 1823 in their phone contacts or clicking the link wa.me/85296171823?text=hi, they will be able to obtain information on COVID-19 as well as the "StayHomeSafe" mobile app and wristband via WhatsApp.

Issued at HKT 17:38

Public hospitals daily update on COVID-19 cases

****

The following is issued on behalf of the Hospital Authority:

As at 9am today (October 9), 16 COVID-19 confirmed patients were discharged from hospital in the last 24 hours. So far, a total of 4 906 patients with confirmed or probable infection have been discharged.

At present, there are 627 negative pressure rooms in public hospitals with 1 119 negative pressure beds activated. A total of 123 confirmed patients are currently hospitalised in 18 public hospitals, among which nine patients are in critical condition, eight are in serious condition and the remaining 106 patients are in stable condition.

The Hospital Authority will maintain close contact with the Centre for Health Protection to monitor the latest developments and to inform the public and healthcare workers on the latest information in a timely manner.

Details of the above-mentioned patients are as follows:

Patient condition	Case numbers
Discharged	2298, 4907, 5004, 5037, 5042, 5048, 5051, 5057, 5071, 5074, 5096, 5098, 5105, 5127, 5128, 5146
Critical	1401, 1989, 3496, 3764, 4706, 4833, 4937, 4990, 5110
Serious	1650, 3904, 4100, 4101, 4433, 4746, 4788, 5088

Issued at HKT 17:45

HAD and Lok Sin Tong arrange one-off free COVID-19 testing service for Thai people in Kowloon City

****

The Government is very concerned about the recent confirmed cases of COVID-19 involving Thai people. In view of a large number of Thai people living and working in Kowloon City District, the Home Affairs Department (HAD) and Lok Sin Tong will join hands to arrange voluntary free COVID-19 virus testing service tomorrow (October 10) and the day after (October 11) for Thai people in Kowloon City.

Thai people can collect specimen bottles tomorrow and the day after from 10am to 5pm from Lok Sin Tong Lee Yin Yee United Centre - Support Service Centre for Ethnic Minorities at 47 Tak Ku Ling Road, Kowloon City and return the specimen bottles to Lok Sin Tong Chan Kwong Hing Memorial Primary Health Centre on G/F, 48 Junction Road, Kowloon City from 9am to 12noon on October 12 and 13. The Government appeals to Thai people to actively participate and return specimen bottles on time to eliminate the transmission link in the community as soon as possible and to seek medical treatment promptly. The Government is truly grateful for Lok Sin Tong's assistance, making it possible to launch the testing scheme within a short time.

The Kowloon City District Office (KCDO) has contacted organisations serving Thai people in the district through Lok Sin Tong to inform them about the testing scheme. Specimen bottles and leaflets on anti-epidemic will be distributed to Thai restaurants and merchants in Kowloon City district tomorrow. To cater for the specific needs of Thai people, Lok Sin Tong will arrange Thai volunteers to provide onsite assistance and the relevant anti-epidemic information and guidelines written in Thai will also be provided.

For details on the testing scheme for Thai people in Kowloon City, please contact the KCDO (hotline: 6201 7660) or Lok Sin Tong (hotline: 2382 0106, with Thai language service).

Issued at HKT 21:32

FEHD encourages bar and pub personnel to undergo virus testing

****

In view of the recent development of the COVID-19 epidemic, the Food and Environmental Hygiene Department (FEHD) today (October 9) announced that the FEHD has arranged testing agency, Prenetics Limited, to deliver specimen bottles at bar areas and a mobile van will be parked near the bar areas for three consecutive nights starting from today to encourage personnel in bars and pubs and their patrons to undergo the voluntary testing.

The testing agency delivered specimen bottles at the Lan Kwai Fong bar area tonight, and the mobile van was parked in the vicinity of Wyndham Street. Specimen bottles will be delivered at bar areas in Tsim Sha Tsui and Wan Chai tomorrow and on Sunday night respectively.

A spokesman for the FEHD said, "The testing agency will be responsible for the provision of one-stop service covering specimen taking and testing. The testing agency will deliver specimen bottles to personnel in bars and pubs for collecting deep throat saliva samples, and then collect the samples in the subsequent one to two days for testing. Moreover, the testing agency will also deliver the specimen bottles to patrons of bars and pubs who are interested in taking the test and they can return their specimen bottles by themselves to the collection mobile van of the testing agency parked at Hoi Chak Street in Quarry Bay from 9am to 5pm between October 10 and 12. Cases with positive results will be relayed to the Centre for Health Protection of the Department of Health for follow-up.

To broaden surveillance at the community level, and incorporate disease prevention and infection control into the new normal of the daily operation of society, the Government has integrated and regularised the Targeted Group Testing Scheme as part of sentinel surveillance. The FEHD announced earlier that it will provide voluntary free virus testing services for high-exposure groups as part of the surveillance and early-warning system. By facilitating contact tracing and epidemiological investigations, it will be conducive to 'early identification, early isolation and early treatment', and can provide data for reference for the overall assessment of the epidemic situation.

The FEHD strongly appeals to personnel in bars and pubs to actively participate in the testing scheme, and continue to comply with the directions made under the Prevention and Control of Disease (Requirements and Directions) (Business and Premises) Regulation (Cap. 599F), to maintain personal and environmental hygiene continuously with a view to ensuring cleanliness of the premises, and to always remind their customers to comply with the requirements of the Prevention and Control of Disease (Prohibition on Group Gathering) Regulation (Cap. 599G).

Issued at HKT 22:43

Government sets up temporary testing centres in Wan Chai and Kwai Tsing

****

The Government will set up a temporary testing centre in each of the four districts, namely Wan Chai, Kwai Tsing, Kowloon City and Yau Tsim Mong in phases starting from tomorrow (October 10) to take specimens from members of the public who are willing to take the test voluntarily. In particular, the Wan Chai Temporary Testing Centre located at Harbour Road Sports Centre will commence operation from 10am tomorrow (October 10) and the Kwai Tsing Temporary Testing Centre located at Shek Lei Community Hall will commence operation at 1pm on Sunday (October 11).

A Government spokesman said, "In view of the worsening epidemic situation in Hong Kong, the Government decided to set up testing centres in locations related to recent community outbreak clusters, which are Wan Chai, Kwai Tsing, Kowloon City and Yau Tsim Mong Districts, to facilitate proactive testing of the public, in order to identify cases and asymptomatic patients as early as possible so as to cut the transmission chains in the community. The temporary district-based testing is voluntary and free of charge. No prior appointment is required. Members of the public who consider themselves as having a higher risk of exposure to the virus may visit any of the testing centres during its opening hours for taking combined nasal and throat swab specimens. The contractors of the testing service will collect specimens from the specimen collection centres and deliver them to laboratories for testing."

Upon arrival at the temporary testing centres, members of the public will be asked to show their Hong Kong Identity (HKID) Card, Hong Kong Birth Certificate or any other valid identity document, and to provide mobile telephone number for registration. After the registration, trained medical or healthcare personnel on duty will collect combined nasal and throat swab specimens of members of the public. People whose test results are negative will be informed by SMS through their registered mobile phone number in around two to three days. If a test result is positive, the case will be referred to the Centre for Health Protection of the Department of Health (DH) for immediate follow-up action.

"Except for children under six years old and people not suitable for the test, all holders of valid HKID cards, birth certificates or any other valid identity document who are asymptomatic can visit the nearest temporary test centre for specimen collection."

Wan Chai Temporary Testing Centre will commence operation from tomorrow (October 10) and will be opened until October 14 tentatively. The centre is located at Harbour Road Sports Centre, 27 Harbour Road, Wan Chai. The centre will be open from 10am to 8pm on October 10 and from 8am to 1.30pm and 2.30pm to 8pm on the following four days (October 11 to 14). The specimen collection and testing services are provided by BGI. The expected daily testing capacity is 1 000 specimens.

Kwai Tsing Temporary Testing Centre will commence operation from October 11 and will be opened until October 14 tentatively. The centre is located at Shek Lei Community Hall, 2 Tai Pak Tin Street, Kwai Chung. The centre will be open from 1pm to 8pm on October 11 and from 8am to 1.30pm and 2.30pm to 8pm on the following three days (October 12 to 14). The specimen collection and testing services are provided by Hong Kong Molecular Pathology Diagnostic Centre. The expected daily testing capacity is 1 000 specimens.

The Government is also working on the setting up of temporary testing centres in Kowloon City and Yau Tsim Mong Districts. Details will be announced in due course. The Government will decide whether it is necessary to extend the operation period of the temporary testing centres after reviewing the usage of the temporary testing centres and public's demand for the testing service.

To ensure the health and safety of the public participating in testing and personnel manning the temporary testing centres, these venues selected for use as temporary testing centres have been assessed and considered suitable by the DH and the Electrical and Mechanical Services Department. Various infection control measures will also be put in place at the centres in accordance with the recommendations of the DH. There will also be an adequate supply of protective equipment for personnel manning the testing centres.

In addition to setting up temporary testing centres, in order to assist members of the public who feel they have a higher risk of exposure and are experiencing mild discomfort to undergo a COVID-19 test, the Hospital Authority (HA) has increased the total number of general outpatient clinics for distribution of the deep throat saliva specimen collection packs to 46 starting from September 28. The specimen collection packs distribution time at the 46 HA general outpatient clinics has been extended to 9am to 1pm and 2pm to 5pm from Monday to Friday starting from today (October 9). Members of the public can obtain the specimen collection packs for free near the entrance of the general outpatient clinics during the aforesaid period.

The spokesman stressed that the above testing services would only involve testing on COVID-19 virus. All testing will be conducted in Hong Kong. Specimens and personal data will not be transported outside Hong Kong and the specimens will be destroyed after testing.

Testing is an integral part of the epidemic control strategy. It helps to achieve the objective of early identification, early isolation and early treatment and to cut silent transmission chain so as to curb the spread of disease in the community. The spokesman appealed to all members of the public who have doubts about their health condition to actively take part in the above testing schemes to protect oneself and others and to fight the virus together.

Issued at HKT 23:59

October 10[10]

CHP investigates six additional confirmed cases of COVID-19

****

The Centre for Health Protection (CHP) of the Department of Health has announced that as of 0.00am, October 10, the CHP was investigating six additional confirmed cases of coronavirus disease 2019 (COVID-19), taking the number of cases to 5 176 in Hong Kong so far (comprising 5 175 confirmed cases and one probable case).

Among the newly reported cases announced, three had a travel history during the incubation period.

The CHP's epidemiological investigations and relevant contact tracing on the confirmed cases are ongoing. For case details and contact tracing information, please see the Annex or the list of buildings with confirmed cases of COVID-19 in the past 14 days and the latest local situation of COVID-19 available on the website "COVID-19 Thematic Website" (www.coronavirus.gov.hk).

A spokesman for the CHP said, "During the CHP's epidemiological investigations and relevant contact tracing on the confirmed cases, we will compile and upload (www.chp.gov.hk/files/pdf/building_list_eng.pdf) a list of buildings that confirmed patients had visited from two days before the onset of symptoms. Given that cases of local infection continue to occur from time to time, members of the public are urged to seek medical attention immediately if they believe that they had visited the same place at an identical time with a confirmed patient and feel unwell subsequently. If they remain asymptomatic but are concerned that they have been infected, they can also visit the Hospital Authority's designated general out-patient clinics (www.ha.org.hk/haho/ho/covid-19/GOPC_extend_EN.pdf) to obtain specimen collection packs and collect deep throat saliva specimens for free COVID-19 testing."

In view of the severe epidemic situation, the CHP called on members of the public to avoid going out, having social contact and dining out. They should put on a surgical mask and maintain stringent hand hygiene when they need to go out. The CHP strongly urged the elderly to stay home as far as possible and avoid going out. They should consider asking their family and friends to help with everyday tasks such as shopping for basic necessities.

[10] https://www.info.gov.hk/gia/general/202010/10.htm

A spokesman for the CHP said, "Given that the situation of COVID-19 infection remains severe and that there is a continuous increase in the number of cases reported around the world, members of the public are strongly urged to avoid all non-essential travel outside Hong Kong.

"The CHP also strongly urges the public to maintain at all times strict personal and environmental hygiene, which is key to personal protection against infection and prevention of the spread of the disease in the community. On a personal level, members of the public should wear a surgical mask when having respiratory symptoms, taking public transport or staying in crowded places. They should also perform hand hygiene frequently, especially before touching the mouth, nose or eyes.

"As for household environmental hygiene, members of the public are advised to maintain drainage pipes properly, regularly pour water into drain outlets (U-traps) and cover all floor drain outlets when they are not in use. After using the toilet, they should put the toilet lid down before flushing to avoid spreading germs."

Moreover, the Government has launched the website "COVID-19 Thematic Website" (www.coronavirus.gov.hk) for announcing the latest updates on various news on COVID-19 infection and health advice to help the public understand the latest updates. Members of the public may also gain access to information via the COVID-19 WhatsApp Helpline launched by the Office of the Government Chief Information Officer. Simply by saving 9617 1823 in their phone contacts or clicking the link wa.me/85296171823?text=hi, they will be able to obtain information on COVID-19 as well as the "StayHomeSafe" mobile app and wristband via WhatsApp.

Issued at HKT 14:00

Public hospitals daily update on COVID-19 cases

****

The following is issued on behalf of the Hospital Authority:

As at 9am today (October 10), seven COVID-19 confirmed patients were discharged from hospital in the last 24 hours. Including a patient (case number: 5166) discharged on October 8, a total of 4 914 patients with confirmed or probable infection have been discharged so far.

At present, there are 636 negative pressure rooms in public hospitals with 1 132 negative pressure beds activated. A total of 123 confirmed patients are currently hospitalised in 18 public hospitals, among which eight patients are in critical condition, eight are in serious condition and the remaining 107 patients are in stable condition.

The Hospital Authority will maintain close contact with the Centre for Health Protection to

monitor the latest developments and to inform the public and healthcare workers on the latest information in a timely manner.

Details of the above-mentioned patients are as follows:

Patient condition	Case numbers
Discharged	5047, 5072, 5080, 5081, 5086, 5087, 5166, 5167
Critical	1989, 3496, 3764, 4706, 4833, 4937, 4990, 5110
Serious	1650, 3904, 4100, 4101, 4433, 4746, 4788, 5088

Issued at HKT 17:00

October 11[11]

CHP investigates seven additional confirmed cases of COVID-19

****

The Centre for Health Protection (CHP) of the Department of Health has announced that as of 0.00am, October 11, the CHP was investigating seven additional confirmed cases of coronavirus disease 2019 (COVID-19), taking the number of cases to 5 183 in Hong Kong so far (comprising 5 182 confirmed cases and one probable case).

Among the newly reported cases announced, three had a travel history during the incubation period. The remaining cases were epidemiologically linked with local cases.

The CHP's epidemiological investigations and relevant contact tracing on the confirmed cases are ongoing. For case details and contact tracing information, please see the Annex or the list of buildings with confirmed cases of COVID-19 in the past 14 days and the latest local situation of COVID-19 available on the website "COVID-19 Thematic Website" (www.coronavirus.gov.hk).

A spokesman for the CHP said, "During the CHP's epidemiological investigations and relevant contact tracing on the confirmed cases, we will compile and upload (www.chp.gov.hk/files/pdf/building_list_eng.pdf) a list of buildings that confirmed patients had visited from two days before the onset of symptoms. Given that cases of local infection continue to occur from time to time, members of the public are urged to seek medical attention immediately if they believe that they had visited the same place at an identical time with a

[11] https://www.info.gov.hk/gia/general/202010/11.htm

confirmed patient and feel unwell subsequently. If they remain asymptomatic but are concerned that they have been infected, they can also visit the Hospital Authority's designated general out-patient clinics (www.ha.org.hk/haho/ho/covid-19/GOPC_extend_EN.pdf) to obtain specimen collection packs and collect deep throat saliva specimens for free COVID-19 testing."

In view of the severe epidemic situation, the CHP called on members of the public to avoid going out, having social contact and dining out. They should put on a surgical mask and maintain stringent hand hygiene when they need to go out. The CHP strongly urged the elderly to stay home as far as possible and avoid going out. They should consider asking their family and friends to help with everyday tasks such as shopping for basic necessities.

The spokesman said, "Given that the situation of COVID-19 infection remains severe and that there is a continuous increase in the number of cases reported around the world, members of the public are strongly urged to avoid all non-essential travel outside Hong Kong.

"The CHP also strongly urges the public to maintain at all times strict personal and environmental hygiene, which is key to personal protection against infection and prevention of the spread of the disease in the community. On a personal level, members of the public should wear a surgical mask when having respiratory symptoms, taking public transport or staying in crowded places. They should also perform hand hygiene frequently, especially before touching the mouth, nose or eyes.

"As for household environmental hygiene, members of the public are advised to maintain drainage pipes properly, regularly pour water into drain outlets (U-traps) and cover all floor drain outlets when they are not in use. After using the toilet, they should put the toilet lid down before flushing to avoid spreading germs."

Moreover, the Government has launched the website "COVID-19 Thematic Website" (www.coronavirus.gov.hk) for announcing the latest updates on various news on COVID-19 infection and health advice to help the public understand the latest updates. Members of the public may also gain access to information via the COVID-19 WhatsApp Helpline launched by the Office of the Government Chief Information Officer. Simply by saving 9617 1823 in their phone contacts or clicking the link wa.me/85296171823?text=hi, they will be able to obtain information on COVID-19 as well as the "StayHomeSafe" mobile app and wristband via WhatsApp.

Issued at HKT 14:00

Public hospitals daily update on COVID-19 cases

****

The following is issued on behalf of the Hospital Authority:

As at 9am today (October 11), five COVID-19 confirmed patients were discharged from hospital in the last 24 hours. So far, a total of 4 919 patients with confirmed or probable infection have been discharged.

At present, there are 636 negative pressure rooms in public hospitals with 1 132 negative pressure beds activated. A total of 124 confirmed patients are currently hospitalised in 18 public hospitals, among which eight patients are in critical condition, nine are in serious condition and the remaining 107 patients are in stable condition.

The Hospital Authority will maintain close contact with the Centre for Health Protection to monitor the latest developments and to inform the public and healthcare workers on the latest information in a timely manner.

Details of the above-mentioned patients are as follows:

Patient condition	Case numbers
Discharged	2006, 3761, 5090, 5162, 5173
Critical	1989, 3496, 3764, 4706, 4833, 4937, 4990, 5110
Serious	1650, 3904, 4100, 4101, 4433, 4746, 4788, 5088, 5152

Issued at HKT 16:30

Government sets up temporary testing centres in Kowloon City and Yau Tsim Mong

****

The Government has been setting up temporary testing centres in four districts, namely Wan Chai, Kwai Tsing, Kowloon City and Yau Tsim Mong in phases starting from yesterday (October 10) to take specimens from members of the public for free. In particular, the Kowloon City Temporary Testing Centre located at Kai Tak Community Hall and the Yau Tsim Mong Temporary Testing Centre located at Henry G. Leong Yaumatei Community Centre will commence operation from 8am tomorrow (October 12).

A Government spokesman said, "In view of the worsening epidemic situation in Hong Kong, the Government decided to set up testing centres in locations related to recent community outbreak clusters, which are Wan Chai, Kwai Tsing, Kowloon City and Yau Tsim Mong Districts, to facilitate proactive testing of the public, in order to identify cases and asymptomatic patients as early as possible so as to cut the transmission chains in the community. The temporary district-based testing is free of charge. No prior appointment is required. Members of the public who consider themselves as having a higher risk of exposure to the virus may visit any of the testing centres during its opening hours for taking combined nasal and throat swab specimens. The contractors of the testing service will collect specimens from the temporary testing centres and deliver them to laboratories for testing."

Upon arrival at the temporary testing centres, members of the public will be asked to show his/her Hong Kong Identity (HKID) Card, Hong Kong Birth Certificate or any other valid identity document, and to provide a local mobile phone number that can receive SMS for registration. After the registration, trained medical or healthcare personnel will collect combined nasal and throat swab specimens of members of the public. People whose test results are negative will be informed by SMS through their registered mobile phone number in around two to three days. If a test result is positive, the case will be referred to the Centre for Health Protection of the Department of Health (DH) for immediate follow-up action.

"Except for children under six years old and people not suitable for the test, all holders of valid HKID cards, birth certificates or any other valid identity document who are asymptomatic can visit the nearest temporary test centre for specimen collection."

Kowloon City Temporary Testing Centre and Yau Tsim Mong Temporary Testing Centre will commence operation from tomorrow and will be opened until October 14 tentatively. The two centres will be open from 8am to 1.30pm and 2.30pm to 8pm every day. Kowloon City Temporary Testing Centre is located at Kai Tak Community Hall, 3 Concorde Road, Kai Tak. Yau Tsim Mong Temporary Testing Centre is located at Henry G Leong Yaumatei Community Centre, 60 Public Square Street, Yau Ma Tei. The specimen collection and testing services for both centres are provided by Hong Kong Molecular Pathology Diagnostic Centre. The expected daily testing capacity is 1 000 specimens for each centre.

Wan Chai Temporary Testing Centre and Kwai Tsing Temporary Testing Centre which have commenced operation yesterday and today respectively will continue to provide service until October 14 tentatively. The two centres will also be open from 8am to 1.30pm and 2.30pm to 8pm every day.

The Government will decide whether it is necessary to extend the operation period of the temporary testing centres after reviewing the usage of the temporary testing centres and public's demand for the testing service.

To ensure the health and safety of the public participating in testing and personnel manning the temporary testing centres, these venues selected for use as temporary testing centres have been assessed and considered suitable by the DH and the Electrical and Mechanical Services Department. Various infection control measures will also be put in place at the centres in accordance with the recommendations of the DH. There will also be an adequate supply of protective equipment for personnel manning the testing centres.

In addition to setting up temporary testing centres, in order to assist members of the public who feel they have a higher risk of exposure and are experiencing mild discomfort to undergo a

COVID-19 test, the Hospital Authority (HA) has increased the total number of general outpatient clinics for distribution of the deep throat saliva specimen collection packs to 46 starting from September 28. The specimen collection packs distribution time at the 46 HA general outpatient clinics has been extended to 9am to 1pm and 2pm to 5pm from Monday to Friday starting from October 9. Members of the public can obtain the specimen collection packs for free near the entrance of the general outpatient clinics during the aforesaid period.

Testing is an integral part of the epidemic control strategy. It helps to achieve the objective of early identification, early isolation and early treatment and to cut silent transmission chain so as to curb the spread of disease in the community. The spokesman appealed to all members of the public who have doubts about their health condition to actively take part in the above testing schemes to protect oneself and others and to fight the virus together.

Issued at HKT 16:46

Temporary testing centres provide free testing service to public

****

As at 8pm today (October 11), specimens had been collected from a total of 1 844 persons at Wan Chai and Kwai Tsing Temporary Testing Centres set up by the Government for COVID-19 nucleic acid test.

Specimens from 619 persons were collected today at the Wan Chai Temporary Testing Centre located at Harbour Road Sports Centre, which opened from from 8am to 1.30pm and 2.30pm to 8pm while specimens from 707 persons were collected today at the Kwai Tsing Temporary Testing Centre located at Shek Lei Community Hall, which opened from 1pm to 8pm.

As at 10pm today, a total of 518 specimens collected under the temporary community testing arrangement had been tested. If there is any specimen tested with positive COVID-19 result, it will be referred to the Public Health Laboratory Services Branch of the Department of Health (DH) for confirmatory test. Confirmed cases will be followed up and announced by the Centre for Health Protection of the DH.

A Government spokesman said that in view of the worsening epidemic situation in Hong Kong, the Government decided to set up one temporary testing centre in each of the four districts, namely Wan Chai, Kwai Tsing, Kowloon City and Yau Tsim Mong Districts, which are related to recent community outbreak clusters. The Wan Chai and Kwai Tsing Temporary Testing Centres commenced operation yesterday and today respectively while the Kowloon City and Yau Tsim Mong Temporary Testing Centres will commence operation at 8am tomorrow (October 12).

The Kowloon City Temporary Testing Centre is located at Kai Tak Community Hall, 3 Concorde Road, Kai Tak. The Yau Tsim Mong Temporary Testing Centre is located at Henry G Leong Yaumatei Community Centre, 60 Public Square Street, Yau Ma Tei.

All four temporary testing centres will be open from 8am to 1.30pm and 2.30pm to 8pm every day, until October 14 tentatively, to provide free specimen collection and testing service to facilitate proactive testing of members of the public, in order to identify cases and asymptomatic patients as early as possible so as to cut the transmission chains in the community.

Moreover, to facilitate more members of the public to receive COVID-19 tests, the deep throat saliva specimen collection packs distribution time at the 46 general outpatient clinics (GOPCs) of the Hospital Authority (HA) has been extended to 9am to 1pm and 2pm to 5pm from Monday to Friday, since October 9. Over 3 000 specimen collection packs were distributed on the first day of extended distribution time in the 46 HA GOPCs. Since July 27, HA GOPCs have distributed over 63 000 specimen collection packs. Over 38 000 specimens were tested by the laboratory, and over 60 were positive for COVID-19.

Furthermore, the second round of testing services provided to frontline staff of catering businesses by the Food and Environmental Hygiene Department (FEHD) under the Targeted Group Testing Scheme commenced on October 1. Up to October 10, over 12 000 specimen bottles have been distributed to catering premises and over 3 800 specimens have been tested. The FEHD has arranged a testing agency to deliver specimen bottles at bar areas and a mobile van will be parked near the bar areas for three consecutive nights starting from October 9 to encourage personnel in bars and pubs and their patrons to undergo the voluntary testing. The testing agency distributed a total of 1 286 specimen bottles in the past two nights. Among them, 991 specimen bottles (included in the over 12 000 specimen bottles mentioned above) were distributed to staff members and 295 were distributed to patrons.

The spokesman appealed to all members of the public who have doubts about their health condition to undergo testing to protect oneself and others and to fight the virus together.

Issued at HKT 23:29

October 12[12]

Public hospitals daily update on COVID-19 cases

****

The following is issued on behalf of the Hospital Authority:

---

[12] https://www.info.gov.hk/gia/general/202010/12.htm

As at 9am today (October 12), two COVID-19 confirmed patients were discharged from hospital in the last 24 hours. So far, a total of 4 921 patients with confirmed or probable infection have been discharged.

At present, there are 623 negative pressure rooms in public hospitals with 1 115 negative pressure beds activated. A total of 129 confirmed patients are currently hospitalised in 18 public hospitals, among which eight patients are in critical condition, nine are in serious condition and the remaining 112 patients are in stable condition.

The Hospital Authority will maintain close contact with the Centre for Health Protection to monitor the latest developments and to inform the public and healthcare workers on the latest information in a timely manner.

Details of the above-mentioned patients are as follows:

Patient condition	Case numbers
Discharged	5106, 5108
Critical	1989, 3496, 3764, 4706, 4833, 4937, 4990, 5110
Serious	1650, 3904, 4100, 4101, 4433, 4746, 4788, 5088, 5152

Issued at HKT 18:32

CHP investigates 11 additional confirmed cases of COVID-19

****

The Centre for Health Protection (CHP) of the Department of Health has announced that as of 0.00am, October 12, the CHP was investigating 11 additional confirmed cases of coronavirus disease 2019 (COVID-19), taking the number of cases to 5 194 in Hong Kong so far (comprising 5 193 confirmed cases and one probable case).

Among the newly reported cases announced, six had a travel history during the incubation period.

The CHP's epidemiological investigations and relevant contact tracing on the confirmed cases are ongoing. For case details and contact tracing information, please see the Annex or the list of buildings with confirmed cases of COVID-19 in the past 14 days and the latest local situation of COVID-19 available on the website "COVID-19 Thematic Website" (www.coronavirus.gov.hk).

A spokesman for the CHP said, "During the CHP's epidemiological investigations and relevant contact tracing on the confirmed cases, we will compile and upload (www.chp.gov.hk/files/pdf/building_list_eng.pdf) a list of buildings that confirmed patients had visited from two days before the onset of symptoms. Given that cases of local infection continue to occur from time to time, members of the public are urged to seek medical attention immediately if they believe that they had visited the same place at an identical time with a confirmed patient and feel unwell subsequently. If they remain asymptomatic but are concerned that they have been infected, they can also visit the Hospital Authority's designated general out-patient clinics (www.ha.org.hk/haho/ho/covid-19/GOPC_extend_EN.pdf) to obtain specimen collection packs and collect deep throat saliva specimens for free COVID-19 testing."

In view of the severe epidemic situation, the CHP called on members of the public to avoid going out, having social contact and dining out. They should put on a surgical mask and maintain stringent hand hygiene when they need to go out. The CHP strongly urged the elderly to stay home as far as possible and avoid going out. They should consider asking their family and friends to help with everyday tasks such as shopping for basic necessities.

The spokesman said, "Given that the situation of COVID-19 infection remains severe and that there is a continuous increase in the number of cases reported around the world, members of the public are strongly urged to avoid all non-essential travel outside Hong Kong.

"The CHP also strongly urges the public to maintain at all times strict personal and environmental hygiene, which is key to personal protection against infection and prevention of the spread of the disease in the community. On a personal level, members of the public should wear a surgical mask when having respiratory symptoms, taking public transport or staying in crowded places. They should also perform hand hygiene frequently, especially before touching the mouth, nose or eyes.

"As for household environmental hygiene, members of the public are advised to maintain drainage pipes properly, regularly pour water into drain outlets (U-traps) and cover all floor drain outlets when they are not in use. After using the toilet, they should put the toilet lid down before flushing to avoid spreading germs."

Moreover, the Government has launched the website "COVID-19 Thematic Website" (www.coronavirus.gov.hk) for announcing the latest updates on various news on COVID-19 infection and health advice to help the public understand the latest updates. Members of the public may also gain access to information via the COVID-19 WhatsApp Helpline launched by the Office of the Government Chief Information Officer. Simply by saving 9617 1823 in their phone contacts or clicking the link wa.me/85296171823?text=hi, they will be able to obtain information on COVID-19 as well as the "StayHomeSafe" mobile app and wristband via WhatsApp.

Issued at HKT 18:41

Princess Margaret Hospital announces incident involving handling of specimens

****

The following is issued on behalf of the Hospital Authority:

The spokesperson for Princess Margaret Hospital (PMH) made the following announcement today (October 12) regarding an incident involving the handling of specimens:

PMH has set up a specimen collection point at the Specialist Out-patient Clinic for PMH patients to submit deep throat saliva specimens for COVID-19 testing. Ten deep throat saliva specimens submitted last Saturday (October 10), which were scheduled to be sent to the PMH laboratory for COVID-19 testing on the same day, were found at the collection point this morning. As the specimens concerned had not been sent to the laboratory for handling immediately, the hospital has contacted all individuals concerned to re-submit deep throat saliva or nasopharyngeal swab specimens to ensure the accuracy of the test results.

The hospital is highly concerned about the incident and apologises to the patients concerned for the inconvenience caused. The hospital has reported the case to the Hospital Authority Head Office via the Advance Incident Reporting System. Meanwhile, the hospital will enhance staff training and review the workflow for handling specimens, and improvement measures will be proposed to prevent similar incidents from happening again.

Issued at HKT 19:04

Temporary testing centres continue to provide free testing service to public

****

As at 8pm today (October 12), specimens had been collected from a total of 4 938 persons at Wan Chai, Kwai Tsing, Kowloon City and Yau Tsim Mong Temporary Testing Centres set up by the Government for COVID-19 nucleic acid tests. The temporary testing centres will continue to provide service to members of the public tomorrow (October 13)

Specimens from 711 persons were collected today at the Wan Chai Temporary Testing Centre located at Harbour Road Sports Centre.

Specimens from 955 persons were collected today at the Kwai Tsing Temporary Testing Centre located at Shek Lei Community Hall.

Specimens from 463 persons were collected today at the Kowloon City Temporary Testing Centre located at Kai Tak Community Hall.

Specimens from 965 persons were collected today at the Yau Tsim Mong Temporary Testing Centre located at Henry G Leong Yaumatei Community Centre.

As at 10pm today, a total of 1 844 specimens collected under the temporary community testing arrangement had been tested. If any specimen tested shows a positive COVID-19 result, the specimen will be referred to the Public Health Laboratory Services Branch of the Department of Health (DH) for a confirmatory test. Confirmed cases will be followed up and announced by the Centre for Health Protection of the DH.

A Government spokesman said that in view of the worsening COVID-19 epidemic situation in Hong Kong, the Government decided to set up one temporary testing centre in each of the four districts, namely Wan Chai, Kwai Tsing, Kowloon City and Yau Tsim Mong Districts, which are related to recent community outbreak clusters.

All four temporary testing centres will be open from 8am to 1.30pm and 2.30pm to 8pm every day until October 14 tentatively, to provide free specimen collection and testing services to facilitate proactive testing of members of the public, in order to identify cases and asymptomatic patients as early as possible so as to cut the transmission chains in the community.

The temporary testing centers will be closed if Tropical Cyclone Warning Signal No. 8 or higher is issued. If Tropical Cyclone Warning Signal No. 8 or higher is cancelled within two hours before the closing time of centres, the centres will not open during the day.

Moreover, to facilitate more members of the public to receive COVID-19 tests, distribution time of the deep throat saliva specimen collection packs at the 46 general outpatient clinics (GOPCs) of the Hospital Authority (HA) has been extended to 9am to 1pm and 2pm to 5pm from Monday to Friday, since October 9. The 46 HA GOPCs distributed a total of over 2 400 specimen collection packs on October 12. Since July 27, HA GOPCs have distributed over 65 000 specimen collection packs. Over 39 000 specimens were tested by the laboratory, and over 60 were positive for COVID-19.

Furthermore, the second round of testing services provided to frontline staff of catering businesses by the Food and Environmental Hygiene Department (FEHD) under the Targeted Group Testing Scheme commenced on October 1. Up to October 11, over 12 900 specimen bottles have been distributed to catering premises and around 4 000 specimens have been tested. The FEHD has arranged a testing agency to deliver specimen bottles at bar areas and a mobile van were parked near the bar areas for three consecutive nights starting from October 9 to encourage personnel in bars and pubs and their patrons to undergo testing. The testing agency distributed a total of over 2 100 specimen bottles in the past three nights. Among them, around 1 770 specimen bottles (included in the over 12 900 specimen bottles mentioned above) were distributed to staff members and around 390 were distributed to patrons.

The spokesman appealed to all members of the public who have doubts about their health condition to undergo testing to protect oneself and others and to fight the virus together.

Issued at HKT 23:24

October 13[13]

Arrangement for free COVID-19 testing service for taxi and public light bus drivers

****

As the No.8 gale or storm signal is now in force, the Transport Department announced that the services of the 11 temporary distribution/collection centres for distribution of swab self-sampling kits and collection of specimens for taxi and public light bus drivers scheduled today (October 13) will be temporarily suspended. If No.8 gale or storm signal is lowered before 2pm, all temporary distribution/collection centres will be reopened within about two hours. If No.8 gale or storm signal is still in force at 2pm, all temporary distribution/collection centres will be closed today.

Issued at HKT 6:04

Suspension of COVID-19 testing service for foreign domestic helpers waiting to join new employers' family

****

Attention duty announcers, radio and TV stations:

Please broadcast the following as soon as possible and repeat it at suitable intervals:

The Labour Department announces that the COVID-19 testing service for foreign domestic helpers (FDHs) who are waiting to join the new employers' family at Harbour Road Sports Centre, as well as the related service of the registration hotline 1836 133 will be suspended as the Tropical Cyclone Warning Signal No. 8 has been issued. The services will be resumed within two hours after the signal was cancelled when weather and traffic permit. FDHs affected by the suspension of services can call the hotline 1836 133 to reschedule the appointment upon the resumption of the hotline service.

Issued at HKT 6:12

---

[13] https://www.info.gov.hk/gia/general/202010/13.htm

HAD's collection point of deep throat saliva samples for Thai people suspended

****

Attention duty announcers of radio and television stations:

Please broadcast the following message as soon as possible and repeat it at suitable intervals:

The Home Affairs Department today (October 13) announced that, as the Tropical Cyclone Warning Signal No. 8 is now in force, the collection point of deep throat saliva samples for COVID-19 testing set up at Lok Sin Tong Chan Kwong Hing Memorial Primary Health Centre on G/F, 48 Junction Road, Kowloon City, for Thai people in Kowloon City district will be suspended today. The date of returning specimen bottles will be postponed to tomorrow (October 14) from 9 am till 12 noon.

Issued at HKT 8:53

CHP investigates eight additional confirmed cases of COVID-19

****

The Centre for Health Protection (CHP) of the Department of Health has announced that as of 0.00am, October 13, the CHP was investigating eight additional confirmed cases of coronavirus disease 2019 (COVID-19), taking the number of cases to 5202 in Hong Kong so far (comprising 5201 confirmed cases and one probable case).

Among the newly reported cases announced, four had a travel history during the incubation period, two are epidemiologically linked with local cases while two are local cases with unknown sources.

One of the cases with unknown sources involves a 68-year-old man (case 5195) who had developed fever on October 5. He consulted a private doctor on October 5 and 8 and then sought medical treatment at the Accident and Emergency (A&E) Department of Tseung Kwan O Hospital on October 11 where he was admitted for further management. A family member who lives with him is also among the newly reported cases announced today.

The other case with unknown sources involves a 48-year-old man (case 5199) who developed fever on October 10. He sought medical treatment at the A&E Department of United Christian Hospital on October 11 and submitted a deep throat saliva sample on the following day. He works at Cityplaza One and last went to work on October 9.

The CHP's epidemiological investigations and relevant contact tracing on the confirmed cases are ongoing. For case details and contact tracing information, please see the Annex or the list of buildings with confirmed cases of COVID-19 in the past 14 days and the latest local situation of COVID-19 available on the website "COVID-19 Thematic Website" (www.coronavirus.gov.hk).

A spokesman for the CHP said, "During the CHP's epidemiological investigations and relevant contact tracing on the confirmed cases, we will compile and upload (www.chp.gov.hk/files/pdf/building_list_eng.pdf) a list of buildings that confirmed patients had visited from two days before the onset of symptoms. Given that cases of local infection continue to occur from time to time, members of the public are urged to seek medical attention immediately if they believe that they had visited the same place at an identical time with a confirmed patient and feel unwell subsequently. If they remain asymptomatic but are concerned that they have been infected, they can also visit the Hospital Authority's designated general out-patient clinics (www.ha.org.hk/haho/ho/covid-19/GOPC_extend_EN.pdf) to obtain specimen collection packs and collect deep throat saliva specimens for free COVID-19 testing."

In view of the severe epidemic situation, the CHP called on members of the public to avoid going out, having social contact and dining out. They should put on a surgical mask and maintain stringent hand hygiene when they need to go out. The CHP strongly urged the elderly to stay home as far as possible and avoid going out. They should consider asking their family and friends to help with everyday tasks such as shopping for basic necessities.

The spokesman said, "Given that the situation of COVID-19 infection remains severe and that there is a continuous increase in the number of cases reported around the world, members of the public are strongly urged to avoid all non-essential travel outside Hong Kong

"The CHP also strongly urges the public to maintain at all times strict personal and environmental hygiene, which is key to personal protection against infection and prevention of the spread of the disease in the community. On a personal level, members of the public should wear a surgical mask when having respiratory symptoms, taking public transport or staying in crowded places. They should also perform hand hygiene frequently, especially before touching the mouth, nose or eyes.

"As for household environmental hygiene, members of the public are advised to maintain drainage pipes properly, regularly pour water into drain outlets (U-traps) and cover all floor drain outlets when they are not in use. After using the toilet, they should put the toilet lid down before flushing to avoid spreading germs."

Moreover, the Government has launched the website "COVID-19 Thematic Website" (www.coronavirus.gov.hk) for announcing the latest updates on various news on COVID-19 infection and health advice to help the public understand the latest updates. Members of the public may also gain access to information via the COVID-19 WhatsApp Helpline launched by the Office of the Government Chief Information Officer. Simply by saving 9617 1823 in their phone contacts or clicking the link wa.me/85296171823?text=hi, they will be able to obtain information on COVID-19 as well as the "StayHomeSafe" mobile app and wristband via WhatsApp.

Issued at HKT 16:00

Four temporary testing centres closed for whole day
****

Attention duty announcers of radio and television stations:

Please broadcast the following message as soon as possible and repeat it at suitable intervals:

The Government today (October 13) announced that, as the Tropical Cyclone Warning Signal No. 8 is still in force, four temporary testing centres located at Harbour Road Sports Centre, Wan Chai District; Shek Lei Community Hall, Kwai Tsing District; Kai Tak Community Hall, Kowloon City District; and Henry G Leong Yaumatei Community Centre, Yau Tsim Mong District, will remain closed today.

Issued at HKT 16:15

Government extends social distancing measures under Prevention and Control of Disease Ordinance
****

The Government announced today (October 13) that the social distancing measures currently in force will be maintained and the directions and specifications under the Prevention and Control of Disease (Requirements and Directions) (Business and Premises) Regulation (Cap. 599F), the Prevention and Control of Disease (Prohibition on Group Gathering) Regulation (Cap. 599G) and the Prevention and Control of Disease (Wearing of Mask) Regulation (Cap. 599I) will be gazetted tomorrow (October 14). The above-mentioned measures will take effect at 0.00am on October 16 for a period of seven days till October 22.

A spokesman for the Food and Health Bureau said, "It is worrying that the seven-day average number of locally confirmed cases continued to increase over the past week, with a number of confirmed cases with unknown sources of infection reported, indicating the existence of silent transmission chains in the community and highly probable rebound in the epidemic situation. Meanwhile, the severe global epidemic situation may also bring public health risks to Hong Kong. Nevertheless, as we have reiterated time and again, under the new normal, we cannot and should not aim at having no confirmed case in the community for an extended period of time.

Although we would much prefer seeing no local cases, it would be unavoidable to have sporadic cases and clusters in the community from time to time as the virus will co-exist with us for quite a long period of time before effective treatment and vaccination become available. In this regard, we will continue to adopt a targeted approach for reducing the risk of the virus entering and spreading within the community as far as practicable, avoid the one-size-fits-all approach when adjusting social distancing measures, and work closely with the relevant trades to strengthen infection control measures at the premises concerned, in order to allow members of the public to maintain social and economic activities to a certain extent as far as practicable under the new normal."

"We understand that members of the public are experiencing anti-epidemic fatigue to different extents and have become less alert in combating the epidemic, after many months of fighting against the disease. However, if each of us as a member of society does not comply strictly with the various epidemic control and social distancing measures and does not remain vigilant in maintaining personal and environmental hygiene, the risk of a rebound of the epidemic would be extremely high and we may well be on the verge of a large-scale community outbreak. As the latest virus strain has higher transmissibility, the epidemic may worsen rapidly in a very short period of time, possibly causing the fourth wave of the local epidemic to arrive early."

Since late August, the Government, having regard to the fact that the epidemic has subsided from its peak in late July, has relaxed or adjusted the various social distancing measures under a refined and sophisticated approach in a gradual and orderly manner, so as to allow social and economic activities to resume as far as possible under the new normal. The measures include relaxing the restriction on the number of persons allowed in group gatherings in public places, extending the hours when dine-in services are allowed in catering premises and relaxing the number of persons allowed to be seated together at one table therein, reopening all catering business and scheduled premises, and allowing team sports at sports premises and public skating rinks.

Taking into account the latest public health risk assessment, starting this Friday (October 16), the Government will maintain all requirements and restrictions applicable to catering business and scheduled premises.

The spokesman added, "As we have stressed time and again, co-operation and self-discipline of members of the public are the keys to the effectiveness of social distancing measures in preventing the spread of the disease in the community and the public's concerted efforts in fighting the epidemic and compliance with requirements and restrictions applicable to individual premises are of utmost importance. Only with the co-operation of society as a whole can we prevent another outbreak in the community and the hard work that the entire society has put in for the past three months from going in vain. Otherwise, when there is another large-scale outbreak in the community, the Government will have no choice but to significantly tighten social distancing measures in order to safeguard public health."

The Government will continue to closely monitor the development of the epidemic situation and review and adjust the various measures in place from time to time while striking a balance among disease prevention and control, economic needs and level of acceptance of the society, and will announce the latest social distancing measures in a timely manner.

The requirements and restrictions under the latest directions and specifications are as follows:

(I) Catering business premises and scheduled premises

The requirements and restrictions applicable to catering business and scheduled premises (see Annex 1 for details) will be maintained during the seven-day period from October 16 to 22, 2020. Amongst others, activities and facilities involving higher health risks such as dancing activities, steam and sauna facilities and ball pits will continue to be suspended or prohibited from opening.

Persons responsible for carrying on catering businesses and managers of scheduled premises that contravene the statutory requirements under Cap. 599F would have committed a criminal offence. Offenders are subject to a maximum fine of $50,000 and imprisonment for six months.

(II) Group gatherings

Unless exempted, the prohibition on group gatherings of more than four persons in public places will continue during the seven-day period from October 16 to 22, 2020.

Any person who participates in a prohibited group gathering; organises a prohibited group gathering; owns, controls or operates the place of such gathering and knowingly allows the taking place of such gathering, commits an offence under Cap. 599G. Offenders are liable to a maximum fine of $25,000 and imprisonment for six months. Persons who participate in a prohibited group gathering may discharge liability for the offence by paying a fixed penalty of $2,000.

(III) Mask-wearing requirement

The mandatory mask-wearing requirement under Cap. 599I will be extended for a period of seven days from October 16 to 22, 2020. During the aforementioned period, a person must wear a mask all the time when the person is boarding or onboard a public transport carrier, is entering or present in an MTR paid area, or is entering or present in a specified public place (i.e. all public places, save for outdoor public places in country parks and special areas as defined in section 2 of the Country Parks Ordinance (Cap. 208).

Under Cap. 599I, if a person does not wear a mask in accordance with the requirement, an authorised person may deny that person from boarding a public transport carrier or entering the area concerned, as well as require that person to wear a mask and disembark from the carrier or leave the said area. A person in contravention of the relevant provision commits an offence and the maximum penalty is a fine at level 2 ($5,000). In addition, authorised public officers may issue fixed penalty notices to persons who do not wear a mask in accordance with the requirement and such persons may discharge liability for the offence by paying a fixed penalty of $2,000.

Issued at HKT 17:24

Public hospitals daily update on COVID-19 cases

****

The following is issued on behalf of the Hospital Authority:

As at 9am today (October 13), 10 COVID-19 confirmed patients were discharged from hospital in the last 24 hours. So far, a total of 4 931 patients with confirmed or probable infection have been discharged.

At present, there are 623 negative pressure rooms in public hospitals with 1 115 negative pressure beds activated. A total of 130 confirmed patients are currently hospitalised in 18 public hospitals, among which 10 patients are in critical condition, eight are in serious condition and the remaining 112 patients are in stable condition.

The Hospital Authority will maintain close contact with the Centre for Health Protection to monitor the latest developments and to inform the public and healthcare workers on the latest information in a timely manner.

Details of the above-mentioned patients are as follows:

Patient condition	Case numbers
Discharged	2709, 5018, 5055, 5068, 5085, 5099, 5107, 5177, 5186, 5190
Critical	1989, 3496, 3764, 4706, 4833, 4937, 4990, 5110, 5152, 5185
Serious	1650, 3904, 4100, 4101, 4433, 4746, 4788, 5088

Issued at HKT 17:25

Operation period of temporary testing centres extended to this Friday

****

The four temporary testing centres set up by the Government in Wan Chai, Kwai Tsing, Kowloon City and Yau Tsim Mong were closed today (October 13) due to the issuance of the Tropical Cyclone Warning Signal No. 8. After reviewing the usage of the temporary testing centres and public's demand for the testing service, the Government has decided to extend the operation period of the four temporary testing centres to October 16. The centres will continue to be open from 8am to 1.30pm and 2.30pm to 8pm every day.

A Government spokesman said that in view of the worsening COVID-19 epidemic situation in Hong Kong, the Government has set up one temporary testing centre in each of the four districts, namely Wan Chai, Kwai Tsing, Kowloon City and Yau Tsim Mong Districts, which are related to recent community outbreak clusters. The temporary testing centres provide free specimen collection and testing services to facilitate proactive testing of members of the public, in order to identify cases and asymptomatic patients as early as possible so as to cut the transmission chains in the community.

As at 10pm today, a total of 4 938 specimens collected under the temporary community testing arrangement had been tested. If any specimen tested shows a positive COVID-19 result, the specimen will be referred to the Public Health Laboratory Services Branch of the Department of Health (DH) for a confirmatory test. Confirmed cases will be followed up and announced by the Centre for Health Protection of the DH.

Moreover, to facilitate more members of the public to receive COVID-19 tests, distribution time of the deep throat saliva specimen collection packs at the 46 general outpatient clinics of the Hospital Authority has been extended to 9am to 1pm and 2pm to 5pm from Monday to Friday, since October 9.

The spokesman appealed to all members of the public who have doubts about their health condition to undergo testing to protect oneself and others and to fight the virus together.

Issued at HKT 22:10

October 14[14]

FEHD and catering businesses join hands to strengthen anti-epidemic measures

****

[14] https://www.info.gov.hk/gia/general/202010/14.htm

The Food and Environmental Hygiene Department (FEHD) met with representatives of the catering businesses, including restaurants, bars, karaoke establishments and nightclubs on October 13, to discuss how the Government and the catering sector could further strengthen anti-epidemic measures in catering premises, and implement various targeted measures to address recommendations made by public health expert advisers on critical control points, with a view to minimising the risk of transmission of COVID-19 in catering premises.

A spokesman for the FEHD said that the trade was reminded again at the meeting to strictly comply with the requirements under relevant anti-epidemic regulations. According to the directions issued by the Secretary for Food and Health in relation to catering business under the Prevention and Control of Disease (Requirements and Directions) (Business and Premises) Regulation (the Regulation) (Cap. 599F) , catering business operators and practitioners have to strictly comply with a series of requirements and restrictions. Among these, selling or supplying food or drink for consumption on the premises from 0.00am to 4.59am must be ceased; the number of customers at any premises must not exceed half of its normal seating capacity; no more than four persons may be seated together at one table at catering premises; tables must be arranged in a way to ensure there is a distance of at least 1.5m or some form of partition which could serve as effective buffer between one table and another table; a mask must be worn at all times within the premises, except when the person is consuming food or drink; and body temperature screening must be conducted before the person is allowed to enter the catering premises and hand sanitisers must be provided. According to the Regulation, directions and the requirements under the Prevention and Control of Disease (Prohibition in Group Gathering) Regulation (Cap. 599G), members of the public also have to comply with the related restriction on group gatherings that no more than four persons may be seated at one table at catering premises.

In order to help catering business operators and practitioners understand the anti-epidemic measures in food premises clearly, the FEHD has uploaded related training materials on anti-epidemic measures onto the FEHD's website (www.fehd.gov.hk/english/licensing/advice_COVID19_FoodPremises.pdf), for hygiene managers and hygiene supervisors of licensed restaurants to familiarise themselves with the measures and strictly implement them in the catering premises.

In addition, in response to expert advisers' advice to improve the ventilation in catering outlets so as to achieve better anti-epidemic effect, the FEHD will make an announcement within this week to launch a webpage for providing a platform for catering outlets to voluntarily report the air change per hour of the ventilation system and the related air disinfection equipment provided as required at their catering premises for public inspection.

At the invitation of the FEHD, the Office of the Government Chief Information Officer (OGCIO) also joined the meeting to introduce to the trade a mobile app under development by the OGCIO on exposure risk notification, which allows catering businesses to participate according to their needs. Members of the public can also participate voluntarily and make records of their own accord, so that it would be easier for them to master their travel history and they could contact the Centre for Health Protection (CHP) themselves if needed. The trade said in the meeting that they will collaborate actively to facilitate the CHP's close contact tracing work. Some bars and karaoke establishments have already called on their customers to fill in electronic health declaration forms to facilitate communication when necessary. The Government and the trade will continue to communicate on operational needs and promote the trade's active participation. In addition, the Government and the trade have also exchanged views on promoting the use of contactless payments in different types of catering outlets.

The spokesman strongly appeals to the frontline staff of catering businesses to actively participate in the Targeted Group Testing Scheme. The deadline for online registration has been extended to October 31. High-exposure groups including restaurant operators, staff and personnel working in FEHD markets, hawker licensees could register through the FEHD website before the deadline for the voluntary testing services. High-exposure groups who had already registered and undergone voluntary testing can register again.

The Government encourages practitioners in bars and pubs and their patrons to undergo virus testing. The testing agency, Prenetics Limited, delivered over 2 100 specimen bottles at bar areas in Lan Kwai Fong, Tsim Sha Tsui and Wan Chai last weekend. Among them, about 1 770 specimen bottles were distributed to staff members while around 390 were distributed to patrons. The testing agency of the FEHD will deliver specimen bottles at bar areas in Soho area, Kennedy Town and Prince Edward this weekend. Details will be announced separately later.

The FEHD will continue to step up inspections at catering outlets and take enforcement actions against offenders. The department will also conduct joint operations with the Police as necessary to ensure that food business operators, practitioners and the patrons strictly comply with the directions under the regulation. Taking enforcement actions at premises that sell liquors as an example, since the re-opening of bars on September 18, the Police have conducted 1 278 inspections and 37 joint operations with the FEHD. Altogether, procedures of prosecution were initiated against operators of about 30 related premises.

The FEHD spokesman appeals to food business operators and practitioners to actively support various anti-epidemic measures, including fully implementing the targeted measures on the critical control points and participation of all bar staff and practitioners in the testing scheme, as well as compliance with the relevant regulations on prevention and control of disease in a concerted and persistent manner, with a view to keeping workers, customers and the public safe.

Issued at HKT 2:18

CHP follows up on preliminary positive case of COVID-19 involving Hong Kong Philharmonic Orchestra musician

****

The Centre for Health Protection (CHP) of the Department of Health today (October 14) continued its investigations into a preliminary positive case of coronavirus disease 2019 (COVID-19), which involves a Hong Kong Philharmonic Orchestra (HK Phil) musician. As a precautionary measure, audience members who attended the HK Phil's concerts on October 9 and 10 are advised to pay attention to their health conditions and undergo virus testing.

The case involves a 35-year-old man who is a wind instrument musician of the HK Phil. He developed a fever on October 11 and sought medical treatment at North Lantau Hospital and Union Hospital respectively on October 12. His respiratory specimen tested preliminarily positive for severe acute respiratory syndrome coronavirus 2 (SARS-CoV-2).

The patient had taken part in the HK Phil's performances at the Concert Hall, Hong Kong Cultural Centre (HKCC), during the evenings of October 9 and 10. As the patient could not wear a mask during the performances, the 90-odd musicians who performed on stage with him were identified as close contacts and are being arranged for quarantine. Initial investigations by the CHP revealed that there were about 50 backstage crew who took part in the same performances. They did not have contact with the patient and had worn masks. The CHP will arrange virus testing for them.

According to the CHP's assessment, as the HKCC had put in place social distancing measures and all audience members were required to put on masks, the audience members of the two concerts are not considered to be close contacts. Nevertheless, for the sake of prudence, the CHP advised audience members who had attended the two concerts to pay attention to their health conditions and seek medical attention immediately if feeling unwell. Those who remain asymptomatic are advised to make use of the existing free COVID-19 testing services, including undergoing testing at the four temporary testing centres set up by the Government in Wan Chai, Kwai Tsing, Kowloon City and Yau Tsim Mong Districts, or to obtain a deep throat saliva specimen collection pack at the general out-patient clinics of the Hospital Authority.

The CHP has advised the Leisure and Cultural Services Department to arrange a thorough cleaning and sterilisation at the venue, and that the Concert Hall be temporarily closed for 14 days. The CHP will distribute specimen collection bottles to the staff of the HKCC and other staff members of the HK Phil.

The patient lives in Tower 2, Phase 1, Coastal Skyline, Tung Chung. His family members who live with him remain asymptomatic and were sent to a quarantine centre. Specimen collection bottles will be distributed at his residence.

The CHP's epidemiological investigations are ongoing.

As the Tropical Cyclone Warning Signal No. 8 was still in force past 7pm yesterday (October 13), the specimen collection service of the Public Health Laboratory Services Branch (PHLSB) under the CHP was suspended and the PHLSB could only maintain limited service, hence no additional confirmed cases of COVID-19 were recorded from the specimens handled yesterday. As of 0.00am, October 14, the number of cases of COVID-19 in Hong Kong maintains at 5,202 in Hong Kong (comprising 5,201 confirmed cases and one probable case).

The CHP's epidemiological investigations and relevant contact tracing on the confirmed cases are ongoing. For case details and contact tracing information, please see the list of buildings with confirmed cases of COVID-19 in the past 14 days and the latest local situation of COVID-19 available on the website "COVID-19 Thematic Website" (www.coronavirus.gov.hk).

A spokesman for the CHP said, "During the CHP's epidemiological investigations and relevant contact tracing on the confirmed cases, we will compile and upload (www.chp.gov.hk/files/pdf/building_list_eng.pdf) a list of buildings that confirmed patients had visited from two days before the onset of symptoms. Given that cases of local infection continue to occur from time to time, members of the public are urged to seek medical attention immediately if they believe that they had visited the same place at an identical time with a confirmed patient and feel unwell subsequently. If they remain asymptomatic but are concerned that they have been infected, they can also visit the Hospital Authority's designated general out-patient clinics (www.ha.org.hk/haho/ho/covid-19/GOPC_extend_EN.pdf) to obtain specimen collection packs and collect deep throat saliva specimens for free COVID-19 testing."

In view of the severe epidemic situation, the CHP called on members of the public to avoid going out, having social contact and dining out. They should put on a surgical mask and maintain stringent hand hygiene when they need to go out. The CHP strongly urged the elderly to stay home as far as possible and avoid going out. They should consider asking their family and friends to help with everyday tasks such as shopping for basic necessities.

The spokesman said, "Given that the situation of COVID-19 infection remains severe and that there is a continuous increase in the number of cases reported around the world, members of the public are strongly urged to avoid all non-essential travel outside Hong Kong.

"The CHP also strongly urges the public to maintain at all times strict personal and environmental hygiene, which is key to personal protection against infection and prevention of the spread of the disease in the community. On a personal level, members of the public should wear a surgical mask when having respiratory symptoms, taking public transport or staying in crowded places. They should also perform hand hygiene frequently, especially before touching the mouth, nose or eyes.

"As for household environmental hygiene, members of the public are advised to maintain drainage pipes properly, regularly pour water into drain outlets (U-traps) and cover all floor drain outlets when they are not in use. After using the toilet, they should put the toilet lid down before flushing to avoid spreading germs."

Moreover, the Government has launched the website "COVID-19 Thematic Website" (www.coronavirus.gov.hk) for announcing the latest updates on various news on COVID-19 infection and health advice to help the public understand the latest updates. Members of the public may also gain access to information via the COVID-19 WhatsApp Helpline launched by the Office of the Government Chief Information Officer. Simply by saving 9617 1823 in their phone contacts or clicking the link wa.me/85296171823?text=hi, they will be able to obtain information on COVID-19 as well as the "StayHomeSafe" mobile app and wristband via WhatsApp.

Issued at HKT 16:09

Public hospitals daily update on COVID-19 cases

****

The following is issued on behalf of the Hospital Authority:

As at 9am today (October 14), one COVID-19 confirmed patient was discharged from hospital in the last 24 hours. So far, a total of 4 932 patients with confirmed or probable infection have been discharged.

At present, there are 623 negative pressure rooms in public hospitals with 1 115 negative pressure beds activated. A total of 137 confirmed patients are currently hospitalised in 18 public hospitals, among which 11 patients are in critical condition, eight are in serious condition and the remaining 118 patients are in stable condition.

The Hospital Authority will maintain close contact with the Centre for Health Protection to monitor the latest developments and to inform the public and healthcare workers on the latest information in a timely manner.

Details of the above-mentioned patients are as follows:

Patient condition	Case numbers
Discharged	5123
Critical	1989, 3496, 3764, 4706, 4833, 4937, 4990, 5110, 5152, 5185, 5195
Serious	1650, 3904, 4100, 4101, 4433, 4746, 4788, 5088

Issued at HKT 16:50

Temporary testing centres continue to provide free testing service to public

****

As at 8pm today (October 14), specimens had been collected from a total of 8 676 persons at Wan Chai, Kwai Tsing, Kowloon City and Yau Tsim Mong Temporary Testing Centres set up by the Government for COVID-19 nucleic acid tests. The temporary testing centres will continue to provide service to members of the public till this Friday (October 16) tentatively.

Specimens from 1 041 persons were collected today at the Wan Chai Temporary Testing Centre located at Harbour Road Sports Centre.

Specimens from 786 persons were collected today at the Kwai Tsing Temporary Testing Centre located at Shek Lei Community Hall.

Specimens from 674 persons were collected today at the Kowloon City Temporary Testing Centre located at Kai Tak Community Hall.

Specimens from 1 237 persons were collected today at the Yau Tsim Mong Temporary Testing Centre located at Henry G Leong Yaumatei Community Centre.

A Government spokesman said that in view of the worsening COVID-19 epidemic situation in Hong Kong, the Government has set up one temporary testing centre in each of the four districts, namely Wan Chai, Kwai Tsing, Kowloon City and Yau Tsim Mong Districts, which are related to recent community outbreak clusters. The temporary testing centres will be open from 8am to 1.30pm and 2.30pm to 8pm till October 16 tentatively, to provide free specimen collection and testing services to facilitate proactive testing of members of the public, in order to identify cases and asymptomatic patients as early as possible so as to cut the transmission chains in the community.

As at 10pm today, a total of 4 938 specimens collected under the temporary community testing arrangement had been tested. If any specimen tested shows a positive COVID-19 result, the specimen will be referred to the Public Health Laboratory Services Branch of the Department of Health (DH) for a confirmatory test. Confirmed cases will be followed up and announced by the Centre for Health Protection of the DH.

Moreover, to facilitate more members of the public to receive COVID-19 tests, distribution time of the deep throat saliva specimen collection packs at the 46 general outpatient clinics (GOPCs) of the Hospital Authority (HA) has been extended to 9am to 1pm and 2pm to 5pm from Monday to Friday. The 46 HA GOPCs distributed a total of over 2 200 specimen collection packs on October 14.

The spokesman appealed to all members of the public who have doubts about their health condition to undergo testing to protect oneself and others and to fight the virus together.

Issued at HKT 22:17

October 15[15]

Hong Kong and Singapore reach in-principle agreement to establish bilateral Air Travel Bubble

****

Hong Kong and Singapore have reached an in-principle agreement to establish a bilateral Air Travel Bubble (ATB). This milestone arrangement will help revive cross-border air travel between the two aviation hubs, in a safe and progressive way.

Hong Kong and Singapore enjoy strong trade, investment, finance, tourism and people-to-people ties. Both cities are major aviation hubs, and the international air route between the two cities was among the busiest in the Asia-Pacific region pre-COVID-19. Travel links between Hong Kong and Singapore are important for both cities.

The in-principle agreement was reached during a videoconference on October 14 between the Secretary for Commerce and Economic Development of the Hong Kong Special Administrative Region Government, Mr Edward Yau, and the Minister for Transport of the Republic of Singapore, Mr Ong Ye Kung.

The key features of the ATB are as follows:

(a) there are no restrictions on travel purpose;

(b) travellers under the ATB will be subject to mutually recognised COVID-19 polymerase chain reaction tests and would need to have negative test results;

(c) travellers under the ATB will not be subject to any quarantine or Stay-Home Notice requirements, or a controlled itinerary;

(d) travellers under the ATB will be required to travel on dedicated flights, i.e. these flights will only serve ATB travellers and no transit passengers or non-ATB travellers will be allowed on board; and

(e) the ATB can be scaled by adjusting the number of dedicated flights upwards or downwards, or even suspended, in line with the latest developments and COVID-19 situation in the two cities.

"I am pleased that both sides have agreed on the key features to underpin the expeditious conclusion of the ATB between two major international aviation hubs in the world. This is a milestone in our efforts to resume normalcy while fighting against the long-drawn battle of COVID-19. Hong Kong and Singapore enjoy long-time close and cordial co-operation on many

---

[15] https://www.info.gov.hk/gia/general/202010/15.htm

fronts. I have every confidence that the ATB arrangement can come to fruition very soon to facilitate resumption of air travel between our two economies," Mr Yau said.

"Both our cities have low incidence of COVID-19 cases and have put in place robust mechanisms to manage and control COVID-19," Mr Ong said. "This has given us the confidence to mutually and progressively open our borders to each other. It is significant that our two regional aviation hubs have decided to collaborate to establish an Air Travel Bubble. It is a safe, careful but significant step forward to revive air travel, and provide a model for future collaboration with other parts of the world."

With a view to achieving early implementation, both governments are committed to fleshing out the full details of the ATB in the coming weeks and look forward to the resumption of travel between both cities, with the necessary safeguards in place to ensure that public health concerns of both sides are addressed.

The launch date of the Hong Kong-Singapore ATB and other implementation details will be announced in due course.

Issued at HKT 14:30

CHP investigates 12 additional confirmed cases of COVID-19
****

The Centre for Health Protection (CHP) of the Department of Health has announced that as of 0.00am, October 15, the CHP was investigating 12 additional confirmed cases of coronavirus disease 2019 (COVID-19), taking the number of cases to 5 214 in Hong Kong so far (comprising 5 213 confirmed cases and one probable case)

Among the newly reported cases announced, eight had a travel history during the incubation period.

The CHP's epidemiological investigations and relevant contact tracing on the confirmed cases are ongoing. For case details and contact tracing information, please see the Annex or the list of buildings with confirmed cases of COVID-19 in the past 14 days and the latest local situation of COVID-19 available on the website "COVID-19 Thematic Website" (www.coronavirus.gov.hk).

In view of the latest epidemic developments in the Mainland, starting today, inbound travellers who have been to Shandong Province in the past 14 days arriving via land boundary control points will be provided with specimen collection containers. They are required to collect their deep throat saliva samples by themselves in accordance with the instructions and return the samples for conducting COVID-19 testing.

A spokesman for the CHP said, "During the CHP's epidemiological investigations and relevant contact tracing on the confirmed cases, we will compile and upload (www.chp.gov.hk/files/pdf/building_list_eng.pdf) a list of buildings that confirmed patients had visited from two days before the onset of symptoms. Given that cases of local infection continue to occur from time to time, members of the public are urged to seek medical attention immediately if they believe that they had visited the same place at an identical time with a confirmed patient and feel unwell subsequently. If they remain asymptomatic but are concerned that they have been infected, they can also visit the Hospital Authority's designated general out-patient clinics (www.ha.org.hk/haho/ho/covid-19/GOPC_extend_EN.pdf) to obtain specimen collection packs and collect deep throat saliva specimens for free COVID-19 testing."

In view of the severe epidemic situation, the CHP called on members of the public to avoid going out, having social contact and dining out. They should put on a surgical mask and maintain stringent hand hygiene when they need to go out. The CHP strongly urged the elderly to stay home as far as possible and avoid going out. They should consider asking their family and friends to help with everyday tasks such as shopping for basic necessities.

The spokesman said, "Given that the situation of COVID-19 infection remains severe and that there is a continuous increase in the number of cases reported around the world, members of the public are strongly urged to avoid all non-essential travel outside Hong Kong.

"The CHP also strongly urges the public to maintain at all times strict personal and environmental hygiene, which is key to personal protection against infection and prevention of the spread of the disease in the community. On a personal level, members of the public should wear a surgical mask when having respiratory symptoms, taking public transport or staying in crowded places. They should also perform hand hygiene frequently, especially before touching the mouth, nose or eyes.

"As for household environmental hygiene, members of the public are advised to maintain drainage pipes properly, regularly pour water into drain outlets (U-traps) and cover all floor drain outlets when they are not in use. After using the toilet, they should put the toilet lid down before flushing to avoid spreading germs."

Moreover, the Government has launched the website "COVID-19 Thematic Website" (www.coronavirus.gov.hk) for announcing the latest updates on various news on COVID-19 infection and health advice to help the public understand the latest updates. Members of the public may also gain access to information via the COVID-19 WhatsApp Helpline launched by the Office of the Government Chief Information Officer. Simply by saving 9617 1823 in their phone contacts or clicking the link wa.me/85296171823?text=hi, they will be able to obtain information on COVID-19 as well as the "StayHomeSafe" mobile app and wristband via WhatsApp.

Issued at HKT 17:22

Public hospitals daily update on COVID-19 cases

****

The following is issued on behalf of the Hospital Authority:

As at 9am today (October 15), 11 COVID-19 confirmed patients were discharged from hospital in the last 24 hours. So far, a total of 4 943 patients with confirmed or probable infection have been discharged.

At present, there are 623 negative pressure rooms in public hospitals with 1 115 negative pressure beds activated. A total of 126 confirmed patients are currently hospitalised in 18 public hospitals, among which 12 patients are in critical condition, six are in serious condition and the remaining 108 patients are in stable condition.

The Hospital Authority will maintain close contact with the Centre for Health Protection to monitor the latest developments and to inform the public and healthcare workers on the latest information in a timely manner.

Details of the above-mentioned patients are as follows:

Patient condition	Case numbers
Discharged	4686, 5097, 5136, 5138, 5139, 5150, 5172, 5183, 5191, 5192, 5202
Critical	1989, 3496, 3764, 4433, 4706, 4833, 4937, 4990, 5110, 5152, 5185, 5195
Serious	1650, 4100, 4101, 4746, 4788, 5088

Issued at HKT 17:42

SCED speaks on "travel bubbles"

****

Following is the transcript of remarks by the Secretary for Commerce and Economic Development, Mr Edward Yau, on "travel bubbles" at a media session today (October 15):

Reporter: Can the "travel bubble" be implemented during November or December this year? Do we have to wait for the border between Hong Kong and Mainland to open first before the "travel bubble" can be officially launched? My second question is what would happen if there are imported cases from Singapore to Hong Kong? What are the protocols to be put in place? Will we have a break or a suspension for the "travel bubble"? My third question is with the "travel bubble" starting to be announced, is it fair to expect that Hong Kong will keep all the borders closed (to all visitors) unless they are residents or they are in the "travel bubble", until a vaccine is proven to work throughout next year?

Secretary for Commerce and Economic Development: For the first question, I think we are doing this initially on a bilateral basis. We have approached or have been approached altogether by 11 countries to start bilateral arrangements to revive travelling. In the process, Singapore and Hong Kong are among the first partners that are able to lock in a mutually agreeable arrangement, whereby after fulfilling certain conditions, essentially mutually recognised COVID-19 tests and bubble flights with no transit passengers coming in ensured, travellers are allowed to come or go under this arrangement. We have to proceed with this on a bilateral basis. Whenever there is a mutual agreement between Hong Kong and our partners, we will proceed along with that. So there is not any magic on the sequencing because different countries might have different considerations of their own and the epidemic situations also vary. We ourselves in July suffered a community outbreak, and it has therefore put back some of the discussions. So we will move along this line: whenever the situation allows and whenever the conditions are mutually agreed, we will proceed on that basis.

Your second question is about what if circumstances turn worse. As I mentioned in one of the five conditions, these arrangements could be adjusted, relaxed if situation improves, reduced in order to minimise risks or suspended in circumstances that we don't feel comfortable. There are mechanisms to handle those (circumstances), and it will be mutually guided by our public health experts as well.

As to your last question, I think nobody throughout the world can say for certain when everything can resume as normal. Somebody said when vaccines come out, we will see light at the end of the tunnel, but to what extent the vaccine will be widely applied to allow us to have that sense of comfort, I think nobody can have a crystal ball on the timing. In the meantime, that's why it is important for us to move at the same time on various ways to revive normal travelling as much as possible, provided that we can track the virus. The set of conditions that has been agreed between Hong Kong and Singapore could be a milestone, where we both feel that by fulfilling these conditions, we would be able to track the virus, through these tests and arrangements, but at the same time, we should make it as facilitating as possible so that travellers can resume some level of travelling without too much hassle. So I think this is a compromise, a balancing act between these two constraints.

Reporter: Mr Yau, can you say at this moment when is the earliest possible date for this "travel bubble" to kick-in? This is my first question. Secondly, would it at all be depending on the virus situation, say, if the epidemic of both places remains the same, or if it spikes up? Would it be too much of a hassle for you to suspend for a week and then bring it back on? How sensitive would the arrangement be to the epidemic situation? Those are my two questions. Thank you.

Secretary for Commerce and Economic Development: For the first question, I think it is an important milestone that we have reached an agreement with the Singapore side to proceed on this framework. The remaining work is to finalise all the details with a view to allowing people to travel through this bubble arrangement as soon as possible. I mentioned in the press release that we hope to use the coming few weeks to put in place all these requirements which involve certain legislative amendments, arrangements with airports and airlines, and also mutual recognition of testing protocol, etc. We hope that all these could be done within the coming few weeks. If we are able to finish it earlier, then, of course, travelling can be resumed much earlier.

For your second question, in establishing the air (travel) bubble, it must be premised on the common objective of the virus being able to be contained through all the control measures, i.e. it is safe and low-risk. So this is the prerequisite, and that's why among the five criteria, we put in certain requirements on that. It is also premised on a situation where both sides feel comfortable with the epidemic situation, particularly the containment on the other side. So these are all factors that we are considering and being kept under review. That's why we have also agreed on an arrangement that this bubble arrangement could be adjusted in the light of the situation. It could be further relaxed if both sides feel more comfortable, or see an obvious improvement in the containment of the virus. But if the circumstances are somehow unable to allow us to do so, then there would be mechanisms for us to adjust it, reduce it, or if really need be, (initiate) a temporary suspension. These are the mechanisms that are based on science, based on the situation, and in fact, also taking on this very important balancing act between containment and facilitation.

Issued at HKT 18:59

Temporary testing centres continue to provide free testing service to public

****

As at 8pm today (October 15), specimens had been collected from a total of 11 865 persons at Wan Chai, Kwai Tsing, Kowloon City and Yau Tsim Mong Temporary Testing Centres set up by the Government for COVID-19 nucleic acid tests. The four temporary testing centres will continue to provide service to members of the public tomorrow (October 16). After reviewing the usage of the temporary testing centres and public's demand for the testing service, the Government has decided to extend the operation period of the Yau Tsim Mong Temporary

Testing Centre to October 18. The other three temporary testing centres will cease operation after October 16.

Specimens from 789 persons were collected today at the Wan Chai Temporary Testing Centre located at Harbour Road Sports Centre.

Specimens from 600 persons were collected today at the Kwai Tsing Temporary Testing Centre located at Shek Lei Community Hall.

Specimens from 495 persons were collected today at the Kowloon City Temporary Testing Centre located at Kai Tak Community Hall.

Specimens from 1 305 persons were collected today at the Yau Tsim Mong Temporary Testing Centre located at Henry G Leong Yaumatei Community Centre.

A Government spokesman said that in view of the worsening COVID-19 epidemic situation in Hong Kong, the Government has set up one temporary testing centre in each of the four districts, namely Wan Chai, Kwai Tsing, Kowloon City and Yau Tsim Mong Districts, which are related to recent community outbreak clusters. The Wan Chai, Kwai Tsing and Kowloon City Temporary Testing Centres will open till October 16 while the Yau Tsim Mong Temporary Testing Centre will continue to open till October 18. The temporary testing centres will be open from 8am to 1.30pm and 2.30pm to 8pm to provide free specimen collection and testing services to facilitate proactive testing of members of the public, in order to identify cases and asymptomatic patients as early as possible so as to cut the transmission chains in the community.

As at 10pm today, a total of 8 676 specimens collected under the temporary community testing arrangement had been tested. If any specimen tested shows a positive COVID-19 result, the specimen will be referred to the Public Health Laboratory Services Branch of the Department of Health (DH) for a confirmatory test. Confirmed cases will be followed up and announced by the Centre for Health Protection of the DH.

Moreover, to facilitate more members of the public to receive COVID-19 tests, distribution time of the deep throat saliva specimen collection packs at the 46 general outpatient clinics (GOPCs) of the Hospital Authority (HA) has been extended to 9am to 1pm and 2pm to 5pm from Monday to Friday. The 46 HA GOPCs distributed a total of over 1 800 specimen collection packs on October 15.

The spokesman appealed to all members of the public who have doubts about their health condition to undergo testing to protect oneself and others and to fight the virus together.

Issued at HKT 23:00

October 16[16]

Specifications under Prevention and Control of Disease (Regulation of Cross-boundary Conveyances and Travellers) Regulation to be gazetted

****

In view of the developments of the COVID-19 epidemic situation worldwide and in Hong Kong, the Government will gazette today (October 16) the latest specifications to include France and Russia as specified places under the Prevention and Control of Disease (Regulation of Cross-boundary Conveyances and Travellers) Regulation (Cap. 599H) starting from October 26 to more effectively combat the epidemic.

A spokesman for the Food and Health Bureau said, "The global epidemic situation is becoming increasingly severe. The daily number of new cases increased from around 70 000 to 100 000 between late March and mid-May, to around 160 000 to 180 000 in late June and to around 220 000 to 290 000 in late July, and further increased to reach a new height of around 240 000 to 320 000 in mid-September and has remained at such a high level since then. In view of the severe global pandemic situation, Hong Kong cannot afford to drop its guard on entry prevention and control measures."

The Government has earlier introduced Cap. 599H to impose testing and quarantine conditions on travellers coming to Hong Kong from very high-risk places to reduce the health risk they may bring to Hong Kong. The Secretary for Food and Health (SFH) has previously published in the Gazette specifications on the relevant measures applicable to 11 specified places (i.e. Bangladesh, Ethiopia, India, Indonesia, Kazakhstan, Nepal, Pakistan, the Philippines, South Africa, the United Kingdom and the United States of America) and adjusted the relevant conditions having regard to the circumstances on the ground since the implementation of the regulation.

Taking into account the latest public health risk assessment, and the changes and developments of the epidemic situation, the SFH will publish in the Gazette new specifications to maintain the conditions imposed and to include France and Russia as specified places with effect from October 26 until further notice.

According to the latest specifications, a traveller who, on the day on which the traveller boarded a civil aviation aircraft that arrives at, or is about to arrive at, Hong Kong (specified aircraft), or during the 14 days before that day, has stayed in one of the aforementioned specified places must provide the following documents:

(1) A test report in English or Chinese issued by a laboratory or healthcare institution bearing the name of the relevant traveller identical to that in his or her valid travel document to show that:

---

[16] https://www.info.gov.hk/gia/general/202010/16.htm

(a) the relevant traveller underwent a nucleic acid test for COVID-19, the sample for which was taken from the relevant traveller within 72 hours before the scheduled time of departure of the specified aircraft;

(b) the test conducted on the sample is a nucleic acid test for COVID-19; and

(c) the result of the test is that the relevant traveller was tested negative for COVID-19; and

(2) If the relevant report is not in English or Chinese or does not contain all of the above information, a written confirmation in English or Chinese issued by the laboratory or healthcare institution bearing the name of the relevant traveller identical to that in his or her valid travel document and setting out all of the above information. The said written confirmation should be presented together with the test report; an

(3) Documentary proof in English or Chinese to show that the laboratory or healthcare institution is ISO 15189 accredited or is recognised or approved by the relevant authority of the government of the place in which the laboratory or healthcare institution is located; and

(4) The relevant traveller has confirmation in English or Chinese of room reservation in a hotel in Hong Kong for not less than 14 days starting on the day of the arrival of the relevant traveller in Hong Kong.

The operator of the specified aircraft must submit to the Department of Health (DH) before the specified aircraft arrives at Hong Kong a document in a form specified by the DH confirming that each relevant traveller has, before being checked in for the flight to Hong Kong on the aircraft, produced for boarding on the aircraft the documentary proof to show that the above conditions are met.

If any condition specified by the SFH is not met in relation to any relevant traveller on the conveyance, each of the operators of the conveyance commits an offence and is liable on conviction to the maximum penalty of a fine at level 5 ($50,000) and imprisonment for six months. If an operator fails to comply with a requirement to provide information, or knowingly or recklessly provides any information that is false or misleading in a material particular, he or she is liable on conviction to the maximum penalty of a fine at level 5 ($50,000) and imprisonment for six months.

As for travellers, if a traveller coming to Hong Kong fails to comply with a requirement to provide information, or knowingly or recklessly provides any information that is false or misleading in a material particular, he or she is liable on conviction to the maximum penalty of a fine at level 3 ($10,000) and imprisonment for six months.

Travellers to Hong Kong should note that they will be mandated to wait for their test results at a designated location after their deep throat saliva samples are collected for conducting testing for COVID-19 at the DH's Temporary Specimen Collection Centre pursuant to the Prevention and Control of Disease Ordinance (Cap. 599). If their test results are negative, they will be allowed to go to the hotel for which they made the reservation to continue the 14-day compulsory quarantine until completion. If their results are positive, the travellers will be transferred to hospital for isolation and treatment.

The Government will continue to monitor closely the situation including the developments of the epidemic situation both globally and locally and changes in the volume of cross-boundary passenger traffic, and may adopt more resolute and severe measures as and when necessary.

Issued at HKT 17:22

Public hospitals daily update on COVID-19 cases

****

The following is issued on behalf of the Hospital Authority:

As at 9am today (October 16), eight COVID-19 confirmed patients were discharged from hospital in the last 24 hours. So far, a total of 4 951 patients with confirmed or probable infection have been discharged.

At present, there are 631 negative pressure rooms in public hospitals with 1 139 negative pressure beds activated. A total of 130 confirmed patients are currently hospitalised in 19 public hospitals, among which 12 patients are in critical condition, six are in serious condition and the remaining 112 patients are in stable condition.

The Hospital Authority will maintain close contact with the Centre for Health Protection to monitor the latest developments and to inform the public and healthcare workers on the latest information in a timely manner.

Details of the above-mentioned patients are as follows:

Patient condition	Case numbers
Discharged	3744, 5095, 5103, 5113, 5130, 5135, 5141, 5148
Critical	1989, 3496, 3764, 4433, 4706, 4833, 4937, 4990, 5110, 5152, 5185, 5195
Serious	1650, 4100, 4101, 4746, 4788, 5088

Issued at HKT 17:50

CHP investigates seven additional confirmed cases of COVID-19

****

The Centre for Health Protection (CHP) of the Department of Health has announced that as of 0.00am, October 16, the CHP was investigating seven additional confirmed cases of coronavirus disease 2019 (COVID-19), taking the number of cases to 5 221 in Hong Kong so far (comprising 5 220 confirmed cases and one probable case).

Among the newly reported cases announced, six had a travel history during the incubation period.

The CHP's epidemiological investigations and relevant contact tracing on the confirmed cases are ongoing. For case details and contact tracing information, please see the Annex or the list of buildings with confirmed cases of COVID-19 in the past 14 days and the latest local situation of COVID-19 available on the website "COVID-19 Thematic Website" (www.coronavirus.gov.hk).

A spokesman for the CHP said, "During the CHP's epidemiological investigations and relevant contact tracing on the confirmed cases, we will compile and upload (www.chp.gov.hk/files/pdf/building_list_eng.pdf) a list of buildings that confirmed patients had visited from two days before the onset of symptoms. Given that cases of local infection continue to occur from time to time, members of the public are urged to seek medical attention immediately if they believe that they had visited the same place at an identical time with a confirmed patient and feel unwell subsequently. If they remain asymptomatic but are concerned that they have been infected, they can also visit the Hospital Authority's designated general out-patient clinics (www.ha.org.hk/haho/ho/covid-19/GOPC_extend_EN.pdf) to obtain specimen collection packs and collect deep throat saliva specimens for free COVID-19 testing."

In view of the severe epidemic situation, the CHP called on members of the public to avoid going out, having social contact and dining out. They should put on a surgical mask and maintain stringent hand hygiene when they need to go out. The CHP strongly urged the elderly to stay home as far as possible and avoid going out. They should consider asking their family and friends to help with everyday tasks such as shopping for basic necessities.

The spokesman said, "Given that the situation of COVID-19 infection remains severe and that there is a continuous increase in the number of cases reported around the world, members of the public are strongly urged to avoid all non-essential travel outside Hong Kong.

"The CHP also strongly urges the public to maintain at all times strict personal and environmental hygiene, which is key to personal protection against infection and prevention of the spread of the disease in the community. On a personal level, members of the public should wear a surgical mask when having respiratory symptoms, taking public transport or staying in

crowded places. They should also perform hand hygiene frequently, especially before touching the mouth, nose or eyes.

"As for household environmental hygiene, members of the public are advised to maintain drainage pipes properly, regularly pour water into drain outlets (U-traps) and cover all floor drain outlets when they are not in use. After using the toilet, they should put the toilet lid down before flushing to avoid spreading germs."

Moreover, the Government has launched the website "COVID-19 Thematic Website" (www.coronavirus.gov.hk) for announcing the latest updates on various news on COVID-19 infection and health advice to help the public understand the latest updates. Members of the public may also gain access to information via the COVID-19 WhatsApp Helpline launched by the Office of the Government Chief Information Officer. Simply by saving 9617 1823 in their phone contacts or clicking the link wa.me/85296171823?text=hi, they will be able to obtain information on COVID-19 as well as the "StayHomeSafe" mobile app and wristband via WhatsApp.

Issued at HKT 18:01

FEHD encourages bar and pub practitioners to undergo virus testing

****

In view of the recent developments of the COVID-19 epidemic, the Food and Environmental Hygiene Department (FEHD) today (October 16) announced that the FEHD will continue to arrange its testing agency, Prenetics Limited, to deliver specimen bottles at bar areas and mobile vans will be parked near the bar areas for three consecutive nights starting from today to encourage practitioners in bars and pubs and their patrons to undergo the voluntary testing.

The testing agency delivered specimen bottles at bar area in Kennedy Town tonight, and mobile vans were parked in the vicinity of Davis Street. Specimen bottles will be delivered at bar areas in Prince Edward and Soho tomorrow and on Sunday night respectively.

The testing agency will be responsible for the provision of one-stop service covering specimen taking and testing. The testing agency will deliver specimen bottles to practitioners in bars and pubs for collecting deep throat saliva samples, and then collect the samples in the subsequent one to two days for testing. Moreover, the testing agency will also deliver the specimen bottles to patrons of bars and pubs who are interested in taking the test and they can return their specimen bottles by themselves to the mobile collection van of the testing agency parked at Hoi Chak Street in Quarry Bay from 9am to 5pm between October 17 and 19. Specimens with preliminary positive results will be relayed to the Public Health Laboratory Services Branch of the Department of Health to re-test and confirm the result. Positive cases will be followed up and announced by the Centre for Health Protection.

The testing agency delivered over 2 100 specimen bottles at bar areas in Lan Kwai Fong, Tsim Sha Tsui and Wan Chai last weekend.

To broaden surveillance at the community level, and incorporate disease prevention and infection control into the new normal of the daily operation of society, the Government has integrated and regularised the Targeted Group Testing Scheme as part of sentinel surveillance. The FEHD announced earlier that the deadline for online registration of the voluntary free virus testing services for high-exposure groups has been extended to October 31. As part of the surveillance and early-warning system, by facilitating contact tracing and epidemiological investigations, the services will be conducive to "early identification, early isolation and early treatment", and can provide data for reference for the overall assessment of the epidemic situation.

A spokesman for the FEHD strongly appeals to practitioners in bars and pubs to actively participate in the testing scheme, and continue to comply with the directions made under the Prevention and Control of Disease (Requirements and Directions) (Business and Premises) Regulation (Cap. 599F), to maintain personal and environmental hygiene continuously with a view to ensuring cleanliness of the premises, and to always remind their customers to comply with the requirements of the Prevention and Control of Disease (Prohibition on Group Gathering) Regulation (Cap. 599G).

Issued at HKT 20:56

Yau Tsim Mong Temporary Testing Centre continues to provide free testing service to public

****

As at 8pm today (October 16), specimens had been collected from a total of 14 824 persons at Wan Chai, Kwai Tsing, Kowloon City and Yau Tsim Mong Temporary Testing Centres set up by the Government for COVID-19 nucleic acid tests. The Yau Tsim Mong Temporary Testing Centre will continue to provide service to members of the public tomorrow (October 17) until October 18.

Specimens from 809 persons were collected today at the Wan Chai Temporary Testing Centre located at Harbour Road Sports Centre.

Specimens from 547 persons were collected today at the Kwai Tsing Temporary Testing Centre located at Shek Lei Community Hall.

Specimens from 496 persons were collected today at the Kowloon City Temporary Testing Centre located at Kai Tak Community Hall.

Specimens from 1 107 persons were collected today at the Yau Tsim Mong Temporary Testing Centre located at Henry G Leong Yaumatei Community Centre.

A Government spokesman said that in view of the worsening COVID-19 epidemic situation in Hong Kong, the Government has set up one temporary testing centre in each of the four districts, namely Wan Chai, Kwai Tsing, Kowloon City and Yau Tsim Mong Districts, which are related to recent community outbreak clusters. After reviewing the usage of the temporary testing centres and public's demand for the testing service, the Government has decided that the Wan Chai, Kwai Tsing and Kowloon City Temporary Testing Centres will cease operation tomorrow while the Yau Tsim Mong Temporary Testing Centre will continue to open till October 18. The Yau Tsim Mong Temporary Testing Centre will be open from 8am to 1.30pm and 2.30pm to 8pm to provide free specimen collection and testing services to facilitate testing of members of the public, in order to identify cases and asymptomatic patients as early as possible so as to cut the transmission chains in the community.

As at 10pm today, a total of 11 865 specimens collected under the temporary community testing arrangement had been tested. If any specimen tested shows a positive COVID-19 result, the specimen will be referred to the Public Health Laboratory Services Branch of the Department of Health (DH) for a confirmatory test. Confirmed cases will be followed up and announced by the Centre for Health Protection of the DH

Moreover, to facilitate more members of the public to receive COVID-19 tests, distribution time of the deep throat saliva specimen collection packs at the 46 general outpatient clinics (GOPCs) of the Hospital Authority (HA) has been extended to 9am to 1pm and 2pm to 5pm from Monday to Friday. The 46 HA GOPCs distributed a total of over 1 600 specimen collection packs on October 16.

The spokesman appealed to all members of the public who have doubts about their health condition to undergo testing to protect oneself and others and to fight the virus together.

Issued at HKT 22:52

October 17[17]

CHP investigates 17 additional confirmed cases of COVID-19

****

The Centre for Health Protection (CHP) of the Department of Health has announced that as of 0.00am, October 17, the CHP was investigating 17 additional confirmed cases of coronavirus disease 2019 (COVID-19), taking the number of cases to 5 238 in Hong Kong so far (comprising 5 237 confirmed cases and one probable case).

All the newly reported cases announced had a travel history during the incubation period.

---

[17] https://www.info.gov.hk/gia/general/202010/17.htm

The CHP's epidemiological investigations and relevant contact tracing on the confirmed cases are ongoing. For case details and contact tracing information, please see the Annex or the list of buildings with confirmed cases of COVID-19 in the past 14 days and the latest local situation of COVID-19 available on the website "COVID-19 Thematic Website" (www.coronavirus.gov.hk)

A spokesman for the CHP said, "During the CHP's epidemiological investigations and relevant contact tracing on the confirmed cases, we will compile and upload (www.chp.gov.hk/files/pdf/building_list_eng.pdf) a list of buildings that confirmed patients had visited from two days before the onset of symptoms. Given that cases of local infection continue to occur from time to time, members of the public are urged to seek medical attention immediately if they believe that they had visited the same place at an identical time with a confirmed patient and feel unwell subsequently. If they remain asymptomatic but are concerned that they have been infected, they can also visit the Hospital Authority's designated general out-patient clinics (www.ha.org.hk/haho/ho/covid-19/GOPC_extend_EN.pdf) to obtain specimen collection packs and collect deep throat saliva specimens for free COVID-19 testing."

In view of the severe epidemic situation, the CHP called on members of the public to avoid going out, having social contact and dining out. They should put on a surgical mask and maintain stringent hand hygiene when they need to go out. The CHP strongly urged the elderly to stay home as far as possible and avoid going out. They should consider asking their family and friends to help with everyday tasks such as shopping for basic necessities.

The spokesman said, "Given that the situation of COVID-19 infection remains severe and that there is a continuous increase in the number of cases reported around the world, members of the public are strongly urged to avoid all non-essential travel outside Hong Kong.

"The CHP also strongly urges the public to maintain at all times strict personal and environmental hygiene, which is key to personal protection against infection and prevention of the spread of the disease in the community. On a personal level, members of the public should wear a surgical mask when having respiratory symptoms, taking public transport or staying in crowded places. They should also perform hand hygiene frequently, especially before touching the mouth, nose or eyes

"As for household environmental hygiene, members of the public are advised to maintain drainage pipes properly, regularly pour water into drain outlets (U-traps) and cover all floor drain outlets when they are not in use. After using the toilet, they should put the toilet lid down before flushing to avoid spreading germs."

Moreover, the Government has launched the website "COVID-19 Thematic Website" (www.coronavirus.gov.hk) for announcing the latest updates on various news on COVID-19 infection and health advice to help the public understand the latest updates. Members of the public may also gain access to information via the COVID-19 WhatsApp Helpline launched by the Office of the Government Chief Information Officer. Simply by saving 9617 1823 in their phone contacts or clicking the link wa.me/85296171823?text=hi, they will be able to obtain information on COVID-19 as well as the "StayHomeSafe" mobile app and wristband via WhatsApp.

Issued at HKT 14:00

Public hospitals daily update on COVID-19 cases
****

The following is issued on behalf of the Hospital Authority:

As at 9am today (October 17), 12 COVID-19 confirmed patient was discharged from hospital in the last 24 hours. So far, a total of 4 963 patients with confirmed or probable infection have been discharged.

At present, there are 623 negative pressure rooms in public hospitals with 1 115 negative pressure beds activated. A total of 125 confirmed patients are currently hospitalised in 19 public hospitals, among which 12 patients are in critical condition, five are in serious condition and the remaining 108 patients are in stable condition.

The Hospital Authority will maintain close contact with the Centre for Health Protection to monitor the latest developments and to inform the public and healthcare workers on the latest information in a timely manner.

Details of the above-mentioned patients are as follows:

Patient condition	Case numbers
Discharged	3434, 3811, 5059, 5088, 5091, 5100, 5116, 5164, 5171, 5193, 5203, 5221
Critical	1989, 3496, 3764, 4433, 4706, 4833, 4937, 4990, 5110, 5152, 5185, 5195
Serious	1650, 4100, 4101, 4746, 4788

Issued at HKT 15:55

FEHD and Police continue to join hands to step up inspections at catering business premises and take stringent enforcement actions relating to anti-epidemic measures

****

The Food and Environmental Hygiene Department (FEHD) and the Police conducted a joint operation at small hours today (October 17) to step up inspections and take stringent enforcement actions at catering business premises including bars and upstairs restaurants in Wan Chai District. The FEHD reminds food business operators and food handlers again to strictly comply with the relevant requirements (including ceasing dining-in from 0.00am to 4.59am) under the Prevention and Control of Disease (Requirements and Directions) (Business and Premises) Regulation (Cap. 599F) (the Regulation), and the public to comply with the restriction in relation to group gatherings under the anti-epidemic regulations and directions when patronising restaurants.

During the operation at small hours today, the FEHD and the Police inspected 10 catering business premises (including bars) and initiated the procedure on prosecution against the operator of 1 upstairs catering business premises in Tang Lung Street and 1 upstairs bar in Jaffe Road respectively for selling or supplying food or drink for consumption on the premises outside permitted hours (i.e. between 0.00am and 4.59am), staff not wearing a mask within the premises, the number of customers exceeding half of its normal seating capacity, distance between tables less than 1.5 metres, etc. Besides, the Police also issued Fixed Penalty Notices to 87 customers inside the upstairs bar for violating the Prevention and Control of Disease (Prohibition on Group Gathering) Regulation (Cap. 599G) on group gathering.

A spokesman for the FEHD said, "According to the directions issued by the Secretary for Food and Health in relation to catering business under the Regulation, food business operators and food handlers have to strictly comply with a series of requirements and restrictions. Among these, selling or supplying food or drink for consumption on the premises from 0.00am to 4.59am must be ceased; the number of customers at any premises must not exceed half of its normal seating capacity; no more than four persons may be seated together at one table at catering premises (no more than two persons may be seated together at one table in bars); tables must be arranged in a way to ensure there is a distance of at least 1.5m or some form of partition which could serve as effective buffer between one table and another table; a mask must be worn at all times within the premises, except when the person is consuming food or drink; and body temperature screening must be conducted before the person is allowed to enter the catering premises and hand sanitisers must be provided. According to the Regulation, directions and the requirements under the Prevention and Control of Disease (Prohibition in Group Gathering) Regulation (Cap. 599G), members of the public also have to comply with the related restriction on group gatherings that no more than four persons may be seated at one table at catering premises."

Under the Regulation, licensees and operators of food business premises must strictly comply with the series of requirements and restrictions. Contravening the requirements and restrictions is a criminal offence. Offenders are subject to a maximum fine of $50,000 and imprisonment for six months. Persons who violate the group gathering restriction of Prevention and Control of

Disease (Prohibition in Group Gathering) Regulation (Cap. 599G) are subject to a fixed penalty of $2,000.

The spokesman said that the FEHD will continue to step up inspections at food business premises across the territory and conduct joint operations with the Police to ensure that food business operators, food handlers and the public strictly comply with the directions under the regulation and will take enforcement actions against offenders so as to minimise the risk of transmission of COVID-19 in catering business premises.

The FEHD spokesman appealed to food business operators and food handlers to comply with the relevant Regulation on prevention and control of disease in a concerted and persistent manner, with a view to keeping workers, customers and the public safe, and to members of the public to comply with the related regulations and directions relating to group gatherings at catering business premises.

Issued at HKT 19:05

Yau Tsim Mong Temporary Testing Centre will continue to provide free testing service to public tomorrow

****

Specimens from 711 persons were collected today (October 17) at the Yau Tsim Mong Temporary Testing Centre located at Henry G Leong Yaumatei Community Centre for COVID-19 nucleic acid tests. Counting the number of specimens collected at the three temporary testing centres that have ceased operation, specimens have been collected from a total of 15 535 persons at the four temporary testing centres set up by the Government.

Tomorrow (October 18) will be the last day for the Yau Tsim Mong Temporary Testing Centre to be open for public service. It will be open from 8am to 1.30pm and 2.30pm to 8pm to provide free specimen collection and testing services to facilitate testing of members of the public, in order to identify cases and asymptomatic patients as early as possible so as to cut the transmission chains in the community.

As at 10pm today, a total of 14 824 specimens collected under the temporary community testing arrangement had been tested. If any specimen tested shows a positive COVID-19 result, the specimen will be referred to the Public Health Laboratory Services Branch of the Department of Health (DH) for a confirmatory test. Confirmed cases will be followed up and announced by the Centre for Health Protection of the DH.

Moreover, to facilitate more members of the public to receive COVID-19 tests, distribution time of the deep throat saliva specimen collection packs at the 46 general outpatient clinics of the Hospital Authority has been extended to 9am to 1pm and 2pm to 5pm from Monday to Friday.

The spokesman appealed to all members of the public who have doubts about their health condition to undergo testing to protect oneself and others and to fight the virus together.

Issued at HKT 22:57

October 18[18]

CHP investigates four additional confirmed cases of COVID-19

****

The Centre for Health Protection (CHP) of the Department of Health has announced that as of 0.00am, October 18, the CHP was investigating four additional confirmed cases of coronavirus disease 2019 (COVID-19), taking the number of cases to 5 242 in Hong Kong so far (comprising 5 241 confirmed cases and one probable case).

Among the newly reported cases announced, two had a travel history during the incubation period. The remaining cases were epidemiologically linked with local cases.

The CHP's epidemiological investigations and relevant contact tracing on the confirmed cases are ongoing. For case details and contact tracing information, please see the Annex or the list of buildings with confirmed cases of COVID-19 in the past 14 days and the latest local situation of COVID-19 available on the website "COVID-19 Thematic Website" (www.coronavirus.gov.hk).

The DH announced that starting from tomorrow (October 19), Rambler Garden Hotel in Tsing Yi will be used as the Holding Centre for Test Results to provide accommodation to inbound travellers whose test results will not be available on the same day (usually passengers arriving in the afternoon or at night). The DH will make flexible arrangements according to the capacity of the facilities and the daily number of passengers arriving on afternoon flights. If necessary, inbound travellers arriving in the afternoon could also be arranged to wait for test results at the Temporary Specimen Collection Centre after collecting their deep throat saliva samples there. The DH also expressed gratitude to Dorsett Tsuen Wan, Hong Kong and its staff for their assistance in fighting the epidemic over the past two months.

A spokesman for the CHP said, "During the CHP's epidemiological investigations and relevant contact tracing on the confirmed cases, we will compile and upload (www.chp.gov.hk/files/pdf/building_list_eng.pdf) a list of buildings that confirmed patients had visited from two days before the onset of symptoms. Given that cases of local infection continue to occur from time to time, members of the public are urged to seek medical attention immediately if they believe that they had visited the same place at an identical time with a confirmed patient and feel unwell subsequently. If they remain asymptomatic but are concerned

[18] https://www.info.gov.hk/gia/general/202010/18.htm

that they have been infected, they can also visit the Hospital Authority's designated general out-patient clinics (www.ha.org.hk/haho/ho/covid-19/GOPC_extend_EN.pdf) to obtain specimen collection packs and collect deep throat saliva specimens for free COVID-19 testing."

In view of the severe epidemic situation, the CHP called on members of the public to avoid going out, having social contact and dining out. They should put on a surgical mask and maintain stringent hand hygiene when they need to go out. The CHP strongly urged the elderly to stay home as far as possible and avoid going out. They should consider asking their family and friends to help with everyday tasks such as shopping for basic necessities.

The spokesman said, "Given that the situation of COVID-19 infection remains severe and that there is a continuous increase in the number of cases reported around the world, members of the public are strongly urged to avoid all non-essential travel outside Hong Kong.

"The CHP also strongly urges the public to maintain at all times strict personal and environmental hygiene, which is key to personal protection against infection and prevention of the spread of the disease in the community. On a personal level, members of the public should wear a surgical mask when having respiratory symptoms, taking public transport or staying in crowded places. They should also perform hand hygiene frequently, especially before touching the mouth, nose or eyes.

"As for household environmental hygiene, members of the public are advised to maintain drainage pipes properly, regularly pour water into drain outlets (U-traps) and cover all floor drain outlets when they are not in use. After using the toilet, they should put the toilet lid down before flushing to avoid spreading germs."

Moreover, the Government has launched the website "COVID-19 Thematic Website" (www.coronavirus.gov.hk) for announcing the latest updates on various news on COVID-19 infection and health advice to help the public understand the latest updates. Members of the public may also gain access to information via the COVID-19 WhatsApp Helpline launched by the Office of the Government Chief Information Officer. Simply by saving 9617 1823 in their phone contacts or clicking the link wa.me/85296171823?text=hi, they will be able to obtain information on COVID-19 as well as the "StayHomeSafe" mobile app and wristband via WhatsApp.

Issued at HKT 14:00

Public hospitals daily update on COVID-19 cases

****

The following is issued on behalf of the Hospital Authority:

As at 9am today (October 18), 10 COVID-19 confirmed patient was discharged from hospital in the last 24 hours. So far, a total of 4 973 patients with confirmed or probable infection have been discharged.

At present, there are 623 negative pressure rooms in public hospitals with 1 115 negative pressure beds activated. A total of 132 confirmed patients are currently hospitalised in 18 public hospitals, among which 12 patients are in critical condition, four are in serious condition and the remaining 116 patients are in stable condition.

The Hospital Authority will maintain close contact with the Centre for Health Protection to monitor the latest developments and to inform the public and healthcare workers on the latest information in a timely manner.

Details of the above-mentioned patients are as follows:

Patient condition	Case numbers
Discharged	2351, 4100, 5137, 5153, 5182, 5184, 5197, 5204, 5207, 5237
Critical	1989, 3496, 3764, 4433, 4706, 4833, 4937, 4990, 5110, 5152, 5185, 5195
Serious	1650, 4101, 4746, 4788

Ends/Sunday, October 18, 2020
Issued at HKT 15:30

Response to enquiries on registration arrangements at temporary testing centre

****

In response to media enquiries about registration arrangements for members of the public at the Yau Tsim Mong Temporary Testing Centre, a Government spokesman today (October 18) gave the following reply:

"To facilitate testing by members of the public, they could visit the temporary testing centre directly for on-site registration without the need for making prior online appointment. An SMS message will be sent to a person's registered mobile number when his or her test result is available.

"If any member of the public could not provide mobile phone numbers, the staff on site would offer assistance in a bid to facilitate him or her to receive the test. Several persons who were unable to provide their mobile phone numbers today had successfully got the tests done under the assistance of the staff. We will review the relevant procedures and guidelines so that the arrangements could be further improved for any similar exercises in the future.

"After the temporary testing centre ceased operation, members of the public may still obtain the deep throat saliva specimen collection packs at the 46 general outpatient clinics of the Hospital Authority for free COVID-19 tests."

Issued at HKT 22:34

Services at temporary testing centres concluded
****

Specimens from 1 267 persons were collected for COVID-19 nucleic acid tests today (October 18) at the Yau Tsim Mong Temporary Testing Centre located at Henry G Leong Yaumatei Community Centre set up by the Government. The centre ceased operation at 8pm. Specimens from a cumulative total of 16 802 persons had been collected from the four temporary testing centres set up by the Government, including the three centres which ceased operation earlier.

As at 10pm today, a total of 15 535 specimens collected under the temporary community testing arrangement had been tested. If any specimen tested shows a positive COVID-19 result, the specimen will be referred to the Public Health Laboratory Services Branch of the Department of Health (DH) for a confirmatory test. Confirmed cases will be followed up and announced by the Centre for Health Protection of the DH.

In view of signs of deterioration of the COVID-19 epidemic situation in Hong Kong in early October, the Government had decided to set up one temporary testing centre in each of the four districts, namely Wan Chai, Kwai Tsing, Kowloon City and Yau Tsim Mong Districts, which were related to recent community outbreak clusters, to provide free specimen collection and testing services to facilitate testing of members of the public, in order to identify cases and asymptomatic patients as early as possible so as to cut the transmission chains in the community.

While the temporary testing centres have ceased operation, members of the public can still receive free COVID-19 tests by collecting deep throat saliva specimen collection packs at the 46 general outpatient clinics of the Hospital Authority. Distribution time of the specimen collection packs has been extended to 9am to 1pm and 2pm to 5pm from Monday to Friday.

A Government spokesman appealed to all members of the public who have doubts about their health condition to undergo testing to protect oneself and others and to fight the virus together.

Issued at HKT 22:44

October 19[19]

CHP investigates 15 additional confirmed cases of COVID-19

****

The Centre for Health Protection (CHP) of the Department of Health has announced that as of 0.00am, October 19, the CHP was investigating 15 additional confirmed cases of coronavirus disease 2019 (COVID-19), taking the number of cases to 5 257 in Hong Kong so far (comprising 5 256 confirmed cases and one probable case).

Among the newly reported cases announced, 14 had a travel history during the incubation period. The remaining case was epidemiologically linked with local case.

The CHP's epidemiological investigations and relevant contact tracing on the confirmed cases are ongoing. For case details and contact tracing information, please see the Annex or the list of buildings with confirmed cases of COVID-19 in the past 14 days and the latest local situation of COVID-19 available on the website "COVID-19 Thematic Website" (www.coronavirus.gov.hk).

A spokesman for the CHP said, "During the CHP's epidemiological investigations and relevant contact tracing on the confirmed cases, we will compile and upload (www.chp.gov.hk/files/pdf/building_list_eng.pdf) a list of buildings that confirmed patients had visited from two days before the onset of symptoms. Given that cases of local infection continue to occur from time to time, members of the public are urged to seek medical attention immediately if they believe that they had visited the same place at an identical time with a confirmed patient and feel unwell subsequently. If they remain asymptomatic but are concerned that they have been infected, they can also visit the Hospital Authority's designated general out-patient clinics (www.ha.org.hk/haho/ho/covid-19/GOPC_extend_EN.pdf) to obtain specimen collection packs and collect deep throat saliva specimens for free COVID-19 testing."

In view of the severe epidemic situation, the CHP called on members of the public to avoid going out, having social contact and dining out. They should put on a surgical mask and maintain stringent hand hygiene when they need to go out. The CHP strongly urged the elderly to stay home as far as possible and avoid going out. They should consider asking their family and friends to help with everyday tasks such as shopping for basic necessities.

[19] https://www.info.gov.hk/gia/general/202010/19.htm

The spokesman said, "Given that the situation of COVID-19 infection remains severe and that there is a continuous increase in the number of cases reported around the world, members of the public are strongly urged to avoid all non-essential travel outside Hong Kong.

"The CHP also strongly urges the public to maintain at all times strict personal and environmental hygiene, which is key to personal protection against infection and prevention of the spread of the disease in the community. On a personal level, members of the public should wear a surgical mask when having respiratory symptoms, taking public transport or staying in crowded places. They should also perform hand hygiene frequently, especially before touching the mouth, nose or eyes.

"As for household environmental hygiene, members of the public are advised to maintain drainage pipes properly, regularly pour water into drain outlets (U-traps) and cover all floor drain outlets when they are not in use. After using the toilet, they should put the toilet lid down before flushing to avoid spreading germs."

Moreover, the Government has launched the website "COVID-19 Thematic Website" (www.coronavirus.gov.hk) for announcing the latest updates on various news on COVID-19 infection and health advice to help the public understand the latest updates. Members of the public may also gain access to information via the COVID-19 WhatsApp Helpline launched by the Office of the Government Chief Information Officer. Simply by saving 9617 1823 in their phone contacts or clicking the link wa.me/85296171823?text=hi, they will be able to obtain information on COVID-19 as well as the "StayHomeSafe" mobile app and wristband via WhatsApp.

Issued at HKT 14:11

Public hospitals daily update on COVID-19 cases

****

The following is issued on behalf of the Hospital Authority:

As at 9am today (October 19), nine COVID-19 confirmed patients were discharged from hospital in the last 24 hours. So far, a total of 4 982 patients with confirmed or probable infection have been discharged.

At present, there are 614 negative pressure rooms in public hospitals with 1 098 negative pressure beds activated. A total of 127 confirmed patients are currently hospitalised in 18 public hospitals, among which 12 patients are in critical condition, five are in serious condition and the remaining 110 patients are in stable condition.

The Hospital Authority will maintain close contact with the Centre for Health Protection to

monitor the latest developments and to inform the public and healthcare workers on the latest information in a timely manner.

Details of the above-mentioned patients are as follows:

Patient condition	Case numbers
Discharged	5104, 5121, 5125, 5142, 5155, 5206, 5208, 5212, 5239
Critical	1989, 3496, 3764, 4433, 4706, 4833, 4937, 4990, 5110, 5152, 5185, 5195
Serious	1650, 4101, 4746, 4788, 5151

Issued at HKT 16:35

CHP's response to media enquiries

****

In response to media enquiries on the quarantine arrangement concerning the 5 217th confirmed case of coronavirus disease 2019 (COVID-19), a spokesman for the Centre for Health Protection (CHP) of the Department of Health (DH) today (October 19) gave the following reply:

The 5 217th case involves a 25-year-old man arriving in Hong Kong from India on October 15. The man had a negative result to a COVID-19 nucleic acid test done at a laboratory recognised by the local government prior to boarding the flight to Hong Kong. Upon arrival in Hong Kong, he provided proof showing his identity as a consular staff in Hong Kong. Personnel of the CHP thus made relevant quarantine and testing arrangements for exempted persons according to the existing mechanism. The man then proceeded to the DH's Temporary Specimen Collection Centre at the Hong Kong International Airport to collect his deep throat saliva specimen and was allowed to leave after completion.

Upon leaving the airport, the man was immediately taken to his residence in a vehicle arranged by the consulate and was placed under medical surveillance for 14 days as required by the DH. Upon testing preliminarily positive on the same day, the CHP immediately transferred him to a public hospital for isolation and treatment. According to the patient, he had stayed at his residence alone upon arrival without leaving.

When following up on this case, the CHP was informed by another relevant government department that the man does not belong to a rank that can be exempted from compulsory quarantine requirements even though he is a consular staff in Hong Kong. Under the prevailing policy, this person who returned from a specified high risk place should have undergone compulsory quarantine at a hotel room.

The department expressed its apologies for the inappropriate quarantine arrangement and has reminded relevant staff to be prudent when handling quarantine exemption arrangements to avoid recurrence of similar incidents.

Issued at HKT 19:15

October 20[20]

Fourth round of COVID-19 testing for RCHEs, RCHDs and nursing homes commences

****

The Social Welfare Department (SWD) said today (October 20) that the fourth round of free COVID-19 testing services will be arranged for staff members of residential care homes for the elderly (RCHEs), residential care homes for persons with disabilities (RCHDs) and nursing homes (including full-time staff, part-time staff, imported staff, relief staff and outsourced contract service workers such as out-patient escort staff) from tomorrow (October 21). This round of testing will last for about three weeks and the SWD appeals to the staff members of the aforementioned institutions for their active participation.

In this exercise, testing will also be arranged on a trial basis for some residents of the aforementioned institutions, namely:

- newly admitted residents;
- residents who need to go out for medical purposes, rehabilitation training, work or other reasons;
- service users of day care/rehabilitation services units attached to residential care homes; and
- other residents who are willing to undergo testing.

Participants have to collect their deep throat saliva specimens by themselves for testing. Specimens tested with a preliminarily positive COVID-19 result will be referred to the Public

[20] https://www.info.gov.hk/gia/general/202010/20.htm

Health Laboratory Services Branch of the Department of Health for confirmatory tests. Confirmed cases will be followed up and announced by the Centre for Health Protection.

Apart from the aforementioned institutions, the SWD has provided free testing services on a voluntary basis for staff of subvented/subsidised welfare service units at a higher risk since September 28. A total of 1 100 welfare units including community care service units for the elderly and persons with disabilities, other residential care service units, child care centres, day training service units for persons with disabilities, etc, have been invited to join the testing in which deep throat saliva specimens are collected. The testing programme is still underway. A spokesman for the SWD appeals again to the units and staff members who have not yet joined the programme for their active participation.

The spokesman said that the testings aim to identify asymptomatic COVID-19 patients as early as possible and minimise the risk of infection for social welfare service users who are physically frail. Staff members and residents of institutions and social welfare organisations are urged to participate in the testing programme for the sake of protecting themselves and others. The spokesman also called on family members of the residents to encourage their relatives residing in the institutions to join the testing programme.

The spokesman emphasised that, as always, personal data of staff members and service users is well protected throughout the testing workflow. The testing service providers do not need, and will not gain access to, the data concerned.

Issued at HKT 15:25

CHP investigates five additional confirmed cases of COVID-19

****

The Centre for Health Protection (CHP) of the Department of Health has announced that as of 0.00am, October 20, the CHP was investigating five additional confirmed cases of coronavirus disease 2019 (COVID-19), taking the number of cases to 5 262 in Hong Kong so far (comprising 5 261 confirmed cases and one probable case).

Among the newly reported cases announced, four had a travel history during the incubation period.

The CHP's epidemiological investigations and relevant contact tracing on the confirmed cases are ongoing. For case details and contact tracing information, please see the Annex or the list of buildings with confirmed cases of COVID-19 in the past 14 days and the latest local situation of COVID-19 available on the website "COVID-19 Thematic Website" (www.coronavirus.gov.hk).

A spokesman for the CHP said, "During the CHP's epidemiological investigations and relevant contact tracing on the confirmed cases, we will compile and upload (www.chp.gov.hk/files/pdf/building_list_eng.pdf) a list of buildings that confirmed patients had visited from two days before the onset of symptoms. Given that cases of local infection continue to occur from time to time, members of the public are urged to seek medical attention immediately if they believe that they had visited the same place at an identical time with a confirmed patient and feel unwell subsequently. If they remain asymptomatic but are concerned that they have been infected, they can also visit the Hospital Authority's designated general out-patient clinics (www.ha.org.hk/haho/ho/covid-19/GOPC_extend_EN.pdf) to obtain specimen collection packs and collect deep throat saliva specimens for free COVID-19 testing."

In view of the severe epidemic situation, the CHP called on members of the public to avoid going out, having social contact and dining out. They should put on a surgical mask and maintain stringent hand hygiene when they need to go out. The CHP strongly urged the elderly to stay home as far as possible and avoid going out. They should consider asking their family and friends to help with everyday tasks such as shopping for basic necessities.

The spokesman said, "Given that the situation of COVID-19 infection remains severe and that there is a continuous increase in the number of cases reported around the world, members of the public are strongly urged to avoid all non-essential travel outside Hong Kong.

"The CHP also strongly urges the public to maintain at all times strict personal and environmental hygiene, which is key to personal protection against infection and prevention of the spread of the disease in the community. On a personal level, members of the public should wear a surgical mask when having respiratory symptoms, taking public transport or staying in crowded places. They should also perform hand hygiene frequently, especially before touching the mouth, nose or eyes.

"As for household environmental hygiene, members of the public are advised to maintain drainage pipes properly, regularly pour water into drain outlets (U-traps) and cover all floor drain outlets when they are not in use. After using the toilet, they should put the toilet lid down before flushing to avoid spreading germs."

Moreover, the Government has launched the website "COVID-19 Thematic Website" (www.coronavirus.gov.hk) for announcing the latest updates on various news on COVID-19 infection and health advice to help the public understand the latest updates. Members of the public may also gain access to information via the COVID-19 WhatsApp Helpline launched by the Office of the Government Chief Information Officer. Simply by saving 9617 1823 in their phone contacts or clicking the link wa.me/85296171823?text=hi, they will be able to obtain information on COVID-19 as well as the "StayHomeSafe" mobile app and wristband via WhatsApp.

Issued at HKT 17:15

Public hospitals daily update on COVID-19 cases

****

The following is issued on behalf of the Hospital Authority:

As at 9am today (October 20), 14 COVID-19 confirmed patients were discharged from hospital in the last 24 hours. So far, a total of 4 996 patients with confirmed or probable infection have been discharged.

At present, there are 614 negative pressure rooms in public hospitals with 1 098 negative pressure beds activated. A total of 127 confirmed patients are currently hospitalised in 18 public hospitals, among which 12 patients are in critical condition, five are in serious condition and the remaining 110 patients are in stable condition.

The Hospital Authority will maintain close contact with the Centre for Health Protection to monitor the latest developments and to inform the public and healthcare workers on the latest information in a timely manner.

Details of the above-mentioned patients are as follows:

Patient condition	Case numbers
Discharged	5118, 5122, 5132, 5134, 5175, 5211, 5219, 5223, 5224, 5225, 5231, 5250, 5251, 5256
Critical	1989, 3496, 3764, 4433, 4706, 4833, 4937, 4990, 5110, 5152, 5185, 5195
Serious	1650, 4101, 4746, 4788, 5151

Issued at HKT 17:41

Transcript of remarks by SFH and SCED at media session

****

Following is the transcript of remarks by the Secretary for Food and Health, Professor Sophia Chan, and the Secretary for Commerce and Economic Development, Mr Edward Yau, at a media session on the latest social distancing measures today (October 20):

Reporter: Firstly, can I ask about the new rule on tour groups? Can the minister tell us, if there are any breaches of the law, who will be punished? Is it the people who have participated in the tours or the people who are running the tour groups? How are you exactly going to enforce the rules? Are you going to increase checks on these tour groups? If there are any infections found in these groups, will there be any punishments, such as suspension of business for 14 days? Any other follow-up infection control measures to be done on those tours? Secondly, can I ask Professor Chan about the latest developments with flu vaccines? We've seen from some reports that there have been a great shortage with flu vaccines, how is the Government going to address this issue? There have been reports about the meeting with sector representatives and doctors yesterday, can you tell us more about what have been discussed, and what will you do to increase the supply? Which group will be prioritised? How can you ensure that everyone who needs the vaccine can get it?

Secretary for Commerce and Economic Development: I think the proposed exemption for the local tour arrangement is premised on the understanding that travel agents, being the organisers of all these exempted group tours, will take the extra steps in protecting public health and minimising the risks. At the same time, people joining these group (tours) will also be assured that they are getting a service better than managing their own. That's why a very important condition on this is for the Travel Industry Council of Hong Kong (TIC), as the industry's representative group, to help us to administer the entire arrangement, through the undertaking signed between the Council and individual travel agents. For individual travel agents, in the undertaking, they will promise to do things, such as heightening the awareness (of public health) by requiring all the participants to wear masks throughout (the tour), or providing sanitisation, doing cleaning and also enforcing these rules.

You asked what (will happen) if someone does not comply (with the rules). Organisers of the group (tours) are accepting customers who come to enjoy a safe and leisurely tour. I believe customers will have every reason to comply. At the same time, for the agents, they can turn away customers who are not willing to comply. The most important responsibility falls on the travel agents. If they violate the undertakings, there would be provisions, including not being allowed to continue with their registration (of local tours) with TIC. That means, they will be deprived of the subsidies that they are supposed to enjoy under the Green Lifestyle Local Tour Incentive Scheme or the "Spend-to-Redeem" programme that is going to be launched by the (Hong Kong) Tourism Board. So there are such arrangements. Most important of all, it's a happy arrangement where customers and travellers will feel safer, travel agents have got something they can promise to deliver, and the whole industry is taking the extra steps to minimise the risk and allow business to carry on.

Secretary for Food and Health: As far as the flu vaccine is concerned, the Government promotes flu vaccination every year, and there are priority groups that we think should take the vaccine.

This year, because of the heightened vigilance and everybody has more awareness, so, as we understand from the private GPs (general practitioners), there are more people who are willing and would like to take vaccines at an early stage.

Normally every year, people would take vaccine in November and December or even later, but this year everybody has been very vigilant and is very careful and trying to take vaccine. We also understand that there are some supply issues in the private sector.

Last night during the meeting, some of the doctors have expressed concerns. The Department of Health has been monitoring the supply of vaccines not only in the public sector, but also in the private sector. They will continue to communicate very closely with vaccine suppliers to understand the situation, and also ensure that there are vaccines provided to private practitioners, especially a number of private practitioners that have participated in the Government's vaccination subsidy programme. They actually will be targeting many of the priority groups set by the Government. So, we will continue to monitor the situation, and also to communicate with the suppliers, to make sure the situation is okay.

We are also considering working with the suppliers to arrange some additional vaccines for the private doctors who have participated in the Government vaccination programme. This is welcomed by the practitioners when we told them this news last night. And of course we also told them if the Government is going to work with the vaccine suppliers, to give them some of the additional vaccine supply, then, first of all, they cannot charge extra to their patients, and secondly, they would have to give those vaccines to priority groups that the Government has designated.

Issued at HKT 19:30

Government to gazette latest legislative amendments, directions and specifications under the Prevention and Control of Disease Ordinance

****

Having regard to the development of the COVID-19 epidemic situation in Hong Kong, the Government will gazette today (October 20) the latest legislative amendments, directions and specifications under the Prevention and Control of Disease Ordinance (Cap. 599) to continue to relax social distancing measures in a gradual and orderly manner

A spokesman for the Food and Health Bureau said, "Although the seven-day average number of locally confirmed cases has dropped gradually after reaching a high level early last week, there were cases with unknown sources of infection among the additional confirmed cases reported last week, indicating the existence of silent transmission chains in the community. Meanwhile, the severe global epidemic situation may also bring public health risks to Hong Kong.

"Nevertheless, as we have reiterated time and again, under the new normal, we cannot and should not aim at having no confirmed case in the community for an extended period of time. Although we would much prefer seeing no local cases, it would be unavoidable to have sporadic cases and clusters in the community from time to time as the virus will co-exist with us for quite a long period of time before effective treatment and vaccination become available. In this regard, we will continue to adopt a targeted approach for reducing the risk of the virus entering and spreading within the community as far as practicable, avoid the one-size-fits-all approach when adjusting social distancing measures, and work closely with the relevant trades to strengthen infection control measures at the premises concerned, in order to allow members of the public to maintain social and economic activities to a certain extent as far as practicable under the new normal."

After taking into account the latest public health risk assessment and having struck a balance with economic needs and level of acceptance of the society, the Government amends the Prevention and Control of Disease (Prohibition on Group Gathering) Regulation (Cap. 599G) to expand the scope of the existing exempted group gatherings to cover local tours and relax the restrictions on the number of persons allowed at wedding ceremonies and meetings that are held in accordance with any Ordinance or other regulatory instrument that governs the operation of the company or its business. The amendments will come into effect on October 23, 2020. For other social distancing measures, apart from minor refinements, the Government will largely maintain the measures currently in place for a period of seven days effective from October 23, 2020 till October 29, 2020.

The spokesman added, "As we have stressed time and again, co-operation and self-discipline of members of the public are the keys to the effectiveness of social distancing measures in preventing the spread of the disease in the community. Only with the co-operation of society as a whole can the Government continue to allow resumption of social and economic activities in a gradual and orderly manner. Therefore, the public's concerted efforts in fighting the epidemic and compliance with requirements and restrictions applicable to individual premises are of utmost importance. Otherwise, when there is another outbreak in the community, the Government will have no choice but to significantly tighten social distancing measures in order to safeguard public health."

Details of the aforementioned social distancing measures which are to take effect from October 23, 2020 are as follows:

(I) Catering business and scheduled premises

(1) The requirements and restrictions applicable to catering business and scheduled premises (see Annex 1 for details) will largely be maintained during the seven-day period from October 23

to 29, 2020. Amongst others, activities and facilities involving higher health risks such as dancing activities, steam and sauna facilities and ball pits will continue to be suspended or prohibited from opening. To provide more opportunities for the general public to exercise to maintain physical and mental health so that the public will be fit to continue to combat the epidemic, the latest directions will allow team sports at swimming pools with the maximum number of persons allowed at more than four persons based on the particular team sports activities.

Persons responsible for carrying on catering businesses and managers of scheduled premises that contravene the statutory requirements under the Prevention and Control of Disease (Requirements and Directions) (Business and Premises) Regulation (Cap. 599F) would have committed a criminal offence. Offenders are subject to a maximum fine of $50,000 and imprisonment for six months.

(II) Group gatherings

(2) Taking into account the public's wish to resume social activities and to allow the travel industry, which has been hard hit by the epidemic, to develop local businesses, the Government amends Cap. 599G to expand the scope of exempted group gatherings (at Annex 3) to allow licensed travel agents to organise local tours involving not more than 30 people. Travel agents must register with the Travel Industry Council of Hong Kong for each tour in advance and undertake to strictly implement a series of anti-epidemic measures, including wearing of masks by participants all the time except when having a meal, restricting the maximum number of persons on a conveyance to 50 per cent of its seat capacity, etc.;

(3) The maximum number of persons at wedding ceremonies, at which no food or drink is served, will increase from 20 to 50.

(4) The maximum number of persons in a room or partitioned area at a meeting that is held in accordance with any Ordinance or other regulatory instrument that governs the operation of the organisation or its business (including shareholders' meeting of listed company), at which no food or drink is served, will increase from 20 to 50.

(5) Unless exempted, the prohibition on group gatherings of more than four persons in public places will continue during the seven-day period from October 23 to 29, 2020.

Any person who participates in a prohibited group gathering; organises a prohibited group gathering; owns, controls or operates the place of such gathering and knowingly allows the taking place of such gathering, commits an offence under Cap. 599G. Offenders are liable to a maximum fine of $25,000 and imprisonment for six months. Persons who participate in a prohibited group gathering may discharge liability for the offence by paying a fixed penalty of $2,000.

(III) Mask-wearing requirement

(6) The mandatory mask-wearing requirement will be extended for a period of seven days from October 23 to 29, 2020. During the aforementioned period, a person must wear a mask all the time when the person is boarding or onboard a public transport carrier, is entering or present in an MTR paid area, or is entering or present in a specified public place (i.e. all public places, save for outdoor public places in country parks and special areas as defined in section 2 of the Country Parks Ordinance (Cap. 208).

Under the Prevention and Control of Disease (Wearing of Mask) Regulation (Cap. 599I), if a person does not wear a mask in accordance with the requirement, an authorised person may deny that person from boarding a public transport carrier or entering the area concerned, as well as require that person to wear a mask and disembark from the carrier or leave the said area. A person in contravention of the relevant provision commits an offence and the maximum penalty is a fine at level 2 ($5,000). In addition, authorised public officers may issue fixed penalty notices to persons who do not wear a mask in accordance with the requirement and such persons may discharge liability for the offence by paying a fixed penalty of $2,000.

Issued at HKT 21:25

Government approves conditional exemption of organising local group tours

****

The Government announced today (October 20) that the Executive Council has approved conditional exemption for licensed travel agents to organise local group tours of not more than 30 persons (inclusive of working staff) under the group gathering restrictions as stipulated in the Prevention and Control of Disease (Prohibition on Group Gathering) Regulation (Cap. 599G)starting from this Friday (October 23). Such local group tours must be in strict compliance with the undertakings on anti-epidemic measures to safeguard public health.

The relevant local group tours must comply with a list of requirements which include:

• prior registration with the Travel Industry Council of Hong Kong (TIC);

• travel agents must sign the Anti-epidemic Undertakings for Local Tours (see Annex), and strictly adhere to various anti-epidemic measures targeting local group tours, which cover the arrangements for tour participants, itineraries, transportation, meals, attractions and working staff of the travel agents to safeguard public health; and

• the local group tour itineraries must cover the designated green spots of the Green Lifestyle Local Tour Incentive Scheme, or any of the some 50 tour itineraries under the "Free Tour" programme launched by the Hong Kong Tourism Board (HKTB).

The Secretary for Commerce and Economic Development, Mr Edward Yau, said, "The tourism industry is one of the hardest hit sectors under the epidemic. Both inbound and outbound tourism have grinded to a complete halt. On the premise that the travel trade would endeavour to safeguard hygiene and health as well as put in place vigorous health protection measures, this conditional exemption arrangement would ensure that the local group tours would be well managed. This will on the one hand extend support to the travel trade and practitioners of the related sectors (e.g. tourist guides and tour escorts, the transport trade or even the catering sector), while on the other hand give the public the confidence to join local group tours during the epidemic."

TIC is responsible for the execution of the arrangement. This includes monitoring the compliance of the undertaking, acting on complaints, and conducting surprise checks on sites.

If a travel agent violates the undertaking, the concerned local group tours will no longer be eligible for incentives under the Green Lifestyle Local Tour Incentive Scheme or HKTB's "Free Tour" programme. The travel agent will also be suspended from registration with TIC for local group tours for a month.

To allow travel agents to make full use of the Green Lifestyle Local Tour Incentive Scheme, Mr Yau said that the Government will extend the application deadline for the Scheme from end of December 2020 to March 7, 2021.

Issued at HKT 22:25

October 21[21]

LCQ19: Coping with seasonal influenza and COVID-19 epidemic

****

Following is a question by Dr the Hon Kwok Ka-ki and a written reply by the Secretary for Food and Health, Professor Sophia Chan, in the Legislative Council today (October 21):

Question:

While the Coronavirus Disease 2019 (COVID-19) epidemic has not yet abated, the winter surge of influenza is approaching. This will undoubtedly aggravate the heavy burden on the healthcare system. In this connection, will the Government inform this Council:

(1) of the separate quantities of injectable vaccines and nasal vaccines procured by the

[21] https://www.info.gov.hk/gia/general/202010/21.htm

Department of Health (DH) respectively for (i) the Vaccination Subsidy Scheme, (ii) the Seasonal Influenza Vaccination School Outreach (Free of Charge) programme in respect of outreach to (a) kindergartens/kindergarten-cum-child care centres/child care centres (kindergartens) and (b) primary schools for schoolchildren's vaccination under this programme, and (iii) the Government Vaccination Programme (including vaccination for residents of residential care homes (RCHs) for the elderly and persons with disabilities), as well as the respective average costs per dose of such vaccines; the rates of changes in the quantities of vaccines procured for this year as compared with those procured in the past three years;

(2) of the new measures put in place by DH to increase the vaccination coverage rates; the respective numbers of kindergartens, primary schools and RCHs which have signed up for the outreach vaccination programmes and the respective numbers of participants involved, and whether it has assessed if the participation in such programmes has been affected by the COVID-19 epidemic; and

(3) given that patients suffering from COVID-19 and those suffering from influenza develop very similar symptoms, whether it knows the measures put in place by the Hospital Authority to quickly differentiate between these two types of patients, so as to give them appropriate treatments and prevent cross-transmission?

Reply:

President,

Vaccination is one of the effective means to prevent seasonal influenza (SI) and its complications. It also reduces the risks of flu-associated in-patient admission and mortality. Therefore, the Government has all along been encouraging the public to receive vaccination as early as possible. In 2020/21, free or subsidised seasonal influenza vaccination (SIV) is provided for eligible groups under the Government Vaccination Programme (GVP), the Vaccination Subsidy Scheme (VSS) and the 2020/21 Seasonal Influenza Vaccination School Outreach (Free of Charge) (School Outreach (Free of Charge)). To enhance the uptake rate among school children, the Department of Health (DH) has regularised the School Outreach Vaccination Pilot Programme for primary schools in 2019/20 and the Pilot Programme for kindergartens, kindergarten-cum-child care centres and child care centres in 2020/21 to cover more primary schools, kindergartens, kindergarten-cum-child care centres and child care centres. DH also actively co-ordinates with schools and private doctors to organise outreach SIV activities in schools. In consultation with DH and the Hospital Authority (HA), the reply to the three parts of the question is as follows:

(1) The quantities of SI vaccines under the various government vaccination schemes procured by DH and the expenditure incurred in this year and the past three years:

Year	Quantities of SI vaccines procured (doses)	Increase compared with last year	Expenditure ($M)
2017/18 (Actual)	527 000	-	28.0
2018/19 (Actual)	654 000	24.1%	30.1
2019/20 (Actual)	815 000*	24.6%	40.8*
2020/21 (Estimate)	878 000	7.7%	83.0

* Including a total of 1 700 nasal vaccine doses actually procured in 2019/20, involving an expenditure of $340,000.

(2) To increase the vaccination coverage rate and raise public awareness on the importance of SIVs, DH has continued to strengthen publicity and educational activities through different channels (including press releases, television/radio, interview with specialists, videos of key opinion leaders, advertisements, social media, thematic websites, Health Education Infoline, posters and pamphlets, etc.) to encourage members of the public, especially those from the high risk groups, to receive vaccination, and to remind people of the possibly more severe condition due to coinfection of SI and Coronavirus Disease 2019 (COVID-19). In view of the global COVID-19 pandemic, in order to reduce the risk of simultaneous outbreak of winter SI and COVID-19, the public should receive vaccination early to enhance personal protection and alleviate the burden to the health care system.

Moreover, DH will publicise the importance and arrangements of vaccination to the organisations that serve the elderly. DH will also disseminate information about the vaccination programmes to the elderly through different elderly websites and organisations, and make use of television/radio, etc. to let the elderly understand the programme arrangements. In order to increase the uptake rate of people from the age group of 50 to 64, DH will invite chambers of commerce/companies/organisations to encourage their members/ staff in the age group of 50 to 64 to receive vaccination.

The various vaccination schemes for 2020/21 has been launched by phases in October 2020. As at October 12, a total of around 450 primary schools and 760 kindergartens/kindergarten-cum-child care centres/child care centres joined the School Outreach (Free of Charge), while around 34 primary schools and 24 kindergartens/kindergarten-cum-child care centres/child care centres arranged outreach vaccination activities under the VSS (School Outreach (Extra Charge Allowed)). The overall school participation is comparable to that of the corresponding period last year.

Moreover, vaccination activities will be arranged by residential care homes under the Residential Care Home Vaccination Programme. Visiting Medical Officers enrolled to the programme will be invited to provide vaccination to eligible persons in residential care homes. The Residential Care Home Vaccination Programme will launch on October 22. DH will closely monitor the participation of residential care homes.

(3) For early identification of COVID-19 cases in the community, HA has reinstated the Triage and Test Centres at 17 Accident and Emergency Departments (AEDs) to provide testing for suspected cases with stable medical conditions. Patients would be arranged to wait for the testing results at designated areas, and are required to wear mask while waiting for their results. Certain hospitals have assigned specific wards as the waiting area or set up tents or cubicles in outdoor area with good air ventilation for the suspected cases to wait for the testing results. All designated waiting areas are in compliance with infection control requirements, such as adoption of unilateral seating and arrangement of seats at least one metre apart.

In addition, HA would arrange deep throat saliva testing for patients attending AEDs or general outpatient clinics (GOPCs) with fever and respiratory symptoms or mild chest infection. To reduce the risk of cross infection, hospitals have also enhanced air ventilation in the waiting areas at AEDs or GOPCs. Meanwhile, all patients are required to wear mask while waiting for medical consultation.

Regarding inpatients, HA has enhanced admission screening to offer testing to all newly admitted patients subject to feasibility since September 9. With a view to further reducing the risk of nosocomial infection, hospitals have also reinforced infection control measures in wards and require inpatients to wear mask when staying in the wards.

Issued at HKT 12:40

LCQ16: Assistance for the unemployed

****

Following is a question by the Hon Vincent Cheng and a written reply by the Secretary for Labour and Welfare, Dr Law Chi-kwong, in the Legislative Council today (October 21):

Question:

As Hong Kong's economy has been hard hit by the Coronavirus Disease 2019 epidemic, the unemployment rate has remained high and stood at 6 per cent in recent months. The number of unemployed persons has reached 200 000-odd, representing an increase by more than 100 000 when compared with the figure six months ago. Some academics have pointed out that given the fluctuating epidemic situation and the fact that the Government has no intention to launch a new round of Employment Support Scheme, the unemployment rate may continue to rise. The Government has implemented a time-limited unemployment support scheme (the support scheme) since June 1 this year, under which the asset limits of the Comprehensive Social Security Assistance (CSSA) applicants who are able-bodied adults are temporarily relaxed. In this connection, will the Government inform this Council:

(1) given that there is only a slight increase of 300-odd cases in the number of CSSA cases under the unemployment category recorded in August when compared with that recorded three months ago, which is far smaller than the increase in the number of unemployed persons in the same period, whether the Government has assessed the reasons for that; if so, of the details

(2) whether it conducted any survey and study in the past six months to look into the difficulties faced by the unemployed and the support they need; if so, of the details; if not, whether it will conduct relevant surveys and studies;

(3) whether it will, in the long term, conduct studies on severance payment, long service payment and unemployment support measures, with a view to enhancing the support and protection for employees; if so, of the details; if not, the reasons for that;

(4) as the Government has claimed that the establishment of a new unemployment assistance system would entail high costs and take a rather long time (nearly 18 months), and that such a system might create an effect that the unemployment rate lingers at 4 per cent to 5 per cent, of the basis for such claim; and

(5) whether it will examine other options (e.g. enhancing the support scheme or the Mandatory Provident Fund system), so as to address the imminent needs of the unemployed; if so, of the details; if not, the reasons for that?

Reply:

President,

Having consulted the relevant policy bureaux and departments, my consolidated response to the Member's questions is set out below:

(1) Having considered the unprecedented challenges posed by the coronavirus disease 2019 in Hong Kong, the Government announced in April 2020 the introduction of a time-limited "Special Scheme of Assistance to the Unemployed" through the Comprehensive Social Security Assistance (CSSA) system. The asset limits for able-bodied applicants under the CSSA Scheme

have been temporarily relaxed for six months by 100 per cent from June 1, 2020. In September 2020, the Government announced the further extension of the special scheme for six months to May 31, 2021. Over the past few months, there has been a significant increase in CSSA unemployment cases with an average of 16 864 cases per month from January to September 2020, representing a 43 per cent increase as compared with the average from January to September 2019. The number of CSSA unemployment cases in September 2020 was 19 024, which was the highest since end-2014. The above shows that CSSA is effectively serving its purpose as the safety net and could help the unemployed who are facing temporary financial hardship.

(2) The Census and Statistics Department conducts the General Household Survey every month to collect information on employment, unemployment and other socio-economic characteristics of the population in Hong Kong. Statistics related to the characteristics of unemployed persons, including age, sex, education attainment, duration of unemployment, industry and occupation before unemployment etc., are published in the Quarterly Report on General Household Survey. The General Household Survey does not collect information on the difficulties faced by unemployed persons or the support they needed.

Besides, the Labour Department (LD) has all along been keeping tabs on the employment support services needs of job seekers through various channels, including annual customer opinion surveys.

(3) and (4) According to the Employment Ordinance (EO), if an employee who has been employed under a continuous contract is dismissed (other than summary dismissal due to serious misconduct) and meets the specified conditions and the qualifying length of service, he/she is entitled to severance payment (SP) (Note 1) or long service payment (LSP) (Note 2). The maximum amount of SP and LSP is $390,000. The above requirements would provide economic support to the employees concerned to help alleviate their financial hardship caused by the loss of employment

Regarding the "offsetting" of SP and LSP by the accrued benefits of employers' mandatory contributions under the Mandatory Provident Fund (MPF) system, the Government is working in full steam to take forward the preparatory work and to draft the enabling legislation. Any reform on the SP and LSP will affect the arrangement for abolition of "offsetting" and will need to be re-examined from the start.

(5) As mentioned in the reply to (1) above, the "Special Scheme of Assistance to the Unemployed" has been extended and will last for 12 months to May 31, 2021. Separately, under the existing CSSA arrangement, the value of an owner-occupied residential property of households with able-bodied persons only will be disregarded for a grace period of the first 12 months.

In light of the deteriorating employment situation, LD raised the ceiling of on-the-job training (OJT) allowance payable to employers under the Employment Programme for the Elderly and Middle-aged, the Youth Employment and Training Programme and the Work Orientation and Placement Scheme in September 2020, with a view to further encouraging employers to hire the elderly and middle-aged, young people and persons with disabilities and provide them with OJT. LD also launched a pilot scheme at the same time to encourage eligible elderly persons, young people and persons with disabilities to undergo and complete OJT under these employment programmes through the provision of a retention allowance, thereby stabilising employment.

The MPF system is designed as a long-term saving scheme for retirement rather than tackling the imminent situation facing the unemployed. The suggestion to allow early withdrawal of MPF accrued benefits for meeting short-term financial needs will weaken the integrity of the MPF system and render it difficult to achieve the purpose of assisting working population to save for their retirement. Based on the same policy considerations, the Government is taking forward the relevant law amendment and drafting work to abolish the "offsetting" of SP and LSP by the accrued benefits of employers' mandatory contributions under the MPF System.

Note 1: Under EO, an employee who has been employed under a continuous contract for a period of not less than 24 months is eligible for SP subject to meeting any one of the following conditions: (1) the employee is dismissed by reason of redundancy; (2) the employment contract of a fixed term expires without being renewed by reason of redundancy; or (3) the employee is laid off.

Note 2: Under EO, an employee who has been employed under a continuous contract for a period of not less than 5 years is eligible for LSP subject to meeting any one of the following conditions: (1) the employee is dismissed by the employer (other than redundancy or summary dismissal due to serious misconduct); (2) the employment contract of a fixed term expires without being renewed; (3) the employee dies; (4) the employee resigns upon granting of a certificate by a registered medical practitioner or a registered Chinese medicine practitioner certifying that he/she is permanently unfit for the present job; or (5) the employee, aged 65 or above, resigns on ground of old age.

Issued at HKT 12:54

LCQ10: Online teaching and learning

****

Following is a question by the Hon Kwok Wai-keung and a written reply by the Secretary for Education, Mr Kevin Yeung, in the Legislative Council today (October 21):

Question:

Earlier on, the findings of a study conducted by a university have indicated that there are huge divides in digital competence performance and family support among secondary and primary school students. Of the students participating in the study, about 10 per cent have no access to desktop or laptop computers or tablets; and among those who have access to such computer devices, over 40 per cent have to share the use of such equipment with other family members. There are comments that during the outbreak of the COVID-19 epidemic in the last school year, online learning became the only channel of teaching and learning for schools, which has highlighted the existence of digital divides among various classes, and the right to learning of students from grass-roots families has been undermined by their lack of digital devices and relevant learning resources. In this connection, will the Government inform this Council:

(1) whether it knows the difficulties and pressure faced by students from grass-roots families and their families when such students undertake online learning; whether it has received relevant requests for assistance, and whether it has assessed the impact of schools switching to online teaching on the learning progress of such students, including whether they lagged behind others in terms of learning progress; if it has assessed and the outcome is in the affirmative, of the extent to which they lagged behind others, and the ways to help them catch up with the progress;

(2) of the (i) details, (ii) state of implementation and (iii) number of beneficiary households since January this year of the existing measures to support students from grass-roots families in undertaking online learning; whether it has plans to devise new measures to provide more students from grass-roots families with adequate mobile computer devices and software as well as stable Internet access services to meet the growing needs for online learning; if so, of the details; if not, the reasons for that;

(3) whether it will consider proactively liaising with non-profit-making organisations and providing them with relevant resources and related support to develop for students more online learning resources and activities that are free of charge; if so, of the details; if not, the reasons for that; and

(4) given the new normal of increasing popularity of online teaching and learning and the impact of the epidemic on the academia, whether it has plans to devise a long-term information technology education policy and provide schools with online teaching and learning strategies, curriculum guides as well as relevant teaching and learning resources; if so, of the details; if not, the reasons for that?

Reply:

President,

Though face-to-face classes in schools were once suspended due to the COVID-19 epidemic, students are able to achieve the goal of "suspending classes without suspending learning" and maintain a certain extent of learning at home through the joint efforts of the Education Bureau (EDB) and schools to flexibly deploy various innovative methods. While schools have now resumed half-day schooling, it is believed that different extents of blended mode of learning, i.e. face-to-face classes, e-learning at home or other modes of learning, may become the new normal in teaching and learning given the volatile development of the epidemic.

During the period of class suspension and when face-to-face classes have not yet fully resumed, schools should continue to support students in their home learning through suitable modes of learning and teaching according to their own circumstances and the needs of students at different stages of learning. The modes of learning and teaching are diversified. Both online and offline learning should focus on encouraging students' self-directed learning at home and cater for students' needs and the school context. e-Learning is only one of the forms of learning. Schools may also encourage students to read extensively, carry out thematic explorations, etc. so as to enhance their ability to engage in self-directed learning and hence achieve the goal of continuous learning at home.

As far as we know, during the period of class suspension, schools generally have undertaken various electronic means, which include producing teaching videos, conducting real-time online teaching, using e-learning platforms/learning management systems to arrange teaching activities, as well as distributing learning and teaching materials to students via emails/intranets, to assist students' learning. Some of the schools have also adopted non-electronic means like encouraging students to read extensively and carry out thematic explorations.

Our reply to the Hon Kwok Wai-keung's question is as follows:

(1) The EDB has been maintaining communication with schools through various channels to better understand the arrangements of and the difficulties encountered by schools in the implementation of "suspending classes without suspending learning" during the period of class suspension, so as to provide appropriate support according to their needs.

Schools will identify students' difficulties and needs in learning through different channels. In view of the situation of some students (including those encountering technical difficulties in online learning), schools have assisted them in keeping up their learning progress by various effective means (such as sending the learning and teaching materials to students by post). Teachers also make phone calls to students from time to time to understand their learning progress and provide them with the necessary support.

For students who have encountered difficulties due to the lack of access to e-learning devices, schools have actively supported them, such as lending them mobile computer devices and assisting them to apply for relevant subsidies. Besides, during the class suspension period, schools have remained open and arranged staff to be on duty to support students who have to return to schools because of individual needs and to answer parents' enquiries. Students and parents with doubts or difficulties may also take the initiative to seek appropriate assistance from the schools. If the EDB receives any requests for assistance from parents or students, it will refer them to the schools concerned for proper follow-up.

The results of a questionnaire survey conducted by the EDB in July this year show that during the period of class suspension, schools have adopted diversified strategies to support students in their home learning, devised and implemented learning plans for different subjects at all levels so that students could continue to learn systematically. As schools and parents are particularly concerned about students' learning progress, schools have adopted different means to track their learning progress during the class suspension period and followed up on the situation after class resumption. Most of the schools considered that the progress of implementation of home learning plans for students could meet the pre-set targets. On the other hand, the EDB has always sought to understand the implementation of learning and teaching as well as student support measures and student learning in schools, through channels such as inspections and school visits; and has been providing professional advice to schools according to the school context to facilitate their continuous development.

(2) The Government is concerned about grass-roots students' e-learning and has implemented various measures to support it. Since the 2010/11 school year, the Student Finance Office of the Working Family and Student Financial Assistance Agency (SFO) and the Social Welfare Department (SWD) have been implementing the Subsidy Scheme for Internet Access Charges, under which Internet access subsidies are disbursed to eligible families to facilitate online learning at home by needy students. The rate of the subsidy is adjusted annually with reference to prevailing market fees of Internet access services. The full rate and half rate of the subsidy in the 2020/21 school year are $1,600 and $800 respectively. The number of beneficiary families under the scheme in the 2019/20 school year is around 171 400.

Through the Community Care Fund (CCF), the EDB has also been implementing a three-year assistance programme on provision of subsidy to needy primary and secondary students (Note) for purchasing mobile computer devices since the 2018/19 school year to relieve the financial burden on students from low-income families under the development of the Bring Your Own Device policy on campus. For students receiving CSSA/full grant, subsidy will be provided to cover the full cost of purchasing the devices. In the 2020/21 school year, the maximum subsidy is $4,740. For students receiving half grant, the subsidy provided is half of the actual cost of the devices up to $2,370. In view of the COVID-19 epidemic, we handle applications flexibly and accept the applications submitted by all public sector primary and secondary schools implementing e-learning for their eligible students before the full resumption of classes. The programme has benefitted about 34 200 students in the 2018/19 and 2019/20 school years. We expect that around 100 000 students from 800 schools will be benefitted in the 2020/21 school year. We will review the CCF assistance programme on provision of subsidy to needy primary and secondary students for purchasing mobile computer devices, including its operation and effectiveness, and will consolidate the relevant experience with a view to enhancing the measures in support of e-learning.

On the other hand, schools could also help needy students who do not have suitable computer devices through other school-based measures such as lending them mobile computer devices for home learning (as schools normally have sufficient quantities of these devices) or assisting them to apply for other assistance programmes.

Moreover, various sectors of the community have joined hands to provide support to needy students. To support students who have difficulties accessing to the Internet for e-learning at home during the class suspension period, the Hong Kong Jockey Club Charities Trust, through two non-government organisations (NGOs), provide internet access support (with mobile data SIM card) for 100 000 local primary and secondary school students for a period of four months.

(3) and (4) To assist schools in adopting e-learning modes to support students' home learning, the EDB has implemented a series of support measures:

(i) Training of teachers:

The EDB has set up a dedicated webpage (www.edb.gov.hk/ited/eh) with videos uploaded, elucidating the skills of using e-learning platforms, flipped classroom approach and real-time online teaching. We have been organising webinars on different topics every week since late January 2020 to share updated information and experiences of online teaching. As at July 2020, dozens of webinars have been organised. We have also launched a new series of webinars since mid-August this year, the themes of which include major findings of focus inspections and good practices of schools, e-teaching pedagogies relating to different subjects, successful experiences of supporting students in home learning, and school leaders making plans in a holistic manner as well as paying attention to students' physical and mental well-being.

(ii) Support services and strategies:

The IT in Education Centres of Excellence set up by the EDB continue to offer remote support services and share student support and home learning strategies according to school-based needs. We also continue to provide advice and support for teachers in need through hotlines, mobile communication applications and online self-learning courses. In March this year, we issued the principles of adopting e-learning to support students' home learning for schools' reference. Recently, we have also consolidated the experiences of the parties concerned, which include the questionnaire survey conducted by the EDB in July this year and the preliminary findings of focus inspections, and updated the aforesaid principles. We informed schools of the principles by issuing letters to them and uploading such principles to the EDB's dedicated webpage (www.edb.gov.hk/ited/eh) in August this year to provide relevant guidelines to schools. Schools should make reference to the implementation principles and support students in their home learning through suitable modes of learning and teaching according to their own circumstances and the needs of students at different stages of learning. We will continue to conduct relevant focus inspections, understand schools' circumstances and share successful experiences with the sector.

(iii) Teaching and learning resources:

In view of the COVID-19 epidemic, we have launched a dedicated webpage "Online Learning 360°" (www.hkedcity.net/home/zh-hant/learning) in collaboration with the Hong Kong Education City (HKEdCity) to consolidate existing e-learning resources and propose learning schedules for the reference of schools, teachers, students and parents. Apart from providing resources for various learning areas through the "EDB One-stop Portal for Learning & Teaching Resources" (www.hkedcity.net/edbosp), the Curriculum Development Institute of the EDB has developed a series of learning and teaching resources covering various subjects at both the primary and secondary levels to support teachers in enhancing students' understanding of how to fight the virus and the related knowledge. Schools can also make use of the assessment tools and assessment items covering Chinese Language, English Language and Mathematics from primary to junior secondary schools provided by the online Student Assessment Repository (STAR) (star.hkedcity.net). During the class suspension period, many IT companies, universities, charitable organisations and NGOs also offered e-learning support to students proactively and allowed the school sector to use their e-learning platforms and resources for free for the benefit of students. Some of the links to the relevant websites were uploaded to the dedicated webpage launched by the EDB during the class suspension period for schools' reference. In addition, the "Resources Depository" (resources.hkedcity.net) set up by the HKEdCity also encourages teachers and related organisations to share quality learning and teaching resources through the platform.

Schools are encouraged to continue to make use of the teaching resources provided by the EDB, including applying for funding under the priority theme of "IT in Education" under the Quality Education Fund. By utilising both the external and internal resources of schools, schools can formulate comprehensive learning and teaching strategies to cater for the learning needs of students. The EDB will continue to review and enhance all relevant measures to further support schools in implementing the blended mode of learning under the new normal.

Note: The beneficiaries are those receiving Comprehensive Social Security Assistance (CSSA) from the SWD or full grant/half grant of the School Textbook Assistance Scheme from the SFO.

Issued at HKT 12:55

CHP investigates eight additional confirmed cases of COVID-19

****

The Centre for Health Protection (CHP) of the Department of Health has announced that as of 0.00am, October 21, the CHP was investigating eight additional confirmed cases of coronavirus disease 2019 (COVID-19), taking the number of cases to 5 270 in Hong Kong so far (comprising 5 269 confirmed cases and one probable case).

Among the newly reported cases announced, seven had a travel history during the incubation period. The remaining case was epidemiologically linked with a local case.

The CHP's epidemiological investigations and relevant contact tracing on the confirmed cases are ongoing. For case details and contact tracing information, please see the Annex or the list of buildings with confirmed cases of COVID-19 in the past 14 days and the latest local situation of COVID-19 available on the website "COVID-19 Thematic Website" (www.coronavirus.gov.hk).

A spokesman for the CHP said, "During the CHP's epidemiological investigations and relevant contact tracing on the confirmed cases, we will compile and upload (www.chp.gov.hk/files/pdf/building_list_eng.pdf) a list of buildings that confirmed patients had visited from two days before the onset of symptoms. Given that cases of local infection continue to occur from time to time, members of the public are urged to seek medical attention immediately if they believe that they had visited the same place at an identical time with a confirmed patient and feel unwell subsequently. If they remain asymptomatic but are concerned that they have been infected, they can also visit the Hospital Authority's designated general out-patient clinics (www.ha.org.hk/haho/ho/covid-19/GOPC_extend_EN.pdf) to obtain specimen collection packs and collect deep throat saliva specimens for free COVID-19 testing."

In view of the severe epidemic situation, the CHP called on members of the public to avoid going out, having social contact and dining out. They should put on a surgical mask and maintain stringent hand hygiene when they need to go out. The CHP strongly urged the elderly to stay home as far as possible and avoid going out. They should consider asking their family and friends to help with everyday tasks such as shopping for basic necessities.

The spokesman said, "Given that the situation of COVID-19 infection remains severe and that there is a continuous increase in the number of cases reported around the world, members of the public are strongly urged to avoid all non-essential travel outside Hong Kong.

"The CHP also strongly urges the public to maintain at all times strict personal and environmental hygiene, which is key to personal protection against infection and prevention of the spread of the disease in the community. On a personal level, members of the public should wear a surgical mask when having respiratory symptoms, taking public transport or staying in crowded places. They should also perform hand hygiene frequently, especially before touching the mouth, nose or eyes.

"As for household environmental hygiene, members of the public are advised to maintain drainage pipes properly, regularly pour water into drain outlets (U-traps) and cover all floor drain outlets when they are not in use. After using the toilet, they should put the toilet lid down before flushing to avoid spreading germs."

Moreover, the Government has launched the website "COVID-19 Thematic Website" (www.coronavirus.gov.hk) for announcing the latest updates on various news on COVID-19 infection and health advice to help the public understand the latest updates. Members of the public may also gain access to information via the COVID-19 WhatsApp Helpline launched by the Office of the Government Chief Information Officer. Simply by saving 9617 1823 in their phone contacts or clicking the link wa.me/85296171823?text=hi, they will be able to obtain information on COVID-19 as well as the "StayHomeSafe" mobile app and wristband via WhatsApp.

Issued at HKT 14:00

Public hospitals daily update on COVID-19 cases
****

The following is issued on behalf of the Hospital Authority:

As at 9am today (October 21), eight COVID-19 confirmed patients were discharged from hospital in the last 24 hours. So far, a total of 5 004 patients with confirmed or probable infection have been discharged.

At present, there are 614 negative pressure rooms in public hospitals with 1 098 negative pressure beds activated. A total of 124 confirmed patients are currently hospitalised in 18 public hospitals, among which 13 patients are in critical condition, five are in serious condition and the remaining 106 patients are in stable condition.

The Hospital Authority will maintain close contact with the Centre for Health Protection to monitor the latest developments and to inform the public and healthcare workers on the latest information in a timely manner.

Details of the above-mentioned patients are as follows:

Patient condition	Case numbers
Discharged	5131, 5168, 5170, 5200, 5201, 5215, 5236, 5258
Critical	1989, 3496, 3764, 4433, 4706, 4732, 4833, 4937, 4990, 5110, 5151, 5185, 5195
Serious	1650, 4101, 4746, 4788, 5152

Issued at HKT 16:47

October 22[22]

Labour Department continues to arrange free COVID-19 testing service for foreign domestic helpers waiting to join new employers' family

****

The Labour Department (LD) announced today (October 22) that the free COVID-19 testing service will continue to be provided for foreign domestic helpers (FDHs) waiting to join their new employers' family from October 27 to November 21, 2020.

An LD spokesman said, "In view of confirmed infection cases of FDHs who had stayed in boarding facilities, the Government provided a free COVID-19 testing service from August 25 to October 15 for FDHs whose previous employment contracts had expired or had been terminated and who were waiting to join the new employers' family. These FDHs are most likely to be staying in boarding facilities while waiting to change employers. To benefit more FDHs, the LD will once again arrange a free COVID-19 testing service for these FDHs. We strongly encourage FDHs staying in boarding facilities while waiting to change employers to actively participate in the free testing to safeguard their health. If an FDH needs to stay in a boarding facility for an extended period of time while waiting to change employer, he or she may retake the test as appropriate, especially before joining the new employer's family. We appeal for employment agencies' active assistance in arranging for FDHs to collect specimen collection packs at the temporary distribution/collection point and to return the specimens for testing. We also advise employers to check that their new FDHs have a valid negative test result before joining the family."

Eligible FDHs may, starting from October 27, collect and return specimen collection packs at the temporary distribution/collection point located at 1/F (footbridge level), Immigration Tower, 7 Gloucester Road, Wan Chai. No prior appointment is required. The temporary distribution/collection point will be open from 11am to 4pm from Monday to Saturday. The testing is free of charge.

When distributing specimen collection packs, duty officers will ask for simple information regarding the eligibility of the FDH for the testing service, e.g. the Hong Kong identity card number and/or passport number, the reference number and limit of stay as shown on the latest

[22] https://www.info.gov.hk/gia/general/202010/22.htm

visa issued by the Immigration Department (ImmD), or the reference number/date of application for a visa/extension of stay as a visitor as shown on documents issued by the ImmD. The FDH should bring along the relevant documents for a smooth identity verification process. He or she will be asked to sign a consent form to give consent to taking the test and confirm his or her eligibility for the testing service. After collecting the specimen collection pack, the FDH is required to register his or her personal information at a government website (www.tgptest.gov.hk, please select "Non-Government Staff - Foreign domestic helpers waiting to join new employers' family") in order to receive SMS notification of the testing result. If necessary, duty officers can assist the FDH in registration. The FDH should self-collect the deep throat saliva specimen and return it to the temporary collection point on the same day of self-collection.

The testing agency will deliver the specimens to the laboratory for testing. The testing agency will not acquire or retain any personal information of the participants. Participants will be notified of a negative test result via SMS. Positive cases will be referred to the Centre for Health Protection of the Department of Health (DH) for follow-up and the DH will contact the participant concerned if it is confirmed to be an infection case.

For enquiries, please contact the LD through the dedicated FDH hotline at 2157 9537 (manned by 1823) or by email to fdh-enquiry@labour.gov.hk.

Issued at HKT 16:50

CHP investigates 11 additional confirmed cases of COVID-19

****

The Centre for Health Protection (CHP) of the Department of Health has announced that as of 0.00am, October 22, the CHP was investigating 11 additional confirmed cases of coronavirus disease 2019 (COVID-19), taking the number of cases to 5 281 in Hong Kong so far (comprising 5 280 confirmed cases and one probable case).

Among the newly reported cases announced, 10 had a travel history during the incubation period.

The CHP's epidemiological investigations and relevant contact tracing on the confirmed cases are ongoing. For case details and contact tracing information, please see the Annex or the list of buildings with confirmed cases of COVID-19 in the past 14 days and the latest local situation of COVID-19 available on the website "COVID-19 Thematic Website" (www.coronavirus.gov.hk).

A spokesman for the CHP said, "During the CHP's epidemiological investigations and relevant contact tracing on the confirmed cases, we will compile and upload (www.chp.gov.hk/files/pdf/building_list_eng.pdf) a list of buildings that confirmed patients had visited from two days before the onset of symptoms. Given that cases of local infection continue to occur from time to time, members of the public are urged to seek medical attention immediately if they believe that they had visited the same place at an identical time with a confirmed patient and feel unwell subsequently. If they remain asymptomatic but are concerned that they have been infected, they can also visit the Hospital Authority's designated general out-patient clinics (www.ha.org.hk/haho/ho/covid-19/GOPC_extend_EN.pdf) to obtain specimen collection packs and collect deep throat saliva specimens for free COVID-19 testing."

In view of the severe epidemic situation, the CHP called on members of the public to avoid going out, having social contact and dining out. They should put on a surgical mask and maintain stringent hand hygiene when they need to go out. The CHP strongly urged the elderly to stay home as far as possible and avoid going out. They should consider asking their family and friends to help with everyday tasks such as shopping for basic necessities.

The spokesman said, "Given that the situation of COVID-19 infection remains severe and that there is a continuous increase in the number of cases reported around the world, members of the public are strongly urged to avoid all non-essential travel outside Hong Kong.

"The CHP also strongly urges the public to maintain at all times strict personal and environmental hygiene, which is key to personal protection against infection and prevention of the spread of the disease in the community. On a personal level, members of the public should wear a surgical mask when having respiratory symptoms, taking public transport or staying in crowded places. They should also perform hand hygiene frequently, especially before touching the mouth, nose or eyes.

"As for household environmental hygiene, members of the public are advised to maintain drainage pipes properly, regularly pour water into drain outlets (U-traps) and cover all floor drain outlets when they are not in use. After using the toilet, they should put the toilet lid down before flushing to avoid spreading germs."

Moreover, the Government has launched the website "COVID-19 Thematic Website" (www.coronavirus.gov.hk) for announcing the latest updates on various news on COVID-19 infection and health advice to help the public understand the latest updates. Members of the public may also gain access to information via the COVID-19 WhatsApp Helpline launched by the Office of the Government Chief Information Officer. Simply by saving 9617 1823 in their phone contacts or clicking the link wa.me/85296171823?text=hi, they will be able to obtain information on COVID-19 as well as the "StayHomeSafe" mobile app and wristband via WhatsApp.

Issued at HKT 17:14

FEHD urges public to postpone grave-sweeping activities and maintain anti-epidemic awareness

****

In view of the latest epidemic development of COVID-19 in Hong Kong, the Food and Environmental Hygiene Department (FEHD) today (October 22) appealed to members of the public to defer their grave-sweeping plans as far as possible to avoid the crowded peak period. Grave sweepers should maintain anti-epidemic awareness, comply with relevant regulations on prevention and control of the disease and keep the environment hygienic.

A spokesman for the FEHD said, "In order to reduce the risk of virus transmission through social contact, members of the public are urged to seriously consider postponing their grave-sweeping plans so as to lessen crowd situations and reduce close contact. People visiting cemeteries and columbaria paying respect to ancestors should avoid group gatherings when grave sweeping, maintain an appropriate social distance with others at all times, and avoid meal gatherings with relatives and friends at worship sites."

The spokesman reminded members of the public that they should seek medical advice promptly and refrain from going grave sweeping if they have a fever or respiratory symptoms. They should maintain good personal hygiene when grave sweeping, wear surgical masks and always keep their hands clean. They are also reminded to keep flammable items (such as alcohol antiseptic sprays and alcohol-based hand sanitisers) away from ignition sources, incense and candles, and furnaces for the sake of safety.

The spokesman urged the public to work together to keep the environment clean to prevent mosquito breeding. Grave sweepers should clear stagnant water and rubbish before leaving. Containers such as lunch boxes, drink cans, plastic bags and buckets for burning incense should also be removed.

During the two weeks before and after the Chung Yeung Festival, the opening hours of public columbaria under the FEHD is extended to 7am to 7pm till November 8. Special cleaning services are provided including disinfection of handrails and lift buttons inside public cemeteries and columbaria, and the deployment of more staff to clear undergrowth and remove rubbish, empty bottles and containers left behind by grave sweepers, remove water in containers and incense burners, and level ground surfaces to prevent accumulation of water. Furthermore, additional litter bins and toilet facilities are also provided.

The FEHD appealed to the public to consider making use of the Internet Memorial Service webpage (www.memorial.gov.hk) and its mobile application to pay tribute to their deceased beloved ones.

Issued at HKT 18:20

Public hospitals daily update on COVID-19 cases

****

The following is issued on behalf of the Hospital Authority:

As at 9am today (October 22), 15 COVID-19 confirmed patients were discharged from hospital in the last 24 hours. So far, a total of 5 019 patients with confirmed or probable infection have been discharged.

At present, there are 614 negative pressure rooms in public hospitals with 1 098 negative pressure beds activated. A total of 116 confirmed patients are currently hospitalised in 18 public hospitals, among which 13 patients are in critical condition, four are in serious condition and the remaining 99 patients are in stable condition.

The Hospital Authority will maintain close contact with the Centre for Health Protection to monitor the latest developments and to inform the public and healthcare workers on the latest information in a timely manner.

Details of the above-mentioned patients are as follows:

Patient condition	Case numbers
Discharged	1650, 4808, 5129, 5133, 5161, 5163, 5165, 5198, 5199, 5209, 5229, 5230, 5235, 5257, 5261
Critical	1989, 3496, 3764, 4433, 4706, 4732, 4833, 4937, 4990, 5110, 5151, 5185, 5195
Serious	4101, 4746, 4788, 5152

Issued at HKT 18:25

Three persons sentenced for breaching compulsory quarantine orders
****

Three persons were sentenced by magistrates' courts today (October 22) for violating the Compulsory Quarantine of Certain Persons Arriving at Hong Kong Regulation (Cap 599C) or the Compulsory Quarantine of Persons Arriving at Hong Kong from Foreign Places Regulation (Cap 599E).

The first case involved a woman aged 48, who was earlier issued a compulsory quarantine order stating that she must conduct quarantine at home for 14 days. Before the expiry of the quarantine order, she left the place of quarantine on July 12 without reasonable excuse nor permission given by an authorised officer. She was charged with contravening sections 8(1) and 8(5) of the Compulsory Quarantine of Certain Persons Arriving at Hong Kong Regulation (Cap 599C) and was sentenced by the West Kowloon Magistrates' Courts today to immediate imprisonment for 10 days.

The second case involved a man aged 20. Before the expiry of the quarantine order, he left the place of quarantine several times on March 23 without reasonable excuse nor permission given by an authorised officer. He was charged with three counts of contravening sections 8(1) and 8(5) of the Compulsory Quarantine of Persons Arriving at Hong Kong from Foreign Places Regulation (Cap 599E) and was sentenced by the Tuen Mun Magistrates' Courts today to eight weeks' imprisonment for each of the three charges, suspended for 24 months.

The third case involved a woman aged 37. Before the expiry of the quarantine order, she left the place of quarantine without reasonable excuse nor permission given by an authorised officer and was stopped by an Immigration Officer at Hong Kong International Airport on September 28. She was also found to have removed her wristband. She was charged with three counts of contravening sections 8(1), 8(4) and 8(5) of the Compulsory Quarantine of Persons Arriving at Hong Kong from Foreign Places Regulation (Cap 599E). She was sentenced by the Kwun Tong Magistrates' Courts today to immediate imprisonment for four weeks for each of the three charges, which are to run concurrently.

Pursuant to the Compulsory Quarantine of Certain Persons Arriving at Hong Kong Regulation (Cap 599C) starting from February 8, save for exempted persons, all persons who have stayed in the Mainland, Macao or Taiwan in the 14 days preceding arrival in Hong Kong, regardless of their nationality or travel documents, will be subject to compulsory quarantine for 14 days. Moreover, pursuant to the Compulsory Quarantine of Persons Arriving at Hong Kong from Foreign Places Regulation (Cap 599E), starting from March 19, all persons arriving from countries or territories outside China would also be subject to compulsory quarantine for 14 days. Breaching a quarantine order is a criminal offence and offenders are subject to a maximum fine of $25,000 and imprisonment for six months.

A spokesman for the Department of Health said the sentence sends a clear message to the community that breaching a compulsory quarantine order is a criminal offence that the Government will not tolerate, and solemnly reminded the public to comply with the compulsory quarantine regulations. As of today, a total of 59 persons have been convicted by the courts for breaching compulsory quarantine orders and have received sentences including immediate imprisonment for up to three months or a fine of $15,000. The spokesman reiterated that resolute actions will be taken against anyone who has breached the relevant regulations.

Issued at HKT 19:08

October 23[23]

Pyrotechnics and Special Effects Operators Subsidy Scheme under AEF opens for applications

****

The Pyrotechnics and Special Effects Operators Subsidy Scheme under the Anti-epidemic Fund (AEF) is open for application from today (October 23) to November 13 at 5pm

The Scheme will provide a one-off subsidy of $7,500 to each eligible special effects operator (SEO) and assistant (SEA) holding at least one valid licence within 2020 (between January 1 and September 30) issued under the Entertainment Special Effects Ordinance (Cap. 560) and its subsidiary legislation, and who have not benefited from the Employment Support Scheme or any other sector-specific subsidy schemes under the AEF. Same practitioners holding different types of SEO/SEA licences should only be eligible to receive a maximum subsidy amount of $7,500.

The application details of the Scheme are available at the Create Hong Kong website (www.createhk.gov.hk).

Issued at HKT 11:00

CHP investigates four additional confirmed cases of COVID-19

****

The Centre for Health Protection (CHP) of the Department of Health has announced that as of 0.00am, October 23, the CHP was investigating four additional confirmed cases of coronavirus disease 2019 (COVID-19), taking the number of cases to 5 285 in Hong Kong so far (comprising 5 284 confirmed cases and one probable case).

Among the newly reported cases announced, three had a travel history during the incubation period. The remaining case was epidemiologically linked with an imported case.

The CHP's epidemiological investigations and relevant contact tracing on the confirmed cases are ongoing. For case details and contact tracing information, please see the Annex or the list of buildings with confirmed cases of COVID-19 in the past 14 days and the latest local situation of COVID-19 available on the website "COVID-19 Thematic Website" (www.coronavirus.gov.hk).

A spokesman for the CHP said, "During the CHP's epidemiological investigations and relevant contact tracing on the confirmed cases, we will compile and upload (www.chp.gov.hk/files/pdf/building_list_eng.pdf) a list of buildings that confirmed patients had visited from two days before the onset of symptoms. Given that cases of local infection continue

[23] https://www.info.gov.hk/gia/general/202010/23.htm

to occur from time to time, members of the public are urged to seek medical attention immediately if they believe that they had visited the same place at an identical time with a confirmed patient and feel unwell subsequently. If they remain asymptomatic but are concerned that they have been infected, they can also visit the Hospital Authority's designated general out-patient clinics (www.ha.org.hk/haho/ho/covid-19/GOPC_extend_EN.pdf) to obtain specimen collection packs and collect deep throat saliva specimens for free COVID-19 testing."

In view of the severe epidemic situation, the CHP called on members of the public to avoid going out, having social contact and dining out. They should put on a surgical mask and maintain stringent hand hygiene when they need to go out. The CHP strongly urged the elderly to stay home as far as possible and avoid going out. They should consider asking their family and friends to help with everyday tasks such as shopping for basic necessities.

The spokesman said, "Given that the situation of COVID-19 infection remains severe and that there is a continuous increase in the number of cases reported around the world, members of the public are strongly urged to avoid all non-essential travel outside Hong Kong.

"The CHP also strongly urges the public to maintain at all times strict personal and environmental hygiene, which is key to personal protection against infection and prevention of the spread of the disease in the community. On a personal level, members of the public should wear a surgical mask when having respiratory symptoms, taking public transport or staying in crowded places. They should also perform hand hygiene frequently, especially before touching the mouth, nose or eyes.

"As for household environmental hygiene, members of the public are advised to maintain drainage pipes properly, regularly pour water into drain outlets (U-traps) and cover all floor drain outlets when they are not in use. After using the toilet, they should put the toilet lid down before flushing to avoid spreading germs."

Moreover, the Government has launched the website "COVID-19 Thematic Website" (www.coronavirus.gov.hk) for announcing the latest updates on various news on COVID-19 infection and health advice to help the public understand the latest updates. Members of the public may also gain access to information via the COVID-19 WhatsApp Helpline launched by the Office of the Government Chief Information Officer. Simply by saving 9617 1823 in their phone contacts or clicking the link wa.me/85296171823?text=hi, they will be able to obtain information on COVID-19 as well as the "StayHomeSafe" mobile app and wristband via WhatsApp.

Issued at HKT 14:00

Public hospitals daily update on COVID-19 cases

****

The following is issued on behalf of the Hospital Authority:

As at 9am today (October 23), 10 COVID-19 confirmed patients were discharged from hospital in the last 24 hours. So far, a total of 5 029 patients with confirmed or probable infection have been discharged.

At present, there are 614 negative pressure rooms in public hospitals with 1 098 negative pressure beds activated. A total of 117 confirmed patients are currently hospitalised in 18 public hospitals, among which 13 patients are in critical condition, three are in serious condition and the remaining 101 patients are in stable condition.

The Hospital Authority will maintain close contact with the Centre for Health Protection to monitor the latest developments and to inform the public and healthcare workers on the latest information in a timely manner.

Details of the above-mentioned patients are as follows:

Patient condition	Case numbers
Discharged	5058, 5126, 5188, 5213, 5226, 5227, 5228, 5269, 5270, 5277
Critical	1989, 3496, 3764, 4433, 4706, 4732, 4833, 4937, 4990, 5110, 5151, 5185, 5195
Serious	4101, 4746, 4788

Ends/Friday, October 23, 2020
Issued at HKT 16:28

Transcript of remarks by SFH at media session

****

Following is the transcript of remarks by the Secretary for Food and Health, Professor Sophia Chan, at a media session after receiving the seasonal influenza vaccination at the Kwai Tsing District Health Centre today (October 23):

Reporter: You said you will closely monitor the effect of the vaccine, what exactly would you do to closely monitor? Will there be follow-ups on people who are vaccinated? How confident are you that the Hong Kong Government can get enough extra vaccines for the high-risk groups, the 100 000 vaccines?

Secretary for Food and Health: We have announced that we will procure additional vaccine of 100 000 doses for the high-risk groups for the VSS (Vaccination Subsidy Scheme) doctors. We understand there is an outcry for more flu vaccines in the private market. It is of our best interest to have these high-risk groups or priority groups to have the vaccine as soon as possible and that is why the Government and the Department of Health have made special arrangements.

Issued at HKT 18:10

Woman sentenced for breaching compulsory quarantine order

****

A 29-year-old woman was sentenced to immediate imprisonment for 14 days by the Kowloon City Magistrates' Courts today (October 23) for violating the Compulsory Quarantine of Certain Persons Arriving at Hong Kong Regulation (Cap 599C) (the Regulation).

The woman was earlier issued a compulsory quarantine order stating that she must conduct quarantine at home for 14 days. Before the expiry of the quarantine order, she left the place of quarantine on May 17 without reasonable excuse nor permission given by an authorised officer. She was charged with contravening sections 8(1) and 8(5) of the Regulation and was sentenced by the Kowloon City Magistrates' Courts today to immediate imprisonment for 14 days.

Pursuant to the Regulation, starting from February 8, save for exempted persons, all persons who have stayed in the Mainland, Macao or Taiwan in the 14 days preceding arrival in Hong Kong, regardless of their nationality or travel documents, will be subject to compulsory quarantine for 14 days. Moreover, pursuant to the Compulsory Quarantine of Persons Arriving at Hong Kong from Foreign Places Regulation (Cap 599E), starting from March 19, all persons arriving from countries or territories outside China would also be subject to compulsory quarantine for 14 days. Breaching a quarantine order is a criminal offence and offenders are subject to a maximum fine of $25,000 and imprisonment for six months.

A spokesman for the Department of Health said the sentence sends a clear message to the community that breaching a compulsory quarantine order is a criminal offence that the Government will not tolerate, and solemnly reminded the public to comply with the Regulation. As of today, a total of 60 persons have been convicted by the courts for breaching compulsory quarantine orders and have received sentences including immediate imprisonment for up to three months or a fine of $15,000. The spokesman reiterated that resolute actions will be taken against anyone who has breached the relevant regulations.

Issued at HKT 18:23

October 24[24]

CHP investigates five additional confirmed cases of COVID-19

****

The Centre for Health Protection (CHP) of the Department of Health has announced that as of 0.00am, October 24, the CHP was investigating five additional confirmed cases of coronavirus disease 2019 (COVID-19), taking the number of cases to 5 290 in Hong Kong so far (comprising 5 289 confirmed cases and one probable case).

Among the newly reported cases announced, four had a travel history during the incubation period.

The CHP's epidemiological investigations and relevant contact tracing on the confirmed cases are ongoing. For case details and contact tracing information, please see the Annex or the list of buildings with confirmed cases of COVID-19 in the past 14 days and the latest local situation of COVID-19 available on the website "COVID-19 Thematic Website" (www.coronavirus.gov.hk).

A spokesman for the CHP said, "During the CHP's epidemiological investigations and relevant contact tracing on the confirmed cases, we will compile and upload (www.chp.gov.hk/files/pdf/building_list_eng.pdf) a list of buildings that confirmed patients had visited from two days before the onset of symptoms. Given that cases of local infection continue to occur from time to time, members of the public are urged to seek medical attention immediately if they believe that they had visited the same place at an identical time with a confirmed patient and feel unwell subsequently. If they remain asymptomatic but are concerned that they have been infected, they can also visit the Hospital Authority's designated general out-patient clinics (www.ha.org.hk/haho/ho/covid-19/GOPC_extend_EN.pdf) to obtain specimen collection packs and collect deep throat saliva specimens for free COVID-19 testing."

[24] https://www.info.gov.hk/gia/general/202010/24.htm

In view of the severe epidemic situation, the CHP called on members of the public to avoid going out, having social contact and dining out. They should put on a surgical mask and maintain stringent hand hygiene when they need to go out. The CHP strongly urged the elderly to stay home as far as possible and avoid going out. They should consider asking their family and friends to help with everyday tasks such as shopping for basic necessities.

The spokesman said, "Given that the situation of COVID-19 infection remains severe and that there is a continuous increase in the number of cases reported around the world, members of the public are strongly urged to avoid all non-essential travel outside Hong Kong

"The CHP also strongly urges the public to maintain at all times strict personal and environmental hygiene, which is key to personal protection against infection and prevention of the spread of the disease in the community. On a personal level, members of the public should wear a surgical mask when having respiratory symptoms, taking public transport or staying in crowded places. They should also perform hand hygiene frequently, especially before touching the mouth, nose or eyes.

"As for household environmental hygiene, members of the public are advised to maintain drainage pipes properly, regularly pour water into drain outlets (U-traps) and cover all floor drain outlets when they are not in use. After using the toilet, they should put the toilet lid down before flushing to avoid spreading germs."

Moreover, the Government has launched the website "COVID-19 Thematic Website" (www.coronavirus.gov.hk) for announcing the latest updates on various news on COVID-19 infection and health advice to help the public understand the latest updates. Members of the public may also gain access to information via the COVID-19 WhatsApp Helpline launched by the Office of the Government Chief Information Officer. Simply by saving 9617 1823 in their phone contacts or clicking the link wa.me/85296171823?text=hi, they will be able to obtain information on COVID-19 as well as the "StayHomeSafe" mobile app and wristband via WhatsApp.

Issued at HKT 17:03

Public hospitals daily update on COVID-19 cases

****

The following is issued on behalf of the Hospital Authority:

As at 9am today (October 24), 12 COVID-19 confirmed patients were discharged from hospital in the last 24 hours. So far, a total of 5 041 patients with confirmed or probable infection have been discharged.

At present, there are 614 negative pressure rooms in public hospitals with 1 098 negative pressure beds activated. A total of 109 confirmed patients are currently hospitalised in 18 public hospitals, among which 12 patients are in critical condition, four are in serious condition and the remaining 93 patients are in stable condition.

The Hospital Authority will maintain close contact with the Centre for Health Protection to monitor the latest developments and to inform the public and healthcare workers on the latest information in a timely manner.

Details of the above-mentioned patients are as follows:

Patient condition	Case numbers
Discharged	5112, 5140, 5154, 5158, 5160, 5169, 5196, 5234, 5242, 5274, 5275, 5285
Critical	1989, 3496, 3764, 4433, 4706, 4732, 4833, 4937, 5110, 5151, 5185, 5195
Serious	4101, 4746, 4788, 4990

Issued at HKT 17:54

October 25[25]

CHP investigates six additional confirmed cases of COVID-19

****

The Centre for Health Protection (CHP) of the Department of Health has announced that as of 0.00am, October 25, the CHP was investigating six additional confirmed cases of coronavirus disease 2019 (COVID-19), taking the number of cases to 5 296 in Hong Kong so far (comprising 5 295 confirmed cases and one probable case).

Among the newly reported cases announced, five had a travel history during the incubation period. The remaining case was a local case with unknown sources.

[25] https://www.info.gov.hk/gia/general/202010/25.htm

The case with unknown sources involves a 42-year-old man (case 5 293) who had developed sore throat on October 20. The patient consulted a private doctor on October 21. He sought medical treatment at Tseung Kwan O (Po Ning Road) General Out-patient Clinic on October 22 and submitted a deep throat saliva sample on the following day. He works at Siu Ying Commercial Building on Queen's Road Central in Sheung Wan and last went to work on October 21.

The CHP's epidemiological investigations and relevant contact tracing on the confirmed cases are ongoing. For case details and contact tracing information, please see the Annex or the list of buildings with confirmed cases of COVID-19 in the past 14 days and the latest local situation of COVID-19 available on the website "COVID-19 Thematic Website" (www.coronavirus.gov.hk).

A spokesman for the CHP said, "During the CHP's epidemiological investigations and relevant contact tracing on the confirmed cases, we will compile and upload (www.chp.gov.hk/files/pdf/building_list_eng.pdf) a list of buildings that confirmed patients had visited from two days before the onset of symptoms. Given that cases of local infection continue to occur from time to time, members of the public are urged to seek medical attention immediately if they believe that they had visited the same place at an identical time with a confirmed patient and feel unwell subsequently. If they remain asymptomatic but are concerned that they have been infected, they can also visit the Hospital Authority's designated general out-patient clinics (www.ha.org.hk/haho/ho/covid-19/GOPC_extend_EN.pdf) to obtain specimen collection packs and collect deep throat saliva specimens for free COVID-19 testing."

In view of the severe epidemic situation, the CHP called on members of the public to avoid going out, having social contact and dining out. They should put on a surgical mask and maintain stringent hand hygiene when they need to go out. The CHP strongly urged the elderly to stay home as far as possible and avoid going out. They should consider asking their family and friends to help with everyday tasks such as shopping for basic necessities.

The spokesman said, "Given that the situation of COVID-19 infection remains severe and that there is a continuous increase in the number of cases reported around the world, members of the public are strongly urged to avoid all non-essential travel outside Hong Kong.

"The CHP also strongly urges the public to maintain at all times strict personal and environmental hygiene, which is key to personal protection against infection and prevention of the spread of the disease in the community. On a personal level, members of the public should wear a surgical mask when having respiratory symptoms, taking public transport or staying in crowded places. They should also perform hand hygiene frequently, especially before touching the mouth, nose or eyes.

"As for household environmental hygiene, members of the public are advised to maintain drainage pipes properly, regularly pour water into drain outlets (U-traps) and cover all floor drain outlets when they are not in use. After using the toilet, they should put the toilet lid down before flushing to avoid spreading germs."

Moreover, the Government has launched the website "COVID-19 Thematic Website" (www.coronavirus.gov.hk) for announcing the latest updates on various news on COVID-19 infection and health advice to help the public understand the latest updates. Members of the public may also gain access to information via the COVID-19 WhatsApp Helpline launched by the Office of the Government Chief Information Officer. Simply by saving 9617 1823 in their phone contacts or clicking the link wa.me/85296171823?text=hi, they will be able to obtain information on COVID-19 as well as the "StayHomeSafe" mobile app and wristband via WhatsApp.

Issued at HKT 14:01

Public hospitals daily update on COVID-19 cases
****

The following is issued on behalf of the Hospital Authority:

As at 9am today (October 25), six COVID-19 confirmed patients were discharged from hospital in the last 24 hours. So far, a total of 5 047 patients with confirmed or probable infection have been discharged.

At present, there are 614 negative pressure rooms in public hospitals with 1 098 negative pressure beds activated. A total of 108 confirmed patients are currently hospitalised in 18 public hospitals, among which 12 patients are in critical condition, four are in serious condition and the remaining 92 patients are in stable condition.

The Hospital Authority will maintain close contact with the Centre for Health Protection to monitor the latest developments and to inform the public and healthcare workers on the latest information in a timely manner.

Details of the above-mentioned patients are as follows:

Patient condition	Case numbers
Discharged	5176, 5179, 5194, 5232, 5244, 5281
Critical	1989, 3496, 3764, 4433, 4706, 4732, 4833, 4937, 5110, 5151, 5185, 5195
Serious	4101, 4746, 4788, 4990

Issued at HKT 16:30

October 26[26]

Transport Department to continue to provide free COVID-19 testing service to taxi and public light bus drivers

****

The Transport Department (TD) announced today (October 26) that starting from tomorrow (October 27), a new round of COVID-19 testing service will be provided to taxi and public light bus (PLB) drivers for a period of two weeks, and encouraged them to participate.

Testing is an integral part of the strategy in preventing and fighting the virus. After the testing services provided in mid-July and early October, the TD will continue to arrange a new round of free testing service for taxi and PLB drivers from tomorrow to November 9. The addresses, opening dates and hours of the 14 temporary testing kit distribution/specimen collection centres are at Annex 1.

Taxi and PLB drivers can visit the specific temporary distribution centre to collect the testing kit upon presenting their valid taxi or PLB driver identity plate. Drivers are required to register their personal information at the government website (www.tgptest.gov.hk), and should self-collect their deep throat saliva specimen and return it to the temporary collection centre on the same day. The testing agency will deliver the specimens collected to the laboratory for testing. As no personal information will be indicated on the specimen bottles, the testing agency will only have records of the barcode number of the specimen bottles and will not collect personal information. Drivers will be notified by the Government of the negative test result by SMS through mobile phone, while cases with positive test results will be relayed to the Centre for Health Protection of the Department of Health for follow-up.

Taxi drivers can collect the "Anti-epidemic Tag for Taxi Drivers" from the relevant taxi trade organisations with the SMS indicating the negative test result and display the tag at a prominent position inside the taxi compartment to enable passengers' checking. The list of taxi trade organisations distributing the "Anti-epidemic Tag for Taxi Drivers" is at Annex 2.

The TD strongly appeals to taxi and PLB drivers to participate in the testing to minimise the spread of the virus in the community. For details of the testing service and the collection of the "Anti-epidemic Tag for Taxi Drivers", please visit the website of the TD (www.td.gov.hk).

[26] https://www.info.gov.hk/gia/general/202010/26.htm

Issued at HKT 10:30

CHP investigates eight additional confirmed cases of COVID-19

****

The Centre for Health Protection (CHP) of the Department of Health has announced that as of 0.00am, October 26, the CHP was investigating eight additional confirmed cases of coronavirus disease 2019 (COVID-19), taking the number of cases to 5 304 in Hong Kong so far (comprising 5 303 confirmed cases and one probable case).

All the newly reported cases announced had a travel history during the incubation period.

The CHP's epidemiological investigations and relevant contact tracing on the confirmed cases are ongoing. For case details and contact tracing information, please see the Annex or the list of buildings with confirmed cases of COVID-19 in the past 14 days and the latest local situation of COVID-19 available on the website "COVID-19 Thematic Website" (www.coronavirus.gov.hk).

A spokesman for the CHP said, "During the CHP's epidemiological investigations and relevant contact tracing on the confirmed cases, we will compile and upload (www.chp.gov.hk/files/pdf/building_list_eng.pdf) a list of buildings that confirmed patients had visited from two days before the onset of symptoms. Given that cases of local infection continue to occur from time to time, members of the public are urged to seek medical attention immediately if they believe that they had visited the same place at an identical time with a confirmed patient and feel unwell subsequently. If they remain asymptomatic but are concerned that they have been infected, they can also visit the Hospital Authority's designated general out-patient clinics (www.ha.org.hk/haho/ho/covid-19/GOPC_extend_EN.pdf) to obtain specimen collection packs and collect deep throat saliva specimens for free COVID-19 testing."

In view of the severe epidemic situation, the CHP called on members of the public to avoid going out, having social contact and dining out. They should put on a surgical mask and maintain stringent hand hygiene when they need to go out. The CHP strongly urged the elderly to stay home as far as possible and avoid going out. They should consider asking their family and friends to help with everyday tasks such as shopping for basic necessities.

The spokesman said, "Given that the situation of COVID-19 infection remains severe and that there is a continuous increase in the number of cases reported around the world, members of the public are strongly urged to avoid all non-essential travel outside Hong Kong.

"The CHP also strongly urges the public to maintain at all times strict personal and environmental hygiene, which is key to personal protection against infection and prevention of the spread of the disease in the community. On a personal level, members of the public should wear a surgical mask when having respiratory symptoms, taking public transport or staying in crowded places. They should also perform hand hygiene frequently, especially before touching the mouth, nose or eyes.

"As for household environmental hygiene, members of the public are advised to maintain drainage pipes properly, regularly pour water into drain outlets (U-traps) and cover all floor drain outlets when they are not in use. After using the toilet, they should put the toilet lid down before flushing to avoid spreading germs."

Moreover, the Government has launched the website "COVID-19 Thematic Website" (www.coronavirus.gov.hk) for announcing the latest updates on various news on COVID-19 infection and health advice to help the public understand the latest updates. Members of the public may also gain access to information via the COVID-19 WhatsApp Helpline launched by the Office of the Government Chief Information Officer. Simply by saving 9617 1823 in their phone contacts or clicking the link wa.me/85296171823?text=hi, they will be able to obtain information on COVID-19 as well as the "StayHomeSafe" mobile app and wristband via WhatsApp.

Issued at HKT 14:00

Public hospitals daily update on COVID-19 cases

****

The following is issued on behalf of the Hospital Authority:

As at 9am today (October 26), three COVID-19 confirmed patients were discharged from hospital in the last 24 hours. So far, a total of 5 050 patients with confirmed or probable infection have been discharged.

At present, there are 614 negative pressure rooms in public hospitals with 1 098 negative pressure beds activated. A total of 111 confirmed patients are currently hospitalised in 18 public hospitals, among which 12 patients are in critical condition, four are in serious condition and the remaining 95 patients are in stable condition.

The Hospital Authority will maintain close contact with the Centre for Health Protection to monitor the latest developments and to inform the public and healthcare workers on the latest information in a timely manner.

Details of the above-mentioned patients are as follows:

Patient condition	Case numbers
Discharged	5156, 5217, 5280

Critical	1989, 3496, 3764, 4433, 4706, 4732, 4833, 4937, 5110, 5151, 5185, 5195
Serious	4101, 4746, 4788, 4990

Issued at HKT 16:21

October 27[27]

CHP investigates five additional confirmed cases of COVID-19

****

The Centre for Health Protection (CHP) of the Department of Health has announced that as of 0.00am, October 27, the CHP was investigating five additional confirmed cases of coronavirus disease 2019 (COVID-19), taking the number of cases to 5 309 in Hong Kong so far (comprising 5 308 confirmed cases and one probable case).

All the newly reported cases announced had a travel history during the incubation period.

The CHP's epidemiological investigations and relevant contact tracing on the confirmed cases are ongoing. For case details and contact tracing information, please see the Annex or the list of buildings with confirmed cases of COVID-19 in the past 14 days and the latest local situation of COVID-19 available on the website "COVID-19 Thematic Website" (www.coronavirus.gov.hk).

In view of the latest epidemic developments in the Mainland, starting tomorrow (October 28), inbound travellers who have been to Xinjiang in the past 14 days arriving via land boundary control points will be provided with specimen collection containers. They are required to collect their deep throat saliva samples by themselves in accordance with the instructions and return the samples for conducting COVID-19 testing. The arrangement of distributing specimen collection containers to inbound travellers who have been to Shandong Province in the past 14 days arriving via land boundary control points, which has come into effect earlier, remains unchanged.

A spokesman for the CHP said, "During the CHP's epidemiological investigations and relevant contact tracing on the confirmed cases, we will compile and upload (www.chp.gov.hk/files/pdf/building_list_eng.pdf) a list of buildings that confirmed patients had visited from two days before the onset of symptoms. Given that cases of local infection continue to occur from time to time, members of the public are urged to seek medical attention immediately if they believe that they had visited the same place at an identical time with a confirmed patient and feel unwell subsequently. If they remain asymptomatic but are concerned

[27] https://www.info.gov.hk/gia/general/202010/27.htm

that they have been infected, they can also visit the Hospital Authority's designated general out-patient clinics (www.ha.org.hk/haho/ho/covid-19/GOPC_extend_EN.pdf) to obtain specimen collection packs and collect deep throat saliva specimens for free COVID-19 testing."

In view of the severe epidemic situation, the CHP called on members of the public to avoid going out, having social contact and dining out. They should put on a surgical mask and maintain stringent hand hygiene when they need to go out. The CHP strongly urged the elderly to stay home as far as possible and avoid going out. They should consider asking their family and friends to help with everyday tasks such as shopping for basic necessities.

The spokesman said, "Given that the situation of COVID-19 infection remains severe and that there is a continuous increase in the number of cases reported around the world, members of the public are strongly urged to avoid all non-essential travel outside Hong Kong.

"The CHP also strongly urges the public to maintain at all times strict personal and environmental hygiene, which is key to personal protection against infection and prevention of the spread of the disease in the community. On a personal level, members of the public should wear a surgical mask when having respiratory symptoms, taking public transport or staying in crowded places. They should also perform hand hygiene frequently, especially before touching the mouth, nose or eyes.

"As for household environmental hygiene, members of the public are advised to maintain drainage pipes properly, regularly pour water into drain outlets (U-traps) and cover all floor drain outlets when they are not in use. After using the toilet, they should put the toilet lid down before flushing to avoid spreading germs."

Moreover, the Government has launched the website "COVID-19 Thematic Website" (www.coronavirus.gov.hk) for announcing the latest updates on various news on COVID-19 infection and health advice to help the public understand the latest updates. Members of the public may also gain access to information via the COVID-19 WhatsApp Helpline launched by the Office of the Government Chief Information Officer. Simply by saving 9617 1823 in their phone contacts or clicking the link wa.me/85296171823?text=hi, they will be able to obtain information on COVID-19 as well as the "StayHomeSafe" mobile app and wristband via WhatsApp.

Issued at HKT 14:00

Specifications under Prevention and Control of Disease (Regulation of Cross-boundary Conveyances and Travellers) Regulation to be gazetted

****

In view of the developments of the COVID-19 epidemic situation worldwide and in Hong Kong, the Government will gazette today (October 27) the latest specifications to include Belgium as a specified place under the Prevention and Control of Disease (Regulation of Cross-boundary Conveyances and Travellers) Regulation (Cap. 599H) starting from November 3 to more effectively combat the epidemic.

A spokesman for the Food and Health Bureau said, "The global epidemic situation is becoming increasingly severe. The daily number of new cases increased from around 70 000 to 100 000 between late March and mid-May, to around 160 000 to 180 000 in late June and to around 220 000 to 290 000 in late July, and further increased to reach a new height of around 340 000 to 460 000 in mid-October. In view of the severe global pandemic situation, Hong Kong cannot afford to drop its guard on entry prevention and control measures."

The Government has earlier introduced Cap. 599H to impose testing and quarantine conditions on travellers coming to Hong Kong from very high-risk places to reduce the health risk they may bring to Hong Kong. The Secretary for Food and Health (SFH) has previously published in the Gazette specifications on the relevant measures applicable to 13 specified places (i.e. Bangladesh, Ethiopia, France, India, Indonesia, Kazakhstan, Nepal, Pakistan, the Philippines, Russia, South Africa, the United Kingdom and the United States of America) and adjusted the relevant conditions having regard to the circumstances on the ground since the implementation of the regulation.

Taking into account the latest public health risk assessment, and the changes and developments of the epidemic situation, the SFH will publish in the Gazette new specifications to maintain the conditions imposed and to include Belgium as specified places with effect from November 3 until further notice.

According to the latest specifications, a traveller who, on the day on which the traveller boarded a civil aviation aircraft that arrives at, or is about to arrive at, Hong Kong (specified aircraft), or during the 14 days before that day, has stayed in one of the aforementioned specified places must provide the following documents:

(1) A test report in English or Chinese issued by a laboratory or healthcare institution bearing the name of the relevant traveller identical to that in his or her valid travel document to show that:

(a) the relevant traveller underwent a nucleic acid test for COVID-19, the sample for which was taken from the relevant traveller within 72 hours before the scheduled time of departure of the specified aircraft;

(b) the test conducted on the sample is a nucleic acid test for COVID-19; and

(c) the result of the test is that the relevant traveller was tested negative for COVID-19; an

(2) If the relevant report is not in English or Chinese or does not contain all of the above information, a written confirmation in English or Chinese issued by the laboratory or healthcare institution bearing the name of the relevant traveller identical to that in his or her valid travel document and setting out all of the above information. The said written confirmation should be presented together with the test report; and

(3) Documentary proof in English or Chinese to show that the laboratory or healthcare institution is ISO 15189 accredited or is recognised or approved by the relevant authority of the government of the place in which the laboratory or healthcare institution is located; and

(4) The relevant traveller has confirmation in English or Chinese of room reservation in a hotel in Hong Kong for not less than 14 days starting on the day of the arrival of the relevant traveller in Hong Kong.

The operator of the specified aircraft must submit to the Department of Health (DH) before the specified aircraft arrives at Hong Kong a document in a form specified by the DH confirming that each relevant traveller has, before being checked in for the flight to Hong Kong on the aircraft, produced for boarding on the aircraft the documentary proof to show that the above conditions are met.

If any condition specified by the SFH is not met in relation to any relevant traveller on the conveyance, each of the operators of the conveyance commits an offence and is liable on conviction to the maximum penalty of a fine at level 5 ($50,000) and imprisonment for six months. If an operator fails to comply with a requirement to provide information, or knowingly or recklessly provides any information that is false or misleading in a material particular, he or she is liable on conviction to the maximum penalty of a fine at level 5 ($50,000) and imprisonment for six months.

As for travellers, if a traveller coming to Hong Kong fails to comply with a requirement to provide information, or knowingly or recklessly provides any information that is false or misleading in a material particular, he or she is liable on conviction to the maximum penalty of a fine at level 3 ($10,000) and imprisonment for six months.

Travellers to Hong Kong should note that they will be mandated to wait for their test results at a designated location after their deep throat saliva samples are collected for conducting testing for COVID-19 at the DH's Temporary Specimen Collection Centre pursuant to the Prevention and Control of Disease Ordinance (Cap. 599). If their test results are negative, they will be allowed to go to the hotel for which they made the reservation to continue the 14-day compulsory quarantine until completion. If their results are positive, the travellers will be transferred to hospital for isolation and treatment.

The Government will continue to monitor closely the situation including the developments of the epidemic situation both globally and locally and changes in the volume of cross-boundary passenger traffic, and may adopt more resolute and severe measures as and when necessary.

Issued at HKT 16:58

Public hospitals daily update on COVID-19 cases

****

The following is issued on behalf of the Hospital Authority:

As at 9am today (October 27), three COVID-19 confirmed patients were discharged from hospital in the last 24 hours. So far, a total of 5 053 patients with confirmed or probable infection have been discharged.

At present, there are 614 negative pressure rooms in public hospitals with 1 098 negative pressure beds activated. A total of 116 confirmed patients are currently hospitalised in 18 public hospitals, among which 11 patients are in critical condition, five are in serious condition and the remaining 100 patients are in stable condition.

The Hospital Authority will maintain close contact with the Centre for Health Protection to monitor the latest developments and to inform the public and healthcare workers on the latest information in a timely manner.

Details of the above-mentioned patients are as follows:

Patient condition	Case numbers
Discharged	5216, 5233, 5238
Critical	1989, 3496, 3764, 4433, 4706, 4732, 4833, 4937, 5110, 5185, 5195
Serious	4101, 4746, 4788, 4990, 5151

Issued at HKT 17:15

Latest service arrangements for LCSD beaches

****

The Leisure and Cultural Services Department (LCSD) announced today (October 27) that, in view of the latest situation of COVID-19, all gazetted beaches under the LCSD will reopen on

November 3. According to arrangements adopted all along in previous years, lifeguard services at the reopened beaches from November to March are as follows:

Deep Water Bay Beach, Clear Water Bay Second Beach, Silverstrand Beach and Golden Beach will provide lifeguard services daily from 8am to 5pm after reopening.

Repulse Bay Beach, Middle Bay Beach, Stanley Main Beach, Big Wave Bay Beach and Silver Mine Bay Beach will reopen, with lifeguard services from 8am to 5pm daily until November 30. (Lifeguard services will be suspended from December 1, 2020, to February 28, 2021.)

Lifeguard services at the remaining 29 beaches will be suspended after reopening until March 31, 2021.

The LCSD appeals to beach users to comply with the Prevention and Control of Disease (Prohibition on Group Gathering) Regulation (Cap 599G). The number of people in group gatherings should not be more than that as stipulated by the law. Members of the public should wear masks at all times when being present in any public place in accordance with the Prevention and Control of Disease (Wearing of Mask) Regulation (Cap 599I). To ensure appropriate distance between users of shower facilities, shower heads which are not within individual cubicles will be open but at 1.5 metres apart. The LCSD will step up cleaning work at the reopened beach facilities. Barbecue sites within gazetted beaches will continue to be closed.

The LCSD calls on members of the public to observe water safety while swimming. People should swim at the beaches only when lifeguard services are available. Please do not enter the water when the red flag is hoisted.

Issued at HKT 18:50

Transcript of remarks by SFH at media session

****

The Secretary for Food and Health, Professor Sophia Chan, and the Deputy Secretary for Food and Health (Health), Mr Howard Chan, met the media today (October 27). Following is the transcript of remarks by Professor Chan at the media session:

Secretary for Food and Health: As we all know, the local epidemic situation showed signs of rebound early this month. We are fortunate that, with the concerted efforts of the Government and the society to fight the virus, the epidemic situation continued to subside over the past two weeks, with the seven-day average number of locally confirmed cases decreasing gradually since mid-October.

But I must point out that there are still sporadic cases especially those with unknown sources of infection reported in different districts in Hong Kong. That shows that there are still community transmission chains. Meanwhile, globally, there are worsening epidemic situations. That may continue to pose some public health risks to Hong Kong although we already have a very stringent control and we have tightened our border control measures.

Under the new normal, we cannot and should not aim to have no confirmed case in the community for an extended period of time. It would be unavoidable that there may be some sporadic cases and small clusters in the community from time to time. I think the most important thing is that we have the capacity and capability to stabilise the situation once there is infection or outbreak.

The Government has adopted a targeted approach for reducing the risk of the virus spreading within the community as far as practicable. So we would avoid the one-size-fits-all approach. We are doing more targeted and sophisticated approaches in order to allow members of the public to maintain social and economic activities to a certain extent as far as practicable under the new normal.

After taking into account the latest public health risk assessment, we are striking a balance with economic needs, the level of acceptance of the society, and the economic situation and job loss situation. The Government decided to continue relaxing social distancing measures imposed under the Prevention and Control of Disease Ordinance in a gradual and also orderly manner.

Starting from this Friday (October 30), the following adjustments will be made to the social distancing measures:

(1) dine-in services would be allowed at all catering business premises until 2am;

(2) the number of persons that may be seated together at one table will be increased from four to six for catering business premises except bars or pubs; and from two to four for bars or pubs and clubs or nightclubs;

(3) members of the public must only take off their masks to consume food or drink at the table but not at any other places within bars or pubs and clubs or nightclubs. In other words, a person must not eat or drink and must wear a mask when he or she is away from the table;

(4) live performances and dancing activities will be allowed to take place in catering business premises and clubs or nightclubs, subject to the implementation of suitable infection prevention and control measures;

(5) members of the public are not required to wear masks when doing exercise in indoor sports premises or public skating rinks; and

(6) the total number of people allowed in catering business premises including bars and pubs, public entertainment venues including theme parks, performance venues, etc, nightclubs, and swimming pools will be increased from 50 per cent to 75 per cent of the capacity of the respective premises.

Apart from the above adjustments, other social distancing measures concerning catering business premises, scheduled premises, group gatherings and mask-wearing requirement will be extended. This latest set of measures will be effective for seven days, from October 30 to November 5.

Moreover, as the Chief Executive mentioned this morning, the Leisure and Cultural Services Department will announce the arrangements of re-opening the beaches under its management later separately.

As we have stressed now time and again, the co-operation and self-discipline of members of the public are keys to the effectiveness of our social distancing measures in the prevention of the spread of the disease in the community. I would like to take the opportunity to appeal to the public again to remain vigilant, observe good personal and environmental hygiene and comply with the requirements and restrictions applicable to individual premises. It is also important for the trade to comply with what they are being asked especially in fulfilling or complying with those critical control points that we have identified, and that our experts have worked with them so that they put in place measures to mitigate and control the risks arising from those critical control points.

Finally, I would also like to say a few words on specifying Belgium under the Prevention and Control of Disease (Regulation of Cross-boundary Conveyances and Travellers) Regulation (Cap. 599H). In view of the severe COVID-19 epidemic situation worldwide, we cannot afford to drop our guard. Therefore, the Government, among these measures, will be gazetting later today specifications to include Belgium as a specified place under Cap. 599H with effect from November 3 with regard to the latest public health risk assessment.

The Government will continue to monitor other countries and their situation very closely, including the developments of the epidemic situations not only globally but also locally and review our various epidemic control measures from time to time so as to make suitable adjustments to the measures taking into consideration of all related factors.

Reporter: Can you give us more details on the Mainland quarantine exemption next month that was announced by the Chief Executive this morning, including how many people will be involved? What circumstances will allow people to qualify? Whether certain people can get priority, and if they will be required to test negative and present a certificate 72 hours before the arrival. Why not Macao? Why isn't Macao involved in this as well?

Second, with enforcement issues at bars where only two people per table are allowed, how will authorities ensure that the new rules will be followed? Have the authorities considered Professor Yuen Kwok-yung's suggestion, using straws to drink alcohol to allow bars to open longer?

My third question is about the rapid testing involving the Airport Authority. How many people will be tested? Is it only for departures or only arrivals or both? Which companies will be involved and how much will it cost? Thank you.

Secretary for Food and Health: First of all, your question about the exemption. We are now working on exempting people, Hong Kong residents coming back from Guangdong Province, from 14-day mandatory quarantine if they have a negative PCR (polymerase chain reaction) test. This is what we are now studying. We do not have further details but this is the general principle because in many places of the Mainland China, if we are talking about the Guangdong Province, their epidemic situation has been stabilised for a very long time. Therefore, people coming from those places are having very, very low risks. Therefore, after the Department of Health have assessed the risk, we can work on the direction on exempting their 14-day mandatory quarantine if they can present a negative test of PCR.

Regarding bars, now we have our Food and Environmental Hygiene Department, which has been working with the trade in order to put in place a number of critical control points and measures that our experts felt that it is important. First of all, it is about the air exchanges. Secondly, they put in place health declarations, so that when people go into the bars, they would leave their contact details and do the health declarations. Thirdly, their staff will be tested. Finally, Professor Yuen has suggested that people, in order to reduce the time of putting off or not wearing masks, may use a straw to drink from the glass. They are continuing to work on that and the trade has been more or less very co-operative, and they will continue to work out these measures so as to mitigate and control the risk arising from the behavior of people at the bars.

Finally, it's the rapid testing. The Airport Authority has been working with some private laboratories in the use of the rapid tests, as well as the PCR tests, starting from this week, probably tomorrow. With this test, we can actually understand more about the validity, sensitivity and specificity of the rapid test because we do not want to have a rapid test that is not valid or that is not sensitive enough to identify the confirmed cases. Therefore, while using rapid tests is the trend and also has its benefits because the PCR tests usually take very long. In the event, or in the future when these cross-boundary travels resume to a more normal situation, the current situation would not be sustainable. Therefore, looking into the use and also validity of these rapid tests is important.

Reporter: Professor Chan, you said that most Mainland Chinese provinces are relatively stable, but Macao has not had a new case in a very long time, so why is it not included as well?

Secretary for Food and Health: We would not rule out Macao. But it is just done in a step-by-step way. I confirm that Macao is also very stable in terms of epidemic situation.

Issued at HKT 18:50

Two persons sentenced for breaching compulsory quarantine order

****

Two persons were sentenced by the Eastern Magistrates' Courts today (October 27) for violating the Compulsory Quarantine of Persons Arriving at Hong Kong from Foreign Places Regulation (Cap 599E) (the Regulation).

The two cases involved a woman aged 60 and a man aged 47. They were earlier issued compulsory quarantine orders separately, stating that they must conduct quarantine at home for 14 days. Before the expiry of the quarantine order, they left the place of quarantine on March 27 without reasonable excuse nor permission given by an authorised officer. The woman and the man were charged with contravening sections 8(1) and 8(5) of the Regulation and were sentenced to immediate imprisonment for 14 days and 20 days respectively.

Pursuant to the Regulation, starting from March 19, save for exempted persons, all persons arriving from countries or territories outside China would be subject to compulsory quarantine for 14 days. Moreover, pursuant to the Compulsory Quarantine of Certain Persons Arriving at Hong Kong Regulation (Cap 599C), starting from February 8, all persons who have stayed in the Mainland, Macao or Taiwan in the 14 days preceding arrival in Hong Kong, regardless of their nationality or travel documents, will also be subject to compulsory quarantine for 14 days. Breaching a quarantine order is a criminal offence and offenders are subject to a maximum fine of $25,000 and imprisonment for six months.

A spokesman for the Department of Health said the sentence sends a clear message to the community that breaching a compulsory quarantine order is a criminal offence that the Government will not tolerate, and solemnly reminded the public to comply with the Regulation. As of today, a total of 62 persons have been convicted by the courts for breaching compulsory quarantine orders and have received sentences including immediate imprisonment for up to three months or a fine of $15,000. The spokesman reiterated that resolute actions will be taken against anyone who has breached the relevant regulations.

Issued at HKT 19:05

Government continues to relax social distancing measures under Prevention and Control of Disease Ordinance in a gradual and orderly manner

****

Having regard to the development of the COVID-19 epidemic situation in Hong Kong, the Government will gazette directions and specifications under the Prevention and Control of Disease (Requirements and Directions) (Business and Premises) Regulation (Cap. 599F), the Prevention and Control of Disease (Prohibition on Group Gathering) Regulation (Cap. 599G) and the Prevention and Control of Disease (Wearing of Mask) Regulation (Cap. 599I) today (October 27) to continue to relax social distancing measures in a gradual and orderly manner. The measures will take effect at 0.00am on October 30 for a period of seven days till November 5.

While the local epidemic situation showed signs of rebound in early October, it continued to subside over the past two weeks, with the seven-day average number of locally confirmed cases coming down gradually since mid-October, given the concerted efforts of the Government and society in fighting the virus. That said, there were still a certain number of cases with unknown sources of infection among the new confirmed cases reported and such cases were distributed across various districts in Hong Kong, indicating the existence of silent transmission chains in the community. Meanwhile, given the very severe and continually worsening global epidemic situation, imported cases would continue to pose public health risks to Hong Kong.

A spokesman for the Food and Health Bureau said, "Under the new normal, we cannot and should not aim at having no confirmed case in the community for an extended period of time. It would be unavoidable to have sporadic cases and clusters in the community from time to time as the virus will co-exist with us for quite a long period of time before effective treatment and vaccination become available. The Government will continue to adopt a targeted approach for reducing the risk of the virus spreading within the community as far as practicable, avoid the one-size-fits-all approach when adjusting social distancing measures, and work closely with the relevant trades to strengthen infection control measures at the premises concerned, in order to allow members of the public to maintain social and economic activities to a certain extent as far as practicable under the new normal."

After taking into account the latest public health risk assessment and having struck a balance with economic needs and level of acceptance of the society, the Government decided to continue relaxing the social distancing measures under the Prevention and Control of Disease Ordinance in a gradual and orderly manner. Since the current epidemic situation has not yet been brought fully under control, community transmission chains still exist and the risk of rebound still remains real, the conditions are not present for the Government to substantially relax the existing social distancing measures at this stage and the Government may only, under a targeted approach, relax to a limited extent the restrictions imposed on individual premises in which infection prevention and control measures can be implemented effectively. It is still considered necessary for us to maintain the restrictions imposed in respect of other kinds of group gatherings in general as infection prevention and control measures may not be as effectively implemented for these gatherings. Meanwhile, having regard to the infection risks brought about by mask-off gatherings in premises such as bars, the Government also decided to restrict the areas in which mask-off activities can take place in those premises, with a view to safeguarding public health.

The Government will continue to closely monitor the development of the epidemic situation, and, depending on whether the epidemic situation can continue to be controlled with the number of confirmed cases stably maintained at a low level, consider the relaxation of social distancing measures to be implemented in the next phase.

Starting from this Friday (October 30), the dine-in hours of catering business premises (including bars and pubs) will be extended to end at 1.59 am (i.e. such premises can provide dine-in service from 0.00am to 1.59am on October 30), the number of persons that may be seated together at one table will be increased from four to six for catering business premises (except bars or pubs) and from two to four for bars or pubs and clubs or nightclubs. Meanwhile, the Government decided to impose a restriction that members of public must only consume food or drink at the table (but not any other places) within bars or pubs and clubs or nightclubs. In other words, a person must not consume food or drink and must wear a mask when he or she is away from the table. Moreover, subject to appropriate infection prevention and control measures being put in place, live performances and dancing activities will be allowed to be conducted in catering business premises and clubs or nightclubs. Members of the public also are not required to wear masks when doing exercise in indoor sports premises and public skating rinks. The total number of people allowed in catering business premises (including bars and pubs), places of public entertainment (including theme parks, performance venues, etc.), clubs or nightclubs, and swimming pools will be increased to 75 per cent of the normal seating capacity or maximum capacity of the premises. Through the above measures, the Government aims to further reduce the risk associated with mask-off activities by strengthening the infection control measures in the premises concerned, so as to allow the resumption of more social and economic activities in an orderly manner as far as practicable.

The spokesman added, "As we have stressed time and again, co-operation and self-discipline of members of the public are the keys to the effectiveness of social distancing measures in preventing the spread of the disease in the community. Only with the co-operation of society as a whole can the Government continue to allow resumption of social and economic activities in a gradual and orderly manner. Therefore, the public's concerted efforts in fighting the epidemic and compliance with requirements and restrictions applicable to individual premises are of utmost importance. Otherwise, when there is another outbreak in the community, the Government will have no choice but to significantly tighten social distancing measures in order to safeguard public health."

Details of the aforementioned social distancing measures (details of the arrangements for premises under Cap. 599F at Annex 1) which are to be effective from October 30, 2020 to November 5, 2020 are as follows:

(I) Catering business and scheduled premises

(1) From 2.00am to 4.59am daily, save for specific premises (details at Annex 2), a person responsible for carrying on a catering business must cease selling or supplying food or drink for consumption on the premises of the business; and close any premises, or part of the premises, on

which food or drink is sold or supplied by the business for consumption on the premises. The premises concerned may still sell or supply food and/or drink for takeaway services and deliveries. A person responsible for carrying on a catering business is also required to put up a notice at the entrance to the catering premises to remind customers that food or drink should not be consumed in areas adjacent to the catering premises;

(2) No more than four persons may be seated together at one table within bars or pubs as well as clubs or nightclubs; no more than six persons may be seated together at one table within other catering business premises;

(3) The total number of people allowed in catering business premise, places of public entertainment, clubs or nightclubs, and swimming pools will be capped at 75 per cent of the normal seating capacity/maximum capacity of the respective premises;

(4) To further reduce the public health risks associated with mask-off activities in bars or pubs as well as clubs or nightclubs, consumption of food or drink will only be allowed at the table;

(5) Live performances and dancing activities will be allowed to take place in catering business premises and clubs or nightclubs, subject to strict compliance of the relevant infection control measures, including mask-on requirement for performers, partitioning to serve as effective buffer between performers and customers/ the audience and no mingling between performers and customers/ the audience before or after the performances;

(6) Members of the public are not required to wear masks when doing exercise in indoor sports premises and public skating rinks; and

(7) Other requirements and restrictions on catering business and scheduled premises will be maintained. Amongst others, facilities involving higher health risks such as steam and sauna facilities and ball pits will continue to be prohibited from opening.

Persons responsible for carrying on catering businesses and managers of scheduled premises that contravene the statutory requirements under the Prevention and Control of Disease (Requirements and Directions) (Business and Premises) Regulation (Cap. 599F) would have committed a criminal offence. Offenders are subject to a maximum fine of $50,000 and imprisonment for six months.

(II) Group gathering

(8) Unless exempted, the prohibition on group gatherings of more than four persons in public places will continue during the seven-day period from October 30 to November 5, 2020.

Any person who participates in a prohibited group gathering; organises a prohibited group gathering; owns, controls or operates the place of such gathering and knowingly allows the taking place of such gathering, commits an offence under Cap. 599G. Offenders are liable to a maximum fine of $25,000 and imprisonment for six months. Persons who participate in a prohibited group gathering may discharge liability for the offence by paying a fixed penalty of $2,000.

(III) Mask-wearing requirement

(9) The mandatory mask-wearing requirement under Cap. 599I will be extended for a period of seven days from October 30 to November 5, 2020. During the aforementioned period, a person must wear a mask all the time when the person is boarding or onboard a public transport carrier, is entering or present in an MTR paid area, or is entering or present in a specified public place (i.e. all public places, save for outdoor public places in country parks and special areas as defined in section 2 of the Country Parks Ordinance (Cap. 208).

Under Cap. 599I, if a person does not wear a mask in accordance with the requirement, an authorised person may deny that person from boarding a public transport carrier or entering the area concerned, as well as require that person to wear a mask and disembark from the carrier or leave the said area. A person in contravention of the relevant provision commits an offence and the maximum penalty is a fine at level 2 ($5,000). In addition, authorised public officers may issue fixed penalty notices to persons who do not wear a mask in accordance with the requirement and such persons may discharge liability for the offence by paying a fixed penalty of $2,000.

Issued at HKT 21:55

October 28[28]

CHP investigates two additional confirmed cases of COVID-19

****

The Centre for Health Protection (CHP) of the Department of Health has announced that as of 0.00am, October 28, the CHP was investigating two additional confirmed cases of coronavirus disease 2019 (COVID-19), taking the number of cases to 5 311 in Hong Kong so far (comprising 5 310 confirmed cases and one probable case).

All the newly reported cases announced had a travel history during the incubation period.

The CHP's epidemiological investigations and relevant contact tracing on the confirmed cases are ongoing. For case details and contact tracing information, please see the Annex or the list of buildings with confirmed cases of COVID-19 in the past 14 days and the latest local situation of COVID-19 available on the website "COVID-19 Thematic Website" (www.coronavirus.gov.hk).

[28] https://www.info.gov.hk/gia/general/202010/28.htm

The DH will conduct an assessment trial on RT-LAMP rapid nucleic acid test at the Hong Kong International Airport (HKIA) starting today. The trial will run in parallel to the existing "reference standard" RT-PCR nucleic acid testing (RT-PCR test) adopted by the Public Health Laboratory Services Branch under DH's CHP. The two-week trial aims to assess the sensitivity and reliability of RT-LAMP technology.

Under the current arrangement, inbound travellers arriving in Hong Kong via HKIA will be required to proceed to the DH's Temporary Specimen Collection Centre (TSCC) set up in the restricted area of HKIA for collecting their deep throat saliva samples immediately upon arrival and submit the samples to DH staff for conducting the RT-PCR test. They will then follow instructions to proceed to the "Rapid Test Zone" inside the TSCC for a briefing and to collect another sample (mouth rinse and gargle) for the RT-LAMP rapid nucleic acid test according to the instructions. The process of collecting a sample for rapid test takes about 30 minutes. The samples will be tested by a local private laboratory.

The parallel run testing is conducted on a voluntary basis and will not affect the progress of the RT-PCR test (i.e. the test result waiting time for inbound travellers will not be affected). The test result will be based on that of the DH's RT-PCR test. During the parallel run trial, the "test and hold" arrangement remains valid and travellers must wait until a negative RT-PCR test result is available before they can proceed to quarantine.

A spokesman for the CHP said, "During the CHP's epidemiological investigations and relevant contact tracing on the confirmed cases, we will compile and upload (www.chp.gov.hk/files/pdf/building_list_eng.pdf) a list of buildings that confirmed patients had visited from two days before the onset of symptoms. Given that cases of local infection continue to occur from time to time, members of the public are urged to seek medical attention immediately if they believe that they had visited the same place at an identical time with a confirmed patient and feel unwell subsequently. If they remain asymptomatic but are concerned that they have been infected, they can also visit the Hospital Authority's designated general out-patient clinics (www.ha.org.hk/haho/ho/covid-19/GOPC_extend_EN.pdf) to obtain specimen collection packs and collect deep throat saliva specimens for free COVID-19 testing."

In view of the severe epidemic situation, the CHP called on members of the public to avoid going out, having social contact and dining out. They should put on a surgical mask and maintain stringent hand hygiene when they need to go out. The CHP strongly urged the elderly to stay home as far as possible and avoid going out. They should consider asking their family and friends to help with everyday tasks such as shopping for basic necessities.

The spokesman said, "Given that the situation of COVID-19 infection remains severe and that there is a continuous increase in the number of cases reported around the world, members of the public are strongly urged to avoid all non-essential travel outside Hong Kong.

"The CHP also strongly urges the public to maintain at all times strict personal and environmental hygiene, which is key to personal protection against infection and prevention of the spread of the disease in the community. On a personal level, members of the public should wear a surgical mask when having respiratory symptoms, taking public transport or staying in

crowded places. They should also perform hand hygiene frequently, especially before touching the mouth, nose or eyes.

"As for household environmental hygiene, members of the public are advised to maintain drainage pipes properly, regularly pour water into drain outlets (U-traps) and cover all floor drain outlets when they are not in use. After using the toilet, they should put the toilet lid down before flushing to avoid spreading germs."

Moreover, the Government has launched the website "COVID-19 Thematic Website" (www.coronavirus.gov.hk) for announcing the latest updates on various news on COVID-19 infection and health advice to help the public understand the latest updates. Members of the public may also gain access to information via the COVID-19 WhatsApp Helpline launched by the Office of the Government Chief Information Officer. Simply by saving 9617 1823 in their phone contacts or clicking the link wa.me/85296171823?text=hi, they will be able to obtain information on COVID-19 as well as the "StayHomeSafe" mobile app and wristband via WhatsApp.

Issued at HKT 14:00

LCQ17: Statistics on the confirmed cases of Coronavirus Disease 2019

****

Following is a question by Dr the Hon Pierre Chan and a written reply by the Secretary for Food and Health, Professor Sophia Chan, in the Legislative Council today (October 28):

Question:

Will the Government inform this Council of the following statistics on the confirmed cases of Coronavirus Disease 2019 (COVID-19) since January this year:

(1) the number of clusters involving five to nine cases, and set out the relevant details in Table 1;

Table 1

Name of cluster	Case numbers	Number of cases

(2) the number of cases with unknown sources;

(3) a breakdown of the numbers of (i) confirmed cases and (ii) death cases by the age group to which the patients belonged (set out in Table 2);

Table 2

Type of cases	Age group										
	0 to 9	10 to 19	20 to 29	30 to 39	40 to 49	50 to 59	60 to 69	70 to 79	80 to 89	90 to 99	100 to 109
(i)											
(ii)											

(4) a breakdown of the numbers of (i) confirmed cases, (ii) death cases, (iii) confirmed cases involving persons aged 60 or above and (iv) death cases involving persons aged 60 or above by the date of confirmation (set out in Table 3);

Table 3

Type of cases	Date of confirmation		
	January 1 to February 29	March 1 to June 30	Since July 1
(i)			
(ii)			
(iii)			
(iv)			

(5) a breakdown of the numbers of confirmed cases involving healthcare personnel and allied health professionals (i.e. (i) doctors, (ii) nurses, (iii) physiotherapists, (iv) occupational therapists, (v) clinical psychologists, (vi) dietitians, (vii) audiologists, (viii) optometrists, (ix) orthoptists, (x) speech therapists, (xi) pharmacists, (xii) dispensers, (xiii) radiographers, (xiv) medical laboratory technologists, (xv) medical social workers, (xvi) prosthetist-orthotists and (xvii) podiatrists) as well as (xviii) supporting healthcare workers by the type of healthcare facilities in which they work (set out in Table 4); and

Table 4

Staff	Public hospitals	Private hospitals	Private clinics
(i)			

...			
(xviii)			

(6) whether it knows the number of cases of compensation claims lodged, since January this year, by employees under the Employees' Compensation Ordinance (Cap. 282) for contracting COVID-19 arising out of and in the course of their employment, together with the following information of such cases:

(i) a breakdown of the number of such cases by the industry in which the employees concerned were engaged,
(ii) the number of cases in which the employers took the initiative to notify the Government of such cases,
(iii) the number and percentage of cases of successful claims,
(iv) the reasons for the claims being unsuccessful, and
(v) the assistance provided by the Government to those employees whose claims for compensations were unsuccessful?

Reply:

President,

Since the outbreak of COVID-19, the Government has been closely monitoring the development of the epidemic situation. Guided by the three key principles of responding promptly, staying alert to the situation and working in an open and transparent manner, and having regard to experts' advice, we have implemented decisive and appropriate measures to safeguard the public's health.

In consultation with the Labour and Welfare Bureau and the Hospital Authority, my reply to the various parts of the question raised by Dr the Hon Pierre Chan is as follows:

(1) As at October 25, 2020, the Centre for Health Protection (CHP) of the Department of Health (DH) recorded a total of 160 clusters of COVID-19 which involved five or more cases. Among them, over 120 clusters involved five to nine cases, most of which involved families, friends or workplace settings.

(2) As at October 25, 2020, the CHP of DH recorded a total 3 849 cases of locally acquired and possibly locally acquired cases of COVID-19, out of which 1 485 were locally acquired and possibly locally acquired cases with unknown sources.

(3) As at October 25, 2020, the 5 296 COVID-19 confirmed cases and 105 death cases in Hong Kong, respectively broken down by the age group to which the patients belonged to are set out in

the table below:

Type of cases	Age groups										
	0 to 9	10 to 19	20 to 29	30 to 39	40 to 49	50 to 59	60 to 69	70 to 79	80 to 89	90 to 99	100 to 109
Confirmed cases	210	379	863	877	807	844	785	321	153	56	1
Death cases	0	0	0	1	0	2	13	27	42	20	0

(4) As at October 25, 2020, the number of COVID-19 confirmed cases, death cases, confirmed cases involving persons aged 60 or above and death cases involving persons aged 60 or above in Hong Kong, respectively broken down by the date of confirmation are set out in the table below:

Type of cases	Date of confirmation		
	January 1 to February 29, 2020	March 1 to June 30, 2020	July 1 to October 25, 2020
Confirmed cases	95	1 111	4 090
Confirmed cases involving persons aged below 60	51	989	2 940
Confirmed cases involving persons aged 60 or above	44	122	1 150
Death cases	3	5	97
Death cases involving persons aged below 60	1	1	1
Death cases involving persons aged 60 or above	2	4	96

(5) As at October 25, 2020, there were 39 confirmed cases which reported to be working at

public hospitals, including two doctors, 11 nurses and 26 staff members from the support or executive ranks. Out of these cases, most of them are believed to be linked to infections in the community and not infection at hospitals.

During the same period, the CHP recorded 23 confirmed cases which reported to be working at private hospitals/private clinics. The CHP does not have a breakdown of the above 23 confirmed cases by types of healthcare personnel and allied health professionals.

(6) As at September 30, 2020, the Labour Department (LD) had received a total of 217 employees' compensation claims with employees suspected to have contracted COVID-19 in employment. Reports by employers to LD had been made for 215 of the claims. The breakdown of reported claims by industry is as follows:

Industry	Number of compensation claims
Public Administration, Social and Personal Services	49
Finance and Insurance, Real Estate, Professional and Business Services	58
Food and Beverage Services	21
Import/Export, Wholesale and Retail Trades, Accommodation Services	10
Transportation, Storage, Postal and Courier Services, Information and Communications	63
Construction	8
Manufacturing	1
Others	7
Total	217

Among the reported cases, one case was settled after the employer had made payment in accordance with the Certificate of Compensation Assessment issued by the Commissioner for Labour. No follow-up action could be taken in 16 cases as the employees withdrew their claims or failed to respond to LD. LD has been following up on the remaining cases.

LD has been proactively following up on employees' compensation claims with employees suspected to have contracted COVID-19 in employment based on information published by the CHP. A note on employees' rights and protection under the Employees' Compensation Ordinance, together with the contact means of LD, has also been distributed through hospitals to all confirmed COVID-19 patients. In case of dispute over employees' compensation cases, LD will obtain medical reports and other relevant information (such as contact tracing reports) and provide its views to the employee and employer concerned on the likelihood of the case being a work injury upon the expert advice of its Occupational Health Officers. If the dispute cannot be resolved through LD, the employee may seek adjudication from the Court. LD will assist the employee in seeking assistance from the Legal Aid Department.

Issued at HKT 16:25

Public hospitals daily update on COVID-19 cases

****

The following is issued on behalf of the Hospital Authority:

As at 9am today (October 28), 10 COVID-19 confirmed patients were discharged from hospital in the last 24 hours. So far, a total of 5 063 patients with confirmed or probable infection have been discharged.

At present, there are 614 negative pressure rooms in public hospitals with 1 098 negative pressure beds activated. A total of 111 confirmed patients are currently hospitalised in 18 public hospitals, among which 10 patients are in critical condition, four are in serious condition and the remaining 97 patients are in stable condition.

The Hospital Authority will maintain close contact with the Centre for Health Protection to monitor the latest developments and to inform the public and healthcare workers on the latest information in a timely manner.

Details of the above-mentioned patients are as follows:

Patient condition	Case numbers
Discharged	5149, 5187, 5220, 5222, 5240, 5255, 5260, 5289, 5306, 5309
Critical	1989, 3496, 3764, 4433, 4706, 4833, 4937, 5110, 5185, 5195
Serious	4101, 4746, 4788, 5151

Issued at HKT 17:26

Latest arrangements for LCSD public services

****

The Leisure and Cultural Services Department (LCSD) announced today (October 28) that in view of the latest situation of COVID-19, the limit on the number of audiences/users in each facility of LCSD performance venues will be relaxed starting from October 30 (Friday), with seating capacity to be increased from 50 to 75 per cent of the original. Consecutive seats will be limited to four. For details, please refer to the notifications of individual venues. The limit on the number of users in other leisure and cultural facilities such as public swimming pools and public libraries will also be suitably relaxed on the same day.

For public programmes to be held at museums, including the Cinema of the Hong Kong Film Archive, the limit on the number of audiences/users and other arrangements will be the same as the above-mentioned performance venues, with capacity increased to 75 per cent.

Visitors to facilities of performance venues and museums will need to use hand sanitiser and will be subject to temperature checks before admission. They also need to wear their own masks. Children under 12 will only be allowed to enter museums and exhibition facilities when accompanied by an adult. Enhanced measures including cleaning and disinfection between sessions will be conducted.

The LCSD will continue to monitor the situation closely and review the arrangements in a timely manner.

Issued at HKT 18:37

FEHD reminds catering business operators and customers to strictly comply with anti-epidemic regulations and measures

****

The Food and Environmental Hygiene Department (FEHD) today (October 28) reminded catering business operators and practitioners to strictly comply with anti-epidemic regulations and make every effort to implement the Government's anti-epidemic measures and the public health experts' various recommendations targeting at critical control points. With Halloween approaching, the FEHD has communicated with trade representatives to remind catering businesses and their customers to comply with various social distancing measures and strongly appealed to them to exercise self-discipline. The trade representatives have indicated that they will fully cooperate. Meanwhile, the FEHD will join hands with the Police closely to step up their respective inspections and to conduct joint operations at various bar areas proactively, in the coming Halloween weekend and on its eve. Stringent enforcement actions will be taken to ensure compliance of relevant regulations, so as to avert the risk of rebound of infection cases.

A spokesman for the FEHD said that in view of the latest situation of COVID-19, the Government announced yesterday (October 27) that it would continue to relax social distancing measures in a gradual and orderly manner. The latest directions issued by the Secretary for Food and Health in relation to catering business premises under the Prevention and Control of Disease (Requirements and Directions) (Business and Premises) Regulation (Cap. 599F) will come into effect on October 30. According to the latest directions, catering business operators and practitioners have to strictly comply with a series of requirements and restrictions. Among these, selling or supplying food or drink for consumption on the premises from 2am to 4.59am must cease; except for bars and pubs which are subject to separate requirement (see the third paragraph), any person within catering premises must wear a mask at any time except when the person is consuming food or drink therein; no more than four persons may be at one table at bars or pubs, while no more than six persons may be at one table in other catering premises; the total number of people allowed in catering business premises will be capped at 75 per cent of the normal seating capacity; tables must be arranged in a way to ensure there is a distance of at least 1.5m or some form of partition which could serve as effective buffer between one table and another table; body temperature screening must be conducted before the person is allowed to enter the catering premises; and hand sanitisers must be provided.

The spokesman particularly emphasised that to further reduce the public health risks arisen from mask-off activities in bars/pubs and night establishments/nightclubs, under the new requirement, any person within such premises must wear a mask at any times except when the person is consuming food or drink at the table therein. If persons responsible for carrying on catering businesses and managers of scheduled premises contravene the requirements under Cap. 599F, they are liable to a maximum fine of $50,000 and imprisonment for six months. The FEHD and the Police may also take enforcement action under the Prevention and Control of Disease (Wearing of Mask) Regulation (Cap. 599I) against persons who fail to wear a mask in accordance with the requirements. Offenders are liable to a maximum fine at level 2 ($5,000) or be issued with a fixed penalty notice ($2,000).

Trade representatives have expressed to the Government that they will fully cooperate with the Government regulations and measures. They will not only make wide appeals to remind their customers to comply with the regulations, but also give their best to persuade their customers to exercise self-discipline. These include advising them not to gather and to wear a mask, at adjoining public places outside the premises, so as to protect personal and public health.

The Government has all along been communicating with public health experts and the catering sector on recommendations made by public health expert advisers on critical control points, and advised the catering businesses to implement various measures with a view to minimising the risk of transmission of COVID-19 within the premises. The FEHD has issued an advisory letter to the trade today on the latest directions and recommendations for catering businesses, including the following measures targeting at critical control points:

(1) arrange for hygiene supervisors/hygiene managers to familiarise themselves with the FEHD's training materials on anti-epidemic measures (www.fehd.gov.hk/english/licensing/advice_COVID19_FoodPremises.pdf) and implement them in their catering premises;

(2) participate actively in the voluntary declaration scheme on air changes in licensed catering premises launched by the FEHD to enable the public to identify catering premises with air changes or air purification devices meeting the recommendations made by public health expert advisers;

(3) pay attention to the compliance of the requirement that customers must wear a mask at any times except when consuming food or drink at the table within bars/pubs (as well as night establishments/nightclubs);

(4) encourage customers entering food premises to fill in electronic health declaration forms self-developed by the trade or use the mobile app on exposure risk notification to be launched by the Government, so as to assist the Centre for Health Protection in the tracing of close contacts; and

(5) adopt contactless payment methods to reduce the risk of virus transmission via contacting cash.

For more details, please visit the FEHD's website (www.fehd.gov.hk/english/licensing/guide_general_reference/CateringBusiness_direction_20201028.html) with a powerpoint and a video from Professor Yuen Kwok-yung of the University of Hong Kong.

The spokesman appealed to the frontline staff of catering businesses to actively participate in the Targeted Group Testing Scheme. The deadline for online registration has been extended to November 30. Restaurant operators may register through the FEHD's website before the deadline for the voluntary testing service. High-exposure groups who had already registered and undergone voluntary testing may register again. For details, please visit the FEHD's website (www.fehd.gov.hk/english/events/covid19_test/info_20200926.html). The FEHD and the bar trade have exchanged views and will take effective measures to increase the participation rate of staff of bar and pubs.

The FEHD spokesman appealed to food business operators and practitioners to fully implement the targeted measures on critical control points, actively participate in the virus testing services for targeted groups and give their best to appeal to customers to fully cooperate with the Government's regulations and measures. All must comply with relevant regulations on prevention and control of disease in a concerted and persistent manner, with a view to keeping their staff, customers and the public safe. Members of the public also have to comply with the related regulations and directions on group gatherings at catering premises.

Issued at HKT 23:41

October 29[29]

CHP investigates three additional confirmed cases of COVID-19

****

The Centre for Health Protection (CHP) of the Department of Health has announced that as of 0.00am, October 29, the CHP was investigating three additional confirmed cases of coronavirus disease 2019 (COVID-19), taking the number of cases to 5 314 in Hong Kong so far (comprising 5 313 confirmed cases and one probable case).

Among the newly reported cases announced, two had a travel history during the incubation period. The remaining case was epidemiologically linked with a local case.

The CHP's epidemiological investigations and relevant contact tracing on the confirmed cases are ongoing. For case details and contact tracing information, please see the Annex or the list of buildings with confirmed cases of COVID-19 in the past 14 days and the latest local situation of COVID-19 available on the website "COVID-19 Thematic Website" (www.coronavirus.gov.hk).

A spokesman for the CHP said, "During the CHP's epidemiological investigations and relevant contact tracing on the confirmed cases, we will compile and upload (www.chp.gov.hk/files/pdf/building_list_eng.pdf) a list of buildings that confirmed patients had visited from two days before the onset of symptoms. Given that cases of local infection continue to occur from time to time, members of the public are urged to seek medical attention immediately if they believe that they had visited the same place at an identical time with a confirmed patient and feel unwell subsequently. If they remain asymptomatic but are concerned that they have been infected, they can also visit the Hospital Authority's designated general out-patient clinics (www.ha.org.hk/haho/ho/covid-19/GOPC_extend_EN.pdf) to obtain specimen collection packs and collect deep throat saliva specimens for free COVID-19 testing."

In view of the severe epidemic situation, the CHP called on members of the public to avoid going out, having social contact and dining out. They should put on a surgical mask and maintain stringent hand hygiene when they need to go out. The CHP strongly urged the elderly to stay home as far as possible and avoid going out. They should consider asking their family and friends to help with everyday tasks such as shopping for basic necessities.

The spokesman said, "Given that the situation of COVID-19 infection remains severe and that there is a continuous increase in the number of cases reported around the world, members of the public are strongly urged to avoid all non-essential travel outside Hong Kong.

[29] https://www.info.gov.hk/gia/general/202010/29.htm

"The CHP also strongly urges the public to maintain at all times strict personal and environmental hygiene, which is key to personal protection against infection and prevention of the spread of the disease in the community. On a personal level, members of the public should wear a surgical mask when having respiratory symptoms, taking public transport or staying in crowded places. They should also perform hand hygiene frequently, especially before touching the mouth, nose or eyes.

"As for household environmental hygiene, members of the public are advised to maintain drainage pipes properly, regularly pour water into drain outlets (U-traps) and cover all floor drain outlets when they are not in use. After using the toilet, they should put the toilet lid down before flushing to avoid spreading germs."

Moreover, the Government has launched the website "COVID-19 Thematic Website" (www.coronavirus.gov.hk) for announcing the latest updates on various news on COVID-19 infection and health advice to help the public understand the latest updates. Members of the public may also gain access to information via the COVID-19 WhatsApp Helpline launched by the Office of the Government Chief Information Officer. Simply by saving 9617 1823 in their phone contacts or clicking the link wa.me/85296171823?text=hi, they will be able to obtain information on COVID-19 as well as the "StayHomeSafe" mobile app and wristband via WhatsApp.

Issued at HKT 14:00

Public hospitals daily update on COVID-19 cases

****

The following is issued on behalf of the Hospital Authority:

As at 9am today (October 29), nine COVID-19 confirmed patients were discharged from hospital in the last 24 hours. Including a patient (case number: 5311) discharged on October 27, a total of 5 073 patients with confirmed or probable infection have been discharged so far.

At present, there are 614 negative pressure rooms in public hospitals with 1 098 negative pressure beds activated. A total of 103 confirmed patients are currently hospitalised in 18 public hospitals, among which nine patients are in critical condition, four are in serious condition and the remaining 90 patients are in stable condition.

The Hospital Authority will maintain close contact with the Centre for Health Protection to monitor the latest developments and to inform the public and healthcare workers on the latest information in a timely manner.

Details of the above-mentioned patients are as follows:

Patient condition	Case numbers
Discharged	5089, 5144, 5178, 5210, 5243, 5252, 5266, 5276, 5294, 5311
Critical	1989, 3496, 4433, 4706, 4833, 4937, 5110, 5185, 5195
Serious	4101, 4746, 4788, 5151

Issued at HKT 17:00

October 30[30]

Hong Kong Customs detects largest-ever counterfeit face mask case

****

Hong Kong Customs mounted a special operation against counterfeit face masks on October 28 and seized about 100 000 suspected counterfeit medical-grade face masks intended to be transshipped overseas via Hong Kong, with an estimated market value of about $3 million. One person was arrested. This is the largest-ever suspected counterfeit face mask case detected by Customs in terms of both quantity and seizure value.

Customs earlier received information alleging that a company was suspected of selling counterfeit face masks. After an investigation with the assistance of the trademark owner, Customs took enforcement action on the above-mentioned date and first seized the batch of suspected counterfeit medical-grade face masks at a storehouse in Yuen Long.

Customs further raided a trading company in connection with the case in San Po Kong and a residential premises in Kowloon City on the same day. A 71-year-old male person-in-charge of the trading company was arrested.

Initial investigations revealed that unscrupulous merchants intended to transship the batch of masks overseas for sale and profit. Customs is looking into the source of the face masks involved in the case. Samples have also been sent to a laboratory for safety testing.

[30] https://www.info.gov.hk/gia/general/202010/30.htm

Investigation is ongoing and the arrested man has been released on bail pending further investigation.

Customs will continue to take stringent enforcement action and maintain close contact with trademark owners in monitoring the market situation with a view to proactively combating counterfeit protective items.

Under the Trade Descriptions Ordinance (TDO), any person who sells or possesses for sale any goods with a forged trade mark commits an offence. The maximum penalty upon conviction is a fine of $500,000 and imprisonment for five years.

Customs has conducted a territory-wide special operation codenamed "Guardian" since January 27 this year to conduct spot checks and enforcement operations on common protective items. More than 6 000 officers have been mobilised to conduct over 38 000 inspections at retail spots. Investigations have been conducted against 17 cases of suspected violations of the TDO and 13 cases of suspected violations of the Consumer Goods Safety Ordinance (CGSO). Eighty persons have been arrested so far and goods suspected of violating the law including nearly 6 million surgical masks, 314 bottles of disinfectant alcohol and 23 bottles of normal saline have been seized.

The "Guardian" operation will continue and Customs will carry on its high-profile law enforcement to combat and prevent violation of relevant ordinances.

Members of the public may report any suspected violation of the TDO or the CGSO to Customs' 24-hour hotline 2545 6182 or its dedicated crime-reporting email account (crimereport@customs.gov.hk).

Issued at HKT 16:12

Public hospitals daily update on COVID-19 cases

****

The following is issued on behalf of the Hospital Authority:

As at 9am today (October 30), nine COVID-19 confirmed patients were discharged from hospital in the last 24 hours. So far, a total of 5 082 patients with confirmed or probable infection have been discharged.

At present, there are 614 negative pressure rooms in public hospitals with 1 098 negative pressure beds activated. A total of 97 confirmed patients are currently hospitalised in 18 public hospitals, among which nine patients are in critical condition, four are in serious condition and the remaining 84 patients are in stable condition.

The Hospital Authority will maintain close contact with the Centre for Health Protection to monitor the latest developments and to inform the public and healthcare workers on the latest information in a timely manner.

Details of the above-mentioned patients are as follows:

Patient condition	Case numbers
Discharged	4915, 5000, 5111, 5115, 5152, 5174, 5247, 5253, 5291
Critical	1989, 3496, 4433, 4706, 4833, 4937, 5110, 5185, 5195
Serious	4101, 4746, 4788, 5151

Issued at HKT 18:12

CHP investigates seven additional confirmed cases of COVID-19

****

The Centre for Health Protection (CHP) of the Department of Health has announced that as of 0.00am, October 30, the CHP was investigating seven additional confirmed cases of coronavirus disease 2019 (COVID-19), taking the number of cases to 5 321 in Hong Kong so far (comprising 5 320 confirmed cases and one probable case).

Among the newly reported cases announced, six had a travel history during the incubation period.

The CHP's epidemiological investigations and relevant contact tracing on the confirmed cases are ongoing. For case details and contact tracing information, please see the Annex or the list of buildings with confirmed cases of COVID-19 in the past 14 days and the latest local situation of COVID-19 available on the website "COVID-19 Thematic Website" (www.coronavirus.gov.hk).

A spokesman for the CHP said, "During the CHP's epidemiological investigations and relevant contact tracing on the confirmed cases, we will compile and upload (www.chp.gov.hk/files/pdf/building_list_eng.pdf) a list of buildings that confirmed patients had visited from two days before the onset of symptoms. Given that cases of local infection continue to occur from time to time, members of the public are urged to seek medical attention immediately if they believe that they had visited the same place at an identical time with a confirmed patient and feel unwell subsequently. If they remain asymptomatic but are concerned

that they have been infected, they can also visit the Hospital Authority's designated general out-patient clinics (www.ha.org.hk/haho/ho/covid-19/GOPC_extend_EN.pdf) to obtain specimen collection packs and collect deep throat saliva specimens for free COVID-19 testing."

In view of the severe epidemic situation, the CHP called on members of the public to avoid going out, having social contact and dining out. They should put on a surgical mask and maintain stringent hand hygiene when they need to go out. The CHP strongly urged the elderly to stay home as far as possible and avoid going out. They should consider asking their family and friends to help with everyday tasks such as shopping for basic necessities.

The spokesman said, "Given that the situation of COVID-19 infection remains severe and that there is a continuous increase in the number of cases reported around the world, members of the public are strongly urged to avoid all non-essential travel outside Hong Kong.

"The CHP also strongly urges the public to maintain at all times strict personal and environmental hygiene, which is key to personal protection against infection and prevention of the spread of the disease in the community. On a personal level, members of the public should wear a surgical mask when having respiratory symptoms, taking public transport or staying in crowded places. They should also perform hand hygiene frequently, especially before touching the mouth, nose or eyes.

"As for household environmental hygiene, members of the public are advised to maintain drainage pipes properly, regularly pour water into drain outlets (U-traps) and cover all floor drain outlets when they are not in use. After using the toilet, they should put the toilet lid down before flushing to avoid spreading germs."

Moreover, the Government has launched the website "COVID-19 Thematic Website" (www.coronavirus.gov.hk) for announcing the latest updates on various news on COVID-19 infection and health advice to help the public understand the latest updates. Members of the public may also gain access to information via the COVID-19 WhatsApp Helpline launched by the Office of the Government Chief Information Officer. Simply by saving 9617 1823 in their phone contacts or clicking the link wa.me/85296171823?text=hi, they will be able to obtain information on COVID-19 as well as the "StayHomeSafe" mobile app and wristband via WhatsApp.

Issued at HKT 18:45

Woman sentenced for breaching compulsory quarantine order

****

A 54-year-old woman was sentenced to immediate imprisonment for eight weeks by the Eastern Magistrates' Courts today (October 30) for violating the Compulsory Quarantine of Certain Persons Arriving at Hong Kong Regulation (Cap 599C) (the Regulation).

The woman was earlier issued a compulsory quarantine order stating that she must conduct quarantine at a hotel for 14 days. Before the expiry of the quarantine order, she left the place of quarantine on August 1 without reasonable excuse nor permission given by an authorised officer. She was charged with contravening sections 8(1) and 8(5) of the Regulation and was sentenced by the Eastern Magistrates' Courts today to immediate imprisonment for eight weeks.

Pursuant to the Regulation, starting from February 8, save for exempted persons, all persons who have stayed in the Mainland, Macao or Taiwan in the 14 days preceding arrival in Hong Kong, regardless of their nationality or travel documents, will be subject to compulsory quarantine for 14 days. Moreover, pursuant to the Compulsory Quarantine of Persons Arriving at Hong Kong from Foreign Places Regulation (Cap 599E), starting from March 19, all persons arriving from countries or territories outside China would also be subject to compulsory quarantine for 14 days. Breaching a quarantine order is a criminal offence and offenders are subject to a maximum fine of $25,000 and imprisonment for six months.

A spokesman for the Department of Health said the sentence sends a clear message to the community that breaching a compulsory quarantine order is a criminal offence that the Government will not tolerate, and solemnly reminded the public to comply with the Regulation. As of today, a total of 63 persons have been convicted by the courts for breaching compulsory quarantine orders and have received sentences including immediate imprisonment for up to three months or a fine of $15,000. The spokesman reiterated that resolute action will be taken against anyone who has breached the relevant regulations.

Issued at HKT 19:05

Public Sector Trial Scheme funds 63 projects for combating COVID-19

****

A spokesman for the Innovation and Technology Commission said today (October 30) that the assessment for the special call under the Public Sector Trial Scheme for projects to combat the COVID-19 epidemic has been completed. A total of 63 projects have been approved with total funding of over $102 million. Trials of the research and development (R&D) outcomes in the public sector have commenced progressively.

Lasting from March 9 to April 10, the special call aimed to support product development and application of technologies for the prevention and control of the epidemic. It was well received with 332 applications. The 63 approved projects, coming from local universities, R&D centres, designated local public research institutes and technology companies conducting R&D activities in Hong Kong, fall under a number of categories relating to epidemic prevention and control, including COVID-19 virus detection or diagnosis methods, masks and other protective equipment, disinfection equipment and products, body temperature checking devices and virus transmission tracking devices.

"The local public sector has rendered strong support for this call. Fifty-seven public organisations are involved in the trials of the approved projects. We will continue to follow up on the progress of the projects for early realisation and commercialisation of the R&D outcomes, thereby bringing about anti-epidemic benefits for the community," the spokesman said.

Fung Kai Care & Attention Home for the Elderly is one of the public organisations joining the trial scheme. The trial project in which it has participated is the Centralized Nano Bubble System for Surface Cleaning and Sanitization. Developed by the Nano and Advanced Materials Institute, the System splits ozone into nano bubbles. Fluid carrying such bubbles can be used for sanitisation and reduction of the spread of bacteria and viruses. The Superintendent of Fung Kai Care & Attention Home for the Elderly, Dr Kwok Man-wah, said, "Fluid carrying ozone nano bubbles is cost-effective and ready for use anytime. It is free of flammable or irritating chemicals, and ideal for disinfecting elderly homes. We are pleased to participate in the trial scheme. By employing the system, we hope to strengthen the protection of the health of our residents and employees amid the epidemic."

The University of Hong Kong is another public organisation participating in the trial scheme, including the trial project of a COVID-19 diagnostic kit developed by ImmunoDiagnostics Limited. The technology company expects that the kit, with a short turnaround time, will be able to assist organisations such as medical institutions and testing laboratories in conducting rapid COVID-19 testing. Professor Chen Zhiwei of the Department of Microbiology of the University of Hong Kong said, "The special call supports various anti-epidemic technologies from laboratories to be applied in the community or clinical settings, bolstering the fight against COVID-19 in Hong Kong. We are delighted to join the trial scheme and look forward to contributing to the fight through sharing of our data and experience."

In addition, the School of Nursing of the University of Hong Kong has taken part in the trial project of a fast-track vented enclosure developed by City University of Hong Kong. Made of breathable protective materials, the enclosure aims to prevent viruses from spreading through air in hospitals, thereby minimising the possibility of cross-infection between medical staff and patients. Professor Janet Wong of the School said, "We are happy to provide a trial site and post-trial comments for the project. We hope the project will further protect the safety of medical staff and benefit the medical sector."

The special call aimed to fund trials of R&D outcomes in the local public sector relating to detection, diagnosis or surveillance of the COVID-19 virus, or reduction of the risks of infection and its spread. The list of the approved projects is available in the annex and on the website of the Innovation and Technology Fund (www.itf.gov.hk/en/funding-programmes/facilitating-technology/psts/psts-covid-19/index.html).

Issued at HKT 19:15

October 31[31]

FEHD and Police continue to work together to step up inspections and take stringent enforcement actions relating to anti-epidemic measures

****

The Food and Environmental Hygiene Department (FEHD) and the Police commenced joint operations during Halloween and on its eve last night (October 30) and at small hours today (October 31) to step up inspections and take stringent enforcement actions at catering business premises including bars in Wan Chai District, Central and Western District, Yau Tsim District and Mong Kok District. Verbal warnings were given to the operators, practitioners and customers of the premises and leaflets were distributed at the initial stage of the operations to remind them to strictly comply with the relevant requirements under the Prevention and Control of Disease (Requirements and Directions) (Business and Premises) Regulation (Cap. 599F) (the Regulation), and to remind the public to comply with the various restrictions in relation to group gatherings and mask-wearing under the anti-epidemic regulations and directions when patronising restaurants. This will help keep the epidemic situation under control and reduce the risk of virus transmission in the community.

During the operations, the FEHD and the Police inspected 89 catering business premises (including bars). A total of 54 verbal warnings were given and different kinds of leaflets were distributed, while procedures on prosecution were initiated against six operators for segregation of tables less than stipulated distance and number of persons at one table in the premises exceeding the requirement stipulated in the Regulation. In addition, procedures on prosecution were initiated by the Police against two bar operators for maintaining dine-in operation during the period between 2am and 3am.

A spokesman for the FEHD said, "According to the latest directions issued by the Secretary for Food and Health in relation to catering business under the Regulation, food business operators and food handlers have to strictly comply with a series of requirements and restrictions. Among these, selling or supplying food or drink for consumption on the premises from 2am to 4.59am must cease; except for bars and pubs which are subject to separate requirement (see the fourth paragraph), any person within catering premises must wear a mask at any time except when the person is consuming food or drink therein; no more than four persons may be at one table at bars or pubs, while no more than six persons may be at one table in other catering premises; the total number of people allowed in catering business premises will be capped at 75 per cent of the normal seating capacity; tables must be arranged in a way to ensure there is a

[31] https://www.info.gov.hk/gia/general/202010/31.htm

distance of at least 1.5m or some form of partition which could serve as effective buffer between one table and another table; body temperature screening must be conducted before the person is allowed to enter the catering premises; and hand sanitisers must be provided."

The spokesman particularly emphasised that the new regulation requires any person within bars/pubs and night establishments/nightclubs must wear a mask at any time except when the person is consuming food or drink at the table therein.

If persons responsible for carrying on catering businesses and managers of scheduled premises contravene the Regulation, they are liable to a maximum fine of $50,000 and imprisonment for six months. The FEHD and the Police may also take enforcement action under the Prevention and Control of Disease (Wearing of Mask) Regulation (Cap. 599I) against persons who fail to wear a mask in accordance with the requirements. Offenders are liable to a maximum fine at level 2 ($5,000) or be issued with a fixed penalty notice ($2,000). Persons who violate the group gathering restriction of Prevention and Control of Disease (Prohibition in Group Gathering) Regulation (Cap. 599G) are subject to a fixed penalty of $2,000.

The spokesman said that the FEHD will continue to step up inspections at food business premises across the territory and conduct joint operations with the Police during Halloween to ensure that food business operators, food handlers and the public strictly comply with the directions under the regulations. Stringent enforcement actions will be taken to ensure compliance of relevant regulations, so as to avert the risk of rebound of COVID-19 infection cases. The enforcement actions on the Halloween Day will be more forceful that those on its eve.

The spokesman appealed to food business operators and practitioners to comply with relevant regulations on prevention and control of disease in a concerted and persistent manner, with a view to keeping their staff, customers and the public safe. Members of the public also have to comply with the related regulations and directions on group gatherings at catering premises.

Issued at HKT 13:31

CHP investigates three additional confirmed cases of COVID-19

****

The Centre for Health Protection (CHP) of the Department of Health has announced that as of 0.00am, October 31, the CHP was investigating three additional confirmed cases of coronavirus disease 2019 (COVID-19), taking the number of cases to 5 324 in Hong Kong so far (comprising 5 323 confirmed cases and one probable case).

All the newly reported cases announced had a travel history during the incubation period.

The CHP's epidemiological investigations and relevant contact tracing on the confirmed cases are ongoing. For case details and contact tracing information, please see the Annex or the list of buildings with confirmed cases of COVID-19 in the past 14 days and the latest local situation of COVID-19 available on the website "COVID-19 Thematic Website" (www.coronavirus.gov.hk).

A spokesman for the CHP said, "During the CHP's epidemiological investigations and relevant contact tracing on the confirmed cases, we will compile and upload (www.chp.gov.hk/files/pdf/building_list_eng.pdf) a list of buildings that confirmed patients had visited from two days before the onset of symptoms. Given that cases of local infection continue to occur from time to time, members of the public are urged to seek medical attention immediately if they believe that they had visited the same place at an identical time with a confirmed patient and feel unwell subsequently. If they remain asymptomatic but are concerned that they have been infected, they can also visit the Hospital Authority's designated general out-patient clinics (www.ha.org.hk/haho/ho/covid-19/GOPC_extend_EN.pdf) to obtain specimen collection packs and collect deep throat saliva specimens for free COVID-19 testing."

In view of the severe epidemic situation, the CHP called on members of the public to avoid going out, having social contact and dining out. They should put on a surgical mask and maintain stringent hand hygiene when they need to go out. The CHP strongly urged the elderly to stay home as far as possible and avoid going out. They should consider asking their family and friends to help with everyday tasks such as shopping for basic necessities.

The spokesman said, "Given that the situation of COVID-19 infection remains severe and that there is a continuous increase in the number of cases reported around the world, members of the public are strongly urged to avoid all non-essential travel outside Hong Kong.

"The CHP also strongly urges the public to maintain at all times strict personal and environmental hygiene, which is key to personal protection against infection and prevention of the spread of the disease in the community. On a personal level, members of the public should wear a surgical mask when having respiratory symptoms, taking public transport or staying in crowded places. They should also perform hand hygiene frequently, especially before touching the mouth, nose or eyes.

"As for household environmental hygiene, members of the public are advised to maintain drainage pipes properly, regularly pour water into drain outlets (U-traps) and cover all floor drain outlets when they are not in use. After using the toilet, they should put the toilet lid down before flushing to avoid spreading germs."

Moreover, the Government has launched the website "COVID-19 Thematic Website" (www.coronavirus.gov.hk) for announcing the latest updates on various news on COVID-19 infection and health advice to help the public understand the latest updates. Members of the public may also gain access to information via the COVID-19 WhatsApp Helpline launched by the Office of the Government Chief Information Officer. Simply by saving 9617 1823 in their phone contacts or clicking the link wa.me/85296171823?text=hi, they will be able to obtain information on COVID-19 as well as the "StayHomeSafe" mobile app and wristband via WhatsApp.

Issued at HKT 14:25

Public hospitals daily update on COVID-19 cases

****

The following is issued on behalf of the Hospital Authority:

As at 9am today (October 31), seven COVID-19 confirmed patients were discharged from hospital in the last 24 hours. So far, a total of 5 089 patients with confirmed or probable infection have been discharged.

At present, there are 615 negative pressure rooms in public hospitals with 1 103 negative pressure beds activated. A total of 97 confirmed patients are currently hospitalised in 19 public hospitals, among which nine patients are in critical condition, four are in serious condition and the remaining 84 patients are in stable condition.

The Hospital Authority will maintain close contact with the Centre for Health Protection to monitor the latest developments and to inform the public and healthcare workers on the latest information in a timely manner.

Details of the above-mentioned patients are as follows:

Patient condition	Case numbers
Discharged	5117, 5157, 5254, 5259, 5283, 5304, 5315
Critical	1989, 3496, 4433, 4706, 4833, 4937, 5110, 5185, 5195
Serious	4101, 4746, 4788, 5151

Issued at HKT 15:55

November 1[32]

Public hospitals daily update on COVID-19 cases

****

The following is issued on behalf of the Hospital Authority:

As at 9am today (November 1), seven COVID-19 confirmed patients were discharged from hospital in the last 24 hours. So far, a total of 5 096 patients with confirmed or probable infection have been discharged.

At present, there are 628 negative pressure rooms in public hospitals with 1 120 negative pressure beds activated. A total of 93 confirmed patients are currently hospitalised in 19 public hospitals, among which nine patients are in critical condition, five are in serious condition and the remaining 79 patients are in stable condition.

The Hospital Authority will maintain close contact with the Centre for Health Protection to monitor the latest developments and to inform the public and healthcare workers on the latest information in a timely manner.

Details of the above-mentioned patients are as follows:

Patient condition	Case numbers
Discharged	3791, 4873, 5214, 5241, 5303, 5310, 5313
Critical	1989, 3496, 4433, 4706, 4833, 4937, 5110, 5185, 5273
Serious	4101, 4746, 4788, 5151, 5195

Issued at HKT 17:27

CHP investigates seven additional confirmed cases of COVID-19

****

[32] https://www.info.gov.hk/gia/general/202011/01.htm

The Centre for Health Protection (CHP) of the Department of Health has announced that as of 0.00am, November 1, the CHP was investigating seven additional confirmed cases of coronavirus disease 2019 (COVID-19), taking the number of cases to 5 331 in Hong Kong so far (comprising 5 330 confirmed cases and one probable case).

Among the newly reported cases announced, six had a travel history during the incubation period.

The CHP's epidemiological investigations and relevant contact tracing on the confirmed cases are ongoing. For case details and contact tracing information, please see the Annex or the list of buildings with confirmed cases of COVID-19 in the past 14 days and the latest local situation of COVID-19 available on the website "COVID-19 Thematic Website" (www.coronavirus.gov.hk).

A spokesman for the CHP said, "During the CHP's epidemiological investigations and relevant contact tracing on the confirmed cases, we will compile and upload (www.chp.gov.hk/files/pdf/building_list_eng.pdf) a list of buildings that confirmed patients had visited from two days before the onset of symptoms. Given that cases of local infection continue to occur from time to time, members of the public are urged to seek medical attention immediately if they believe that they had visited the same place at an identical time with a confirmed patient and feel unwell subsequently. If they remain asymptomatic but are concerned that they have been infected, they can also visit the Hospital Authority's designated general out-patient clinics (www.ha.org.hk/haho/ho/covid-19/GOPC_extend_EN.pdf) to obtain specimen collection packs and collect deep throat saliva specimens for free COVID-19 testing."

In view of the severe epidemic situation, the CHP called on members of the public to avoid going out, having social contact and dining out. They should put on a surgical mask and maintain stringent hand hygiene when they need to go out. The CHP strongly urged the elderly to stay home as far as possible and avoid going out. They should consider asking their family and friends to help with everyday tasks such as shopping for basic necessities.

The spokesman said, "Given that the situation of COVID-19 infection remains severe and that there is a continuous increase in the number of cases reported around the world, members of the public are strongly urged to avoid all non-essential travel outside Hong Kong.

"The CHP also strongly urges the public to maintain at all times strict personal and environmental hygiene, which is key to personal protection against infection and prevention of the spread of the disease in the community. On a personal level, members of the public should wear a surgical mask when having respiratory symptoms, taking public transport or staying in crowded places. They should also perform hand hygiene frequently, especially before touching the mouth, nose or eyes.

"As for household environmental hygiene, members of the public are advised to maintain drainage pipes properly, regularly pour water into drain outlets (U-traps) and cover all floor drain outlets when they are not in use. After using the toilet, they should put the toilet lid down before flushing to avoid spreading germs."

Moreover, the Government has launched the website "COVID-19 Thematic Website" (www.coronavirus.gov.hk) for announcing the latest updates on various news on COVID-19 infection and health advice to help the public understand the latest updates. Members of the public may also gain access to information via the COVID-19 WhatsApp Helpline launched by the Office of the Government Chief Information Officer. Simply by saving 9617 1823 in their phone contacts or clicking the link wa.me/85296171823?text=hi, they will be able to obtain information on COVID-19 as well as the "StayHomeSafe" mobile app and wristband via WhatsApp.

Issued at HKT 17:59

November 2[33]

CHP investigates six additional confirmed cases of COVID-19

****

The Centre for Health Protection (CHP) of the Department of Health has announced that as of 0.00am, November 2, the CHP was investigating six additional confirmed cases of coronavirus disease 2019 (COVID-19), taking the number of cases to 5 337 in Hong Kong so far (comprising 5 336 confirmed cases and one probable case).

Among the newly reported cases announced, three had a travel history during the incubation period, one was a local case with unknown sources while the other two were epidemiologically linked with a local case.

The case with unknown sources involves a 26-year-old woman (case 5 332) who had developed fever on October 28. The patient consulted a private doctor on the same day and was referred to the Accident and Emergency Department (A&ED) of Alice Ho Miu Ling Nethersole Hospital (AHNH). She submitted a deep throat saliva sample on October 31. She works at 1 Heung Yip Road, Wong Chuk Hang and last went to work on October 28. She had been to Seaview Holiday Resort in Mui Wo with seven friends between October 25 and 27.

The two cases which were epidemiologically linked with case 5 332 involve a 26-year-old man (case 5 336) and a 15-year-old boy (case 5 337). Case 5 336 had stayed with case 5 332 in Seaview Holiday Resort between October 25 and 27 who developed cough and runny nose on October 30. He was identified as a symptomatic close contact by the CHP during contact tracing and was arranged to A&ED of AHNH on October 31. Case 5 337 is a relative of case 5 332 who had contact with her on October 27 and developed cough on October 31 and sought medical attention at A&ED of AHNH on November 1.

[33] https://www.info.gov.hk/gia/general/202011/02.htm

The CHP's epidemiological investigations and relevant contact tracing on the confirmed cases are ongoing. The CHP will distribute specimen collection bottles to the residences of the patients and places where the patients had visited during their communicable periods. Bottles will also be distributed to staff and residents of the Seaview Holiday Resort, the company where case 5 332 works in and the school where case 5 337 studies at.

For case details and contact tracing information, please see the Annex or the list of buildings with confirmed cases of COVID-19 in the past 14 days and the latest local situation of COVID-19 available on the website "COVID-19 Thematic Website" (www.coronavirus.gov.hk).

A spokesman for the CHP said, "During the CHP's epidemiological investigations and relevant contact tracing on the confirmed cases, we will compile and upload (www.chp.gov.hk/files/pdf/building_list_eng.pdf) a list of buildings that confirmed patients had visited from two days before the onset of symptoms. Given that cases of local infection continue to occur from time to time, members of the public are urged to seek medical attention immediately if they believe that they had visited the same place at an identical time with a confirmed patient and feel unwell subsequently. If they remain asymptomatic but are concerned that they have been infected, they can also visit the Hospital Authority's designated general out-patient clinics (www.ha.org.hk/haho/ho/covid-19/GOPC_extend_EN.pdf) to obtain specimen collection packs and collect deep throat saliva specimens for free COVID-19 testing."

In view of the severe epidemic situation, the CHP called on members of the public to avoid going out, having social contact and dining out. They should put on a surgical mask and maintain stringent hand hygiene when they need to go out. The CHP strongly urged the elderly to stay home as far as possible and avoid going out. They should consider asking their family and friends to help with everyday tasks such as shopping for basic necessities.

The spokesman said, "Given that the situation of COVID-19 infection remains severe and that there is a continuous increase in the number of cases reported around the world, members of the public are strongly urged to avoid all non-essential travel outside Hong Kong.

"The CHP also strongly urges the public to maintain at all times strict personal and environmental hygiene, which is key to personal protection against infection and prevention of the spread of the disease in the community. On a personal level, members of the public should wear a surgical mask when having respiratory symptoms, taking public transport or staying in crowded places. They should also perform hand hygiene frequently, especially before touching the mouth, nose or eyes.

"As for household environmental hygiene, members of the public are advised to maintain drainage pipes properly, regularly pour water into drain outlets (U-traps) and cover all floor drain outlets when they are not in use. After using the toilet, they should put the toilet lid down before flushing to avoid spreading germs."

Moreover, the Government has launched the website "COVID-19 Thematic Website" (www.coronavirus.gov.hk) for announcing the latest updates on various news on COVID-19 infection and health advice to help the public understand the latest updates. Members of the public may also gain access to information via the COVID-19 WhatsApp Helpline launched by the Office of the Government Chief Information Officer. Simply by saving 9617 1823 in their phone contacts or clicking the link wa.me/85296171823?text=hi, they will be able to obtain information on COVID-19 as well as the "StayHomeSafe" mobile app and wristband via WhatsApp.

Issued at HKT 14:00

Public hospitals daily update on COVID-19 cases

****

The following is issued on behalf of the Hospital Authority:

As at 9am today (November 2), four COVID-19 confirmed patients were discharged from hospital in the last 24 hours. Including the two patients (case numbers: 5124 and 5328) discharged on October 31, a total of 5 102 patients with confirmed or probable infection have been discharged so far.

At present, there are 636 negative pressure rooms in public hospitals with 1 144 negative pressure beds activated. A total of 94 confirmed patients are currently hospitalised in 19 public hospitals, among which nine patients are in critical condition, five are in serious condition and the remaining 80 patients are in stable condition.

The Hospital Authority will maintain close contact with the Centre for Health Protection to monitor the latest developments and to inform the public and healthcare workers on the latest information in a timely manner.

Details of the above-mentioned patients are as follows:

Patient condition	Case numbers
Discharged	5124, 5147, 5189, 5249, 5325, 5328
Critical	1989, 3496, 4433, 4706, 4833, 4937, 5110, 5185, 5273
Serious	4101, 4746, 4788, 5151, 5195

Issued at HKT 17:15

November 3[34]

Employers should not dismiss foreign domestic helpers who have contracted COVID-19

****

The Government today (November 3) reminded employers that they should not dismiss foreign domestic helpers (FDHs) who have contracted COVID-19 and should continue to observe the requirements under the Employment Ordinance (EO) and the Standard Employment Contract (SEC) amidst the COVID-19 pandemic.

A Government spokesman said, "We would like to remind employers that they should not terminate or repudiate an employment contract with an FDH who has contracted COVID-19. Under the EO, an employer is prohibited from terminating the contract of employment of an employee on his or her paid sickness day, except in cases of summary dismissal due to the latter's serious misconduct. An employer who contravenes relevant provisions of the EO commits an offence and is liable to prosecution and, upon conviction, to a maximum fine of $100,000. Employers are also reminded of possible breach of contract if they repudiate the employment contract with their FDHs, or possible violation of the Disability Discrimination Ordinance (DDO) if they treat their FDHs less favourably (e.g. by dismissing them) because the FDHs have been infected with or recovered from COVID-19. Upon the recovery of the FDHs from COVID-19, employers are advised to arrange for their FDHs to start or resume work and maintain a cordial employment relationship with their FDHs."

The spokesman continued, "When handling matters on employment with FDHs, employers should observe their obligations and requirements under the EO and the SEC. Where applicable, the employer should grant sick leave and sickness allowance to the eligible FDH in accordance with the EO. Where a sick FDH has not accumulated sufficient paid sickness days to cover the period of his or her sick leave, we appeal to the employer to be compassionate and consider granting the FDH paid sick leave. According to Clause 9(a) of the SEC, in the event that the FDH is ill or suffers personal injury during the period of employment (except for the period during which the FDH leaves Hong Kong of his or her own volition and for his or her own personal purposes), regardless of whether this arises out of employment, the employer shall provide free medical treatment to the FDH."

At the same time, employers should take note of and comply with the relevant measures implemented by the Government in response to the pandemic, including the requirement that all persons (including FDHs) arriving in Hong Kong from all places outside China must be subject to compulsory quarantine of 14 days under the Compulsory Quarantine of Persons Arriving at Hong Kong from Foreign Places Regulation (Cap. 599E), and the relevant requirements of the specifications under the Prevention and Control of Disease (Regulation of Cross-boundary Conveyances and Travellers) Regulation (Cap. 599H), namely that if a traveller (including an FDH) has stayed in a specified place (including Indonesia and the Philippines) during the 14

[34] https://www.info.gov.hk/gia/general/202011/03.htm

days before arriving in Hong Kong, he or she must provide, before boarding a flight to Hong Kong, a test report issued by a laboratory or healthcare institution recognised or approved by the government of that place as proof that he or she has undergone a nucleic acid test for COVID-19, the sample for which was taken within 72 hours before the scheduled time of departure of the flight to Hong Kong, and that the test result is negative, as well as confirmation of room reservation in a hotel in Hong Kong for not less than 14 days starting on the day of his or her arrival in Hong Kong. The Government again reminded employers to make relevant arrangements and bear the costs of the relevant nucleic acid test, the accommodation expenses and the food allowance during the FDH's compulsory quarantine.

On the other hand, the Government reminded FDHs not to abuse the arrangement for premature contract termination in order to change employers (commonly known as job-hopping). The Immigration Department (ImmD) has been expediting the processing of employment visa applications submitted by FDHs who are in Hong Kong, especially applications for change of employer from those whose employment contracts have expired normally. At the same time, to combat job-hopping, the ImmD will, during case assessment, continue to closely scrutinise the details of applicants, such as the number and reasons for their premature contract termination in the past 12 months. For suspected job-hopping cases, the ImmD will refuse the employment visa applications and require the applicants to leave Hong Kong.

Employers may visit the Labour Department's dedicated FDH Portal (www.fdh.labour.gov.hk) for further information on the obligations and rights of employers and FDHs under the EO and the SEC relating to COVID-19. For information relating to COVID-19 and the DDO, employers may visit the Equal Opportunities Commission's website (www.eoc.org.hk/EOC/Upload/UserFiles/File/FAQ_COVID-19_Foreign_Domestic_Workers_and_Employers_english.pdf).

Issued at HKT 16:30

HA announces enhanced arrangement for greater convenience in testing

****

The following is issued on behalf of the Hospital Authority:

The Hospital Authority (HA) today (November 3) announced that the COVID-19 test services provided by General Out-patient Clinics (GOPCs) and Accident and Emergency (A&E) Departments will be further enhanced to identify cases of infection earlier and minimise the risk of community transmission.

"The time slots for distribution of specimen collection packs will be increased at 46 GOPCs, assisting individuals who perceive themselves as having a higher risk of exposure and who experience mild discomfort to undergo a COVID-19 test. Apart from services on Monday to Friday, members of the public can obtain the specimen collection packs from specific GOPCs during the service hours (9am to 1pm) on Saturdays, Sundays and public holidays, starting from this weekend," the HA spokesperson said.

Regarding the arrangement for specimen submission, the GOPCs will extend the specimen collection hours, beginning this Thursday (November 5), to 9am to 1pm and 2pm to 3pm from Monday to Friday, as well as 9am to 11am on Saturdays. Submission of specimens will also be available between 9am and 11am on Sundays and public holidays at some GOPCs. Details of the collection and submission times and clinics are provided in the attachment

In addition, three GOPCs (namely Sai Wan Ho General Out-patient Clinic, Ap Lei Chau General Out-patient Clinic and Yuen Long Jockey Club Health Centre) will pilot the use of vending machines to help members of the public to obtain specimen collection packs with greater convenience.

"The vending machines will be placed outside the usual service areas to minimise the impact on the clinics' operation and can be used more easily by the public," the spokesperson said.

The HA will closely monitor the utilisation of the vending machines by the general public. If space and operation allow, more clinics will install vending machines to facilitate easy collection of specimen packs by the general public. The clinics can then focus manpower on providing the normal services.

"In addition, according to the latest scientific evidence and expert opinions, deep throat saliva collected under the principle of no food or drink, no mouth rinsing and no brushing teeth within two hours is equally effective as specimen collection in the early morning for a COVID-19 test," the spokesman said.

"Patients provided with specimen collection packs after A&E attendance can submit their specimens anytime on the same day, if the specimens are collected after two hours without eating, drinking, mouth rinsing and brushing teeth. The arrangement can help shorten the time lag for confirming patient infection and expedite the removal of invisible transmission links in the community."

The HA has updated the "Patient Information Sheet on Deep Throat Saliva Collection". Staff of hospitals and clinics will provide the patients with the updated information on collection points and times.

Issued at HKT 16:47

Specifications under Prevention and Control of Disease (Regulation of Cross-boundary Conveyances and Travellers) Regulation to be gazetted

****

In view of the global development and severity of the COVID-19 epidemic situation, the Government announced today (November 3) that it will gazette the specifications under the Prevention and Control of Disease (Regulation of Cross-boundary Conveyances and Travellers) Regulation (Cap. 599H) to include Turkey as a specified place starting from November 13 to more effectively combat the epidemic, and impose conditions based on public health grounds on travellers who have visited any country outside China (excluding very high-risk areas currently specified under Cap. 599H) within 14 days before arrival in Hong Kong starting from November 13, in order to reduce the risk of spreading COVID-19 to household members during home quarantine of imported cases.

A spokesman for the Food and Health Bureau said, "The global epidemic situation is becoming increasingly severe. The daily number of new cases increased from around 70 000 to 100 000 between late March and mid-May, to around 160 000 to 180 000 in late June and to around 220 000 to 290 000 in late July, and further increased to reach a new height of around 550 000 in October. In view of the severe global pandemic situation, Hong Kong cannot afford to drop its guard on entry prevention and control measures."

Travellers who visited very high-risk places

The Government has earlier introduced Cap. 599H to impose testing and quarantine conditions on travellers coming to Hong Kong from very high-risk places to reduce the health risk they may bring to Hong Kong. The Secretary for Food and Health (SFH) has previously published in the Gazette specifications on the relevant measures applicable to 14 specified places (i.e. Bangladesh, Belgium, Ethiopia, France, India, Indonesia, Kazakhstan, Nepal, Pakistan, the Philippines, Russia, South Africa, the United Kingdom and the United States of America) and adjusted the relevant conditions having regard to the circumstances on the ground since the implementation of the regulation.

Taking into account the latest public health risk assessment, and the changes and developments of the epidemic situation, the SFH will publish in the Gazette new specifications to maintain the conditions imposed and to include Turkey as a specified place. The relevant specifications will come into effect on November 13 and remain until further notice.

According to the latest specifications, a traveller who, on the day on which the traveller boarded a civil aviation aircraft that arrives at, or is about to arrive at, Hong Kong (specified aircraft), or during the 14 days before that day, has stayed in one of the aforementioned specified places must provide the following documents:

(1) A test report in English or Chinese issued by a laboratory or healthcare institution bearing the name of the relevant traveller from the aforementioned specified places identical to that in his or her valid travel document to show that:

(a) the relevant traveller from the aforementioned specified places underwent a nucleic acid test for COVID-19, the sample for which was taken from the relevant traveller from the aforementioned specified places within 72 hours before the scheduled time of departure of the specified aircraft;

(b) the test conducted on the sample is a nucleic acid test for COVID-19; and

(c) the result of the test is that the relevant traveller from the aforementioned specified places was tested negative for COVID-19; and

(2) If the relevant report is not in English or Chinese or does not contain all of the above information, a written confirmation in English or Chinese issued by the laboratory or healthcare institution bearing the name of the relevant traveller from the aforementioned specified places identical to that in his or her valid travel document and setting out all of the above information. The said written confirmation should be presented together with the test report; and

(3) Documentary proof in English or Chinese to show that the laboratory or healthcare institution is ISO 15189 accredited or is recognised or approved by the relevant authority of the government of the place in which the laboratory or healthcare institution is located; and

(4) The relevant traveller from the aforementioned specified places has confirmation in English or Chinese of room reservation in a hotel in Hong Kong for not less than 14 days starting on the day of the arrival in Hong Kong of the relevant traveller from the aforementioned specified places.

Travellers who visited any country outside China

A traveller who, on the day on which the traveller boarded a specified aircraft, or during the 14 days before that day, has stayed in a specified place outside China (excluding very high-risk areas specified otherwise), must provide confirmation in English or Chinese of room reservation in a hotel in Hong Kong for not less than 14 days starting on the day of the arrival in Hong Kong of the relevant traveller from the rest of the world. The relevant specifications will come into effect on November 13 and remain until further notice.

The operator of the specified aircraft should submit to the Department of Health (DH) before the specified aircraft arrives at Hong Kong a document in a form specified by the DH confirming that each relevant traveller from the rest of the world has, before being checked in for the flight to Hong Kong on the aircraft, produced for boarding on the aircraft the above document.

A person who is in transit in Hong Kong and a person exempted by the Chief Secretary for Administration from compulsory quarantine under section 4(1) of either the Compulsory

Quarantine of Certain Persons Arriving at Hong Kong Regulation (Cap. 599C) or the Compulsory Quarantine of Persons Arriving at Hong Kong from Foreign Places Regulation (Cap. 599E) will not be affected.

Government to strengthen law enforcement

If any condition specified by the SFH is not met in relation to any relevant traveller on the conveyance, each of the operators of the conveyance commits an offence and is liable on conviction to the maximum penalty of a fine at level 5 ($50,000) and imprisonment for six months. If an operator fails to comply with a requirement to provide information, or knowingly or recklessly provides any information that is false or misleading in a material particular, he or she is liable on conviction to the maximum penalty of a fine at level 5 ($50,000) and imprisonment for six months.

As for travellers, if a traveller coming to Hong Kong fails to comply with a requirement to provide information, or knowingly or recklessly provides any information that is false or misleading in a material particular, he or she is liable on conviction to the maximum penalty of a fine at level 3 ($10,000) and imprisonment for six months.

Travellers to Hong Kong should note that they will be mandated to wait for their test results at a designated location after their deep throat saliva samples are collected for conducting testing for COVID-19 at the DH's Temporary Specimen Collection Centre pursuant to the Prevention and Control of Disease Regulation (Cap. 599A). If their test results are negative, they will be allowed to go to the hotel for which they made the reservation to continue the 14-day compulsory quarantine until completion. If their results are positive, the travellers will be transferred to hospital for isolation and treatment.

The Government will continue to monitor closely the situation including the developments of the epidemic situation both globally and locally and changes in the volume of cross-boundary passenger traffic, and will not hesitate to adopt more resolute and severe measures as and when necessary.

Issued at HKT 18:20

EDB to arrange COVID-19 testing for all teachers and staff in kindergartens and primary, secondary and special schools

****

The Education Bureau (EDB) today (November 3) announced that starting from next Monday (November 9), the COVID-19 Targeted Group Testing Scheme (TGTS) for staff of boarding sections of special schools will be stepped up. More comprehensive surveillance will also be put in place to arrange free-of-charge testing for all teachers and staff in kindergartens (including kindergarten-cum-child care centres) and primary, secondary and special schools in batches with a view to safeguarding the health of school staff and students.

A spokesman for the EDB said, "Testing is an integral part of the strategy in preventing and fighting the virus. To step up virus testing to achieve the objective of 'early identification, early isolation and early treatment', the Government has continued to implement the TGTS, including arranging free testing for individual high-risk groups such as staff of boarding sections of special schools in July this year. In addition, the Government launched the Universal Community Testing Programme in September, in which the EDB arranged some schools as testing centres and also encouraged school staff, students and parents to participate actively in the testing to safeguard the health of all school staff and students."

The spokesman said, "Given the volatile development of the epidemic and the need to cope with the fourth wave of the epidemic which might emerge this autumn and winter with greater severity, we must remain vigilant. In line with the Government's epidemic prevention and infection control measures, the EDB will step up the TGTS for special schools by arranging regular testing for all staff of boarding sections of special schools once every three weeks."

The spokesman added, "Taking into consideration that schools are places where people gather and school staff are high-exposure groups, as a precautionary measure, the EDB will extend the TGTS to conduct extensive and continuous surveillance at the level of teachers and staff of kindergartens (including kindergarten-cum-child care centres) and primary and secondary schools during autumn and winter. This will not only help detect confirmed cases and cut the transmission chains in the community, but also provide data for reference for the overall assessment of the epidemic situation."

The spokesman said testing would be conducted on a voluntary basis. Taking schools as a unit, the EDB will sample about 2 per cent of teaching and non-teaching staff in Hong Kong for a deep throat saliva (DTS) test on each school day. The number of schools sampled may be adjusted according to the data obtained with a view to conducting testing for all 130 000 school staff in Hong Kong.

The school staff and staff of boarding sections of special schools joining the TGTS should register relevant information at the government website (www.tgptest.gov.hk) and collect the DTS specimens by themselves. They should return the specimen bottles to schools on the specified dates for the testing contractor to conduct the testing. The specimen bottles will not indicate any personal information and hence the testing contractor will not collect any personal information. The staff concerned will be informed of the testing results by short messaging service. For those cases that test positive, they will be referred to the Centre for Health Protection (CHP) of the Department of Health for follow-up action.

The spokesman said, "As there are more close contacts with group gatherings in schools, we strongly appeal to schools to join hands with us and encourage all school staff and staff of boarding sections of special schools to actively participate in the COVID-19 testing to safeguard the health of individuals, students and other teaching staff so as to minimise the risk of transmission in schools and the community."

The spokesman stressed that the TGTS mainly targets school staff and staff of boarding sections of special schools who have not had any signs of illness. If any school staff are feeling unwell (even the symptoms may be very mild), they must not return to the school and should seek medical advice promptly to receive appropriate diagnoses and treatments. For school staff and students who perceive themselves to have a higher risk of infection and experience mild discomfort, the EDB also encourages them to receive testing at the general out-patient clinics or Accident and Emergency Departments operated by the Hospital Authority. The EDB urges all parties in schools to continue to observe the "Health Protection Measures for Schools" issued earlier by the EDB and the "Health Advice to Schools for the Prevention of Coronavirus Disease (COVID-19)" issued by the CHP to put in place all the anti-epidemic preventive measures.

Issued at HKT 18:27

CHP investigates nine additional confirmed cases of COVID-19
****

The Centre for Health Protection (CHP) of the Department of Health has announced that as of 0.00am, November 3, the CHP was investigating nine additional confirmed cases of coronavirus disease 2019 (COVID-19), taking the number of cases to 5 346 in Hong Kong so far (comprising 5 345 confirmed cases and one probable case).

Among the newly reported cases announced, six had a travel history during the incubation period.

The CHP's epidemiological investigations and relevant contact tracing on the confirmed cases are ongoing. For case details and contact tracing information, please see the Annex or the list of buildings with confirmed cases of COVID-19 in the past 14 days and the latest local situation of COVID-19 available on the website "COVID-19 Thematic Website" (www.coronavirus.gov.hk).

Meanwhile, starting from Thursday (November 5), the collection hours for deep throat saliva samples for COVID-19 testing in the 13 designated chest clinics or social hygiene/dermatological clinics under the DH will be extended to 9am to 1pm and 2pm to 3pm from Monday to Friday, and will remain as 9am to 11am on Saturdays, Sundays and public holidays.

A spokesman for the CHP said, "During the CHP's epidemiological investigations and relevant contact tracing on the confirmed cases, we will compile and upload (www.chp.gov.hk/files/pdf/building_list_eng.pdf) a list of buildings that confirmed patients had visited from two days before the onset of symptoms. Given that cases of local infection continue to occur from time to time, members of the public are urged to seek medical attention immediately if they believe that they had visited the same place at an identical time with a confirmed patient and feel unwell subsequently. If they remain asymptomatic but are concerned that they have been infected, they can also visit the Hospital Authority's designated general out-patient clinics (www.ha.org.hk/haho/ho/covid-19/GOPC_extend_EN.pdf) to obtain specimen collection packs and collect deep throat saliva specimens for free COVID-19 testing."

In view of the severe epidemic situation, the CHP called on members of the public to avoid going out, having social contact and dining out. They should put on a surgical mask and maintain stringent hand hygiene when they need to go out. The CHP strongly urged the elderly to stay home as far as possible and avoid going out. They should consider asking their family and friends to help with everyday tasks such as shopping for basic necessities.

The spokesman said, "Given that the situation of COVID-19 infection remains severe and that there is a continuous increase in the number of cases reported around the world, members of the public are strongly urged to avoid all non-essential travel outside Hong Kong.

"The CHP also strongly urges the public to maintain at all times strict personal and environmental hygiene, which is key to personal protection against infection and prevention of the spread of the disease in the community. On a personal level, members of the public should wear a surgical mask when having respiratory symptoms, taking public transport or staying in crowded places. They should also perform hand hygiene frequently, especially before touching the mouth, nose or eyes.

"As for household environmental hygiene, members of the public are advised to maintain drainage pipes properly, regularly pour water into drain outlets (U-traps) and cover all floor drain outlets when they are not in use. After using the toilet, they should put the toilet lid down before flushing to avoid spreading germs."

Moreover, the Government has launched the website "COVID-19 Thematic Website" (www.coronavirus.gov.hk) for announcing the latest updates on various news on COVID-19 infection and health advice to help the public understand the latest updates. Members of the public may also gain access to information via the COVID-19 WhatsApp Helpline launched by the Office of the Government Chief Information Officer. Simply by saving 9617 1823 in their phone contacts or clicking the link wa.me/85296171823?text=hi, they will be able to obtain information on COVID-19 as well as the "StayHomeSafe" mobile app and wristband via WhatsApp.

Issued at HKT 18:40

Public hospitals daily update on COVID-19 cases

****

The following is issued on behalf of the Hospital Authority:

As at 9am today (November 3), seven COVID-19 confirmed patients were discharged from hospital in the last 24 hours. So far, a total of 5 109 patients with confirmed or probable infection have been discharged.

At present, there are 625 negative pressure rooms in public hospitals with 1 121 negative pressure beds activated. A total of 93 confirmed patients are currently hospitalised in 19 public hospitals, among which nine patients are in critical condition, four are in serious condition and the remaining 80 patients are in stable condition.

The Hospital Authority will maintain close contact with the Centre for Health Protection to monitor the latest developments and to inform the public and healthcare workers on the latest information in a timely manner.

Details of the above-mentioned patients are as follows:

Patient condition	Case numbers
Discharged	5145, 5205, 5279, 5287, 5301, 5316, 5329
Critical	1989, 3496, 4433, 4706, 4833, 4937, 5110, 5185, 5273
Serious	4101, 4746, 4788, 5151

Issued at HKT 19:00

Government extends social distancing measures under Prevention and Control of Disease Ordinance

****

The Government will gazette directions and specifications under the Prevention and Control of Disease (Requirements and Directions) (Business and Premises) Regulation (Cap. 599F), the Prevention and Control of Disease (Prohibition on Group Gathering) Regulation (Cap. 599G) and the Prevention and Control of Disease (Wearing of Mask) Regulation (Cap. 599I) today (November 3) to maintain the social distancing measures currently in place. These measures will take effect at 0.00am on November 6 for a period of seven days till November 12.

A spokesman for the Food and Health Bureau said, "The local epidemic situation has continued to subside since mid-October, with the seven-day average number of locally confirmed cases staying at a low level. That said, new confirmed cases with unknown sources of infection have still been identified over the past week, indicating the existence of silent transmission chains in the community. In addition, it is worrying that the number of locally acquired cases has shown an increasing trend in recent days and that we are seeing small cluster outbreaks as a result of anti-epidemic fatigue and frequent social activities in the community. Meanwhile, the global epidemic situation has continued to worsen, with the number of new confirmed cases hitting a daily record high. The past 14 days have seen 80 imported cases involving new sources of infection. While we have enhanced the testing and quarantine requirements for travellers coming to Hong Kong, imported cases would continue to pose discernible public health risks to Hong Kong.

"Having regard to the fact that the epidemic continued to subside in October, we have relaxed the various social distancing measures under a refined and sophisticated approach in a gradual and orderly manner over the past weeks. The relaxation includes that under the latest round of measures which took effect last Friday, i.e. further extending the hours when dine-in services are allowed in catering business premises and relaxing the number of persons allowed to be seated together at one table therein, raising the total number of people allowed in catering business premises and some scheduled premises, resuming live performances and dancing activities in catering business premises and clubs or nightclubs, and allowing members of the public to do exercise in indoor sports premises and public skating rinks without wearing masks. While our intention is to allow members of the public to further resume social and economic activities as far as practicable under the new normal, with the relaxation of social distancing measures members of the public appeared to become less alert in combating the epidemic, especially during recent festive celebrations when non-compliance with infection control-related requirements and restrictions at some premises was observed. As the number of locally acquired cases has shown an increasing trend in recent days, indicating that the local epidemic situation has not yet fully come under control, it is difficult for us to further relax existing social distancing measures at this stage."

Taking into account the latest public health risk assessment, starting from this Friday (November 6), apart from refinements to the social distancing restrictions for spectator stands at public skating rinks, sports premises and swimming pools, the Government will maintain all other requirements and restrictions applicable to catering business and scheduled premises. The Government will continue to closely monitor the development of the epidemic situation and consider if there is room for relaxing social distancing measures in the next stage, subject to whether the epidemic situation is continually under control and the number of locally confirmed cases is maintained at a low level. If the epidemic situation fluctuates persistently and even shows signs of a rebound, the Government does not rule out tightening again the existing anti-epidemic measures including social distancing measures. As a rebound in the epidemic situation may bring about early the fourth wave of the local epidemic, which would likely coincide with the peak of the winter influenza season, such tightening of anti-epidemic measures may need to be pursued within a shorter period of time and to a larger extent as compared with the previous wave.

The spokesman added, "As we have stressed time and again, co-operation and self-discipline of members of the public are the keys to the effectiveness of social distancing measures in preventing the spread of the disease in the community. The public's concerted efforts in fighting the epidemic, staying vigilant in maintaining personal and environmental hygiene, and compliance with requirements and restrictions applicable to individual premises are of utmost importance. Otherwise, when there is another outbreak in the community, the Government will have no choice but to significantly tighten social distancing measures. At the same time, the Government continues to strengthen prevention and control measures in various areas. Amongst others, the preparations for setting up community testing centres are being made and the Government continues to enhance testing arrangements to assist members of the public to undergo testing in a more convenient and timely manner. We also call on the public to proactively get tested as soon as possible when having mild symptoms, so as to allow early identification of asymptomatic carriers in the community which will help further stabilise the epidemic situation."

Details of the aforementioned social distancing measures which are to be effective during the seven-day period from November 6 to 12, 2020, are as follows:

(I) Catering business and scheduled premises

(1) The requirements and restrictions applicable to catering business and scheduled premises (see Annex 1 for details) will be largely maintained during the seven-day period from November 6 to 12, 2020. Amongst others, facilities involving higher health risks such as steam and sauna facilities and ball pits will continue to be prohibited from opening. In addition, social distancing restrictions applicable to spectator stands at public skating rinks, sports premises and swimming pools will be aligned with those applicable to other places of public entertainment such as cinemas and performing venues, i.e. seats to be occupied must not exceed 75 per cent of the total seating capacity of the spectator stands, and no more than four consecutive seats in the same row may be occupied.

Persons responsible for carrying on catering businesses and managers of scheduled premises that contravene the statutory requirements under Cap. 599F would have committed a criminal offence. Offenders are subject to a maximum fine of $50,000 and imprisonment for six months.

(II) Group gatherings

(2) Unless exempted, the prohibition on group gatherings of more than four persons in public places will continue during the seven-day period from November 6 to 12, 2020.

Any person who participates in a prohibited group gathering; organises a prohibited group gathering; owns, controls or operates the place of such a gathering; and knowingly allows the taking place of such a gathering commits an offence under Cap. 599G. Offenders are liable to a maximum fine of $25,000 and imprisonment for six months. Persons who participate in a prohibited group gathering may discharge liability for the offence by paying a fixed penalty of $2,000.

(III) Mask-wearing requirement

(3) The mandatory mask-wearing requirement will be extended for a period of seven days from November 6 to 12, 2020. During the aforementioned period, a person must wear a mask all the time when the person is boarding or on board a public transport carrier, is entering or present in an MTR paid area, or is entering or present in a specified public place (i.e. all public places, save for outdoor public places in country parks and special areas as defined in section 2 of the Country Parks Ordinance (Cap. 208)).

Under Cap. 599I, if a person does not wear a mask in accordance with the requirement, an authorised person may deny that person from boarding a public transport carrier or entering the area concerned, as well as require that person to wear a mask and disembark from the carrier or leave the said area. A person in contravention of the relevant provision commits an offence and the maximum penalty is a fine at level 2 ($5,000). In addition, authorised public officers may issue fixed penalty notices to persons who do not wear a mask in accordance with the requirement and such persons may discharge liability for the offence by paying a fixed penalty of $2,000.

Issued at HKT 20:03

November 4[35]

CHP investigates three additional confirmed cases of COVID-19

****

The Centre for Health Protection (CHP) of the Department of Health has announced that as of 0.00am, November 4, the CHP was investigating three additional confirmed cases of coronavirus disease 2019 (COVID-19), taking the number of cases to 5 349 in Hong Kong so far (comprising 5 348 confirmed cases and one probable case).

Among the newly reported cases announced, one had a travel history during the incubation period. The other two were epidemiologically linked with a local case.

[35] https://www.info.gov.hk/gia/general/202011/04.htm

The CHP's epidemiological investigations and relevant contact tracing on the confirmed cases are ongoing. For case details and contact tracing information, please see the Annex or the list of buildings with confirmed cases of COVID-19 in the past 14 days and the latest local situation of COVID-19 available on the website "COVID-19 Thematic Website" (www.coronavirus.gov.hk)

A spokesman for the CHP said, "During the CHP's epidemiological investigations and relevant contact tracing on the confirmed cases, we will compile and upload (www.chp.gov.hk/files/pdf/building_list_eng.pdf) a list of buildings that confirmed patients had visited from two days before the onset of symptoms. Given that cases of local infection continue to occur from time to time, members of the public are urged to seek medical attention immediately if they believe that they had visited the same place at an identical time with a confirmed patient and feel unwell subsequently. If they remain asymptomatic but are concerned that they have been infected, they can also visit the Hospital Authority's designated general out-patient clinics (www.ha.org.hk/haho/ho/covid-19/GOPC_extend_EN.pdf) to obtain specimen collection packs and collect deep throat saliva specimens for free COVID-19 testing."

In view of the severe epidemic situation, the CHP called on members of the public to avoid going out, having social contact and dining out. They should put on a surgical mask and maintain stringent hand hygiene when they need to go out. The CHP strongly urged the elderly to stay home as far as possible and avoid going out. They should consider asking their family and friends to help with everyday tasks such as shopping for basic necessities.

The spokesman said, "Given that the situation of COVID-19 infection remains severe and that there is a continuous increase in the number of cases reported around the world, members of the public are strongly urged to avoid all non-essential travel outside Hong Kong

"The CHP also strongly urges the public to maintain at all times strict personal and environmental hygiene, which is key to personal protection against infection and prevention of the spread of the disease in the community. On a personal level, members of the public should wear a surgical mask when having respiratory symptoms, taking public transport or staying in crowded places. They should also perform hand hygiene frequently, especially before touching the mouth, nose or eyes.

"As for household environmental hygiene, members of the public are advised to maintain drainage pipes properly, regularly pour water into drain outlets (U-traps) and cover all floor drain outlets when they are not in use. After using the toilet, they should put the toilet lid down before flushing to avoid spreading germs."

Moreover, the Government has launched the website "COVID-19 Thematic Website" (www.coronavirus.gov.hk) for announcing the latest updates on various news on COVID-19 infection and health advice to help the public understand the latest updates. Members of the public may also gain access to information via the COVID-19 WhatsApp Helpline launched by the Office of the Government Chief Information Officer. Simply by saving 9617 1823 in their phone contacts or clicking the link wa.me/85296171823?text=hi, they will be able to obtain information on COVID-19 as well as the "StayHomeSafe" mobile app and wristband via WhatsApp.

Issued at HKT 14:15

FEHD actively promotes participation of bar and pub staff in virus testing

****

The Food and Environmental Hygiene Department (FEHD) today (November 4) announced that to actively promote the participation of bar and pub staff in the voluntary free COVID-19 testing, the FEHD and its testing agency, Prenetics Limited, will take the initiative to contact operators of bars and pubs to arrange testing services.

The FEHD met or communicated with a number of representatives of the bar and pub industry last week. All parties appreciated the fact that implementing effective anti-epidemic measures on critical control points could effectively help reduce the risk of virus transmission. The trade representatives also pledged to cooperate with the FEHD and the testing agency on the virus testing services for staff of bars and pubs.

The testing agency will be responsible for the provision of one-stop service covering specimen collection and testing. The testing agency will deliver specimen bottles to operators of bars and pubs for collecting deep throat saliva samples of their staff, and then collect the samples in the subsequent one to two days for testing. To boost the participation rate of the bar and pub targeted group, the testing agency will proactively visit various bars and pubs for two consecutive weeks starting this Friday (November 6) to carry out the work. Bar and pub operators may also call the testing agency's hotline (3008 8319) for enquiries or follow-up arrangements if necessary.

In addition, starting November 6, the testing agency will again arrange mobile vans to be parked in the following bar areas from Friday to Sunday nights for two consecutive weeks to distribute specimen bottles to bar and pub patrons:

November 6	near The Centrium, 60 Wyndham Street, Central
November 7	near 25 Kimberley Road, Tsim Sha Tsui
November 8	near 88 Lockhart Road, Wan Chai
November 13	near 38-40 Davis Street, Kennedy Town
November 14	near CTMA Centre, Sai Yeung Choi Street South, Mong Kok
November 15	near 36 Staunton street, Central

Patrons may return their specimen bottles by themselves to the mobile collection van of the testing agency parked at Hoi Chak Street in Quarry Bay from 9am to 5pm between November 7 and 17. Specimens with preliminary positive results will be relayed to the Public Health Laboratory Services Branch of the Department of Health to re-test and confirm the result. Positive cases will be followed up and announced by the Centre for Health Protection

Since October 1, the testing agency has delivered over 8 300 specimen bottles at over 420 bars and pubs, and collected about 5 400 specimens for testing.

An FEHD spokesman said that laying a solid foundation on anti-epidemic measures as early as possible could help the industry rise above the challenges of the epidemic situation steadily in the future. The spokesman strongly appealed to bar and pub operators to actively arrange for their staff to participate in the testing scheme, and continue to comply with the directions made under the Prevention and Control of Disease (Requirements and Directions) (Business and Premises) Regulation (Cap. 599F), to maintain personal and environmental hygiene continuously with a view to ensuring cleanliness of the premises, and to always remind their customers to comply with the requirements of the Prevention and Control of Disease (Prohibition on Group Gathering) Regulation (Cap. 599G).

Issued at HKT 14:52

LCQ22: Statistics and dissemination of information on epidemic
****

Following is a question by the Hon Chung Kwok-pan and a written reply by the Acting Secretary for Food and Health, Dr Chui Tak-yi, in the Legislative Council today (November 4):

Question:

The Centre for Health Protection has, to date, recorded over 5 000 as well as over 100 confirmed and fatal cases of coronavirus disease 2019 (COVID-19) respectively. Regarding the statistics and dissemination of information on the epidemic, will the Government inform this Council:

(1) of a breakdown of the total number of confirmed cases to date by the age group to which the patients belonged; the respective age groups with the highest recovery rate and highest mortality rate;

(2) as the findings of overseas medical studies have reportedly shown that obese people and elderly persons, upon contracting COVID-19, have a comparatively higher incidence of hospitalisation, developing severe symptoms and death (e.g. the mortality rate of patients aged above 65 is more than 90 times of those aged 18 to 29), whether the authorities have conducted

similar statistical analyses on the local confirmed cases; if so, of the details; and

(3) as some medical experts have pointed out that there may be a new wave of the epidemic outbreak in the winter, whether the authorities will consider providing the public with more information relating to the epidemic, such as the correlation between age and health condition and the morbidity and mortality rates, so that members of the public (in particular those belonging to high-risk groups) can take precautionary measures early?

Reply:

President,

Since the outbreak of COVID-19, the Government has been closely monitoring the development of the epidemic situation. Guided by the three key principles of responding promptly, staying alert to the situation and working in an open and transparent manner, and having regard to experts' advice, we have implemented decisive and appropriate measures to safeguard the public's health.

In consultation with the Hospital Authority (HA), my reply to the various parts of the question raised by the Hon Chung Kwok-pan is as follows:

(1) As at November 1, 2020, 5 331 confirmed cases of COVID-19 were reported in Hong Kong. The relevant number of confirmed cases, death cases and discharged cases respectively broken down by the age group to which the patients belonged to are set out in the table below. In view that the epidemic is still ongoing, the calculation of death rate and recovery rate may lead to bias in the analysis. Thus, the relevant figures cannot be provided.

	Age groups										
Type of cases	0 to 9	10 to 19	20 to 29	30 to 39	40 to 49	50 to 59	60 to 69	70 to 79	80 to 89	90 to 99	100 to 109
Confirmed cases (see Note 1 and 2)	214	383	869	890	811	847	785	322	153	56	1
Death cases	0	0	0	1	0	2	13	27	42	20	0
Discharged cases	210	376	856	864	796	835	752	272	105	35	1

Note 1: Including 1 probable case.
Note 2: 31 cases were not admitted to hospital, and one of them was a death case.

(2) Among the studies on COVID-19 supported by the Health and Medical Research Fund administered by the Food and Health Bureau, there are two projects titled "Nowcasting COVID-19 transmission dynamics, severity, and the effectiveness of control measures" and "Comprehensive clinical, virological, microbiological, immunological and laboratory monitoring of patients hospitalised with Coronavirus Diseases (COVID-19)" which estimate the fatality risk of different age groups and investigate the association among virus shedding, host factors, and clinical outcomes. The two projects will last for one year.

Among the studies, the project "Nowcasting COVID-19 transmission dynamics, severity, and the effectiveness of control measures" provides online a real-time snapshot on the age distribution of confirmed COVID-19 cases in Hong Kong (https://covid19.sph.hku.hk/). With respect to reported cases, so far over half of the cases were found in individuals from 20 to 59 years old, followed by elders of 60 years old or above with fewer cases found in young adults aged below 20 and children.

Moreover, the Centre for Health Protection (CHP) of the Department of Health (DH) has launched the "COVID-19 Thematic Website" (www.coronavirus.gov.hk/eng/index.html). It publishes daily on the thematic website the latest information related to COVID-19, including the number of confirmed cases, date of onset, case classification, etc.

(3) To enable members of the public to be well-informed about the development of the epidemic and get themselves prepared to fight the virus, the Government has launched the "COVID-19 Thematic Website" as a one-stop platform to integrate the latest information on COVID-19, as well as set up an Interactive Map Dashboard (https://chp-dashboard.geodata.gov.hk/covid-19/en.html) to consolidate information on the epidemic. Furthermore, the CHP and HA have been announcing the daily number of cases fulfilling the reporting criteria since January, and making regular reports to the public on the latest local epidemic situation via press conferences.

The CHP has issued guidelines reminding members of the public to observe good personal and environmental hygiene and disseminated health messages to them on preventing communicable diseases, social distancing, early testing and adapting to the new normal, etc. through various channels, including Announcements in the Public Interest on both television and radio stations, Facebook page, Instagram platform, YouTube channel and newspapers, etc. The CHP has also produced various health education materials for distribution in the community and maintained close liaison with different stakeholders.

Furthermore, to enable ethnic minorities (EM) to keep abreast of the health information announced by the Government, the main content of the "COVID-19 Thematic Website" has been translated into different languages, including Hindi, Nepali, Urdu, Thai, Bahasa Indonesia,

Tagalog, Sinhala, Bengali and Vietnamese. The CHP also promotes health messages to EM through EM groups and relevant organisations and religious groups, and provides health education materials on anti-epidemic measures to EM organisations for publication of newsletters and dissemination of information.

Issued at HKT 16:33

LCQ1: Anti-epidemic work in private buildings
****

Following is a question by the Hon Tony Tse and a reply by the Secretary for Development, Mr Michael Wong, in the Legislative Council today (November 4):

Question:

The Government indicated in April this year that it would commission consultancy firms to proactively inspect the external drainage pipes of 20 000 target private domestic and composite buildings across the territory (the inspection scheme) in order to reduce the risk of epidemic spreading. The Government has also allocated funding under the Anti-epidemic Fund for the creation of time-limited jobs to undertake the relevant tasks. Some members of the public have criticised the inspection scheme for not covering the repair works for problematic drainage pipes and the inadequacies in the number of buildings covered and the scope of inspection items. Regarding the anti-epidemic work in private buildings, will the Government inform this Council:

(1) of the implementation status of the inspection scheme, including the respective numbers of jobs created in various trades, the number of buildings inspected, the major problems uncovered in the drainage pipes, and the follow-up actions taken, so far; the total estimated expenditure and the anticipated completion date of the inspection scheme;

(2) whether it will expand the inspection scheme, including increasing the number of buildings covered and conducting more extensive epidemic prevention inspections on other common areas and facilities of the buildings (including lift lobbies, main gates, refuse chambers and ventilation systems); if not, of the reasons for that; an

(3) whether it will provide subsidies for private building owners who have financial difficulties to help them meet the expenses arising from repairing drainage pipes and enhancing the overall epidemic prevention standards and facilities of their buildings; if not, of the reasons for that?

Reply:

President,

Owners should take primary responsibility for the proper maintenance of their private properties, including regular inspection and maintenance of the drainage systems of their buildings to ensure that they are functioning well with a view to creating a safe and healthy living environment. Nevertheless, in face of the heightened public concerns about building drainage systems under the COVID-19, and the increasing unemployment rate in the construction industry due to economic downturn, the Government has launched a 24-month special measure through the second round of the Anti-epidemic Fund (AEF) to inspect the external drainage systems of buildings (the inspection scheme).

The inspection scheme upholds the concept of "prevention is better than cure". The consultants engaged by the Buildings Department (BD) will, as a large-scale "health check", proactively inspect the external drainage systems of around 20 000 private residential or composite buildings across the territory. If the drainage systems are found to be defective upon inspection, the BD may serve orders under the Buildings Ordinance (BO) (Cap 123) to the owners concerned requiring them to arrange necessary further investigations and/or repairs.

To step up public education and publicity, when inspecting the external drainage systems of buildings, staff of the BD's consultants will also dispatch relevant materials to owners or occupiers. The consultants will also provide telephone enquiry services to owners.

My reply to the three parts of the question is as follows:

(1) The estimated expenditure of the inspection scheme is around $300 million. Some 500 jobs for the construction industry, comprising 320 professional and technical jobs and 160 clerical jobs are expected to be created. The BD will also employ 36 professional, technical and clerical staff to implement the inspection scheme and undertake follow-up actions under the BO. Currently, the inspection scheme has created about 80 jobs for the construction industry and the BD has employed 20 staff. The remaining jobs will be created gradually as the BD awards more consultancy contracts for the inspection scheme. Furthermore, it is estimated that 2 000 repair works projects of various scale would be brought to the industry as individual buildings would need to repair the external drainage systems of their buildings subsequent to the implementation of the inspection scheme.

The inspection scheme has been implemented since June this year. The inspection of the 20 000 private residential or composite buildings is expected to be completed in the first quarter of 2022, and the related follow-up actions six months after. As at the end of September this year, the BD's consultants have inspected about 1 100 buildings. Defects at external drainage pipes, including leaking or broken drainage pipes, mis-connection of drainage pipes, etc., were found in some buildings. The BD is now reviewing the consultants' reports and will take appropriate actions under the BO, such as issuing drainage repair orders requiring owners concerned to carry out the necessary repair works depending on case circumstances.

(2) The inspection scheme has currently covered all private residential or composite buildings exceeding three storeys in height across the territory. Generally speaking, as the titles of private buildings not exceeding three storeys in height are in fewer hands or even solely owned, arrangement of personnel to inspect the building external drainage systems is easier. Commercial or industrial buildings are used for operating businesses. Generally speaking, inspection for such buildings could be relatively easily arranged amongst themselves through property management. The Government currently has no plan to expand the inspection scheme to other types of buildings such as commercial or industrial buildings.

The inspection scheme is targeted at the external drainage systems as disrepair at the external walls may not be detected by residents, and the external drainage systems could create significant impacts on building hygiene. Other common areas and facilities at the buildings, such as lift lobbies, main gates and refuse rooms could be inspected more readily. Regular cleaning and disinfection of the relevant areas and facilities is the most effective way to prevent them from becoming a medium for spreading virus. After all, the inspection scheme has to be targeted so that it could be commenced timely and completed in time to swiftly address public concerns on building drainage systems.

Apart from the inspection scheme, the BD under the AEF has a series of tasks, including to select, on top of the original 300 target buildings annually, 50 additional Category 2 buildings under the Operation Building Bright 2.0 between third quarter of 2020 and second quarter of 2021 for exercising its statutory power to conduct prescribed inspection and repair works under the Mandatory Building Inspection Scheme in default of the owners concerned; to expedite the discharge of non-compliant drainage repair orders and the cases of mis-connection of drainage systems; to enhance the efficiency of professional investigations on cases of water seepage in buildings, and to organise more public education and publicity activities, etc. Under the AEF, the BD will recruit a total of about 120 contract staff to meet the needs of the various tasks.

(3) Owners should take primary responsibility for the proper maintenance of their properties. Nevertheless, the Government recognises that some owners may have genuine difficulties in fulfilling their responsibility in maintaining their properties due to lack of financial means, technical knowledge and/or organisation ability. Therefore, apart from taking enforcement action to ensure that building owners would discharge their statutory responsibilities, the Government has also provided financial assistance to owners of private buildings to maintain and repair their buildings, including building drainage systems through various assistance and loan schemes. Key assistance and loan schemes comprise "Operation Building Bright 2.0", "Building Maintenance Grant Scheme for Needy Owners", "Building Safety Loan Scheme", and Urban Renewal Authority's "Home Renovation Interest-free Loan" and "Common Area Repair Works Subsidy".

These schemes can effectively assist needy owners to inspect and repair the drainage systems of their buildings.

Thank you, President.

Issued at HKT 17:00

Mobile vans to distribute and collect virus testing specimen bottles in Mui Wo and Tai Wai

****

In view of the recent development of the COVID-19 epidemic and based on risk assessment, the Government announced today (November 4) that a testing agency, Prenetics Limited, will be arranged to distribute and collect specimen bottles by mobile vans in Mui Wo and Tai Wai for three consecutive days from tomorrow (November 5), with a view to enabling and encouraging the residents of these districts or individuals who perceive themselves as having a higher risk of exposure to undergo virus testing.

The testing agency will go to Mui Wo and Tai Wai tomorrow to distribute and collect specimen bottles with the mobile vans parked at Mui Wo Recreation Centre and near Exit D of Tai Wai MTR station respectively. Members of the public may collect and return the specimen bottles free of charge from 10am to 5pm between November 5 and 7.

A Government spokesman said, "The testing agency will distribute specimen bottles to members of the public for deep throat saliva samples and then collect these samples at the same spot for testing. Positive cases identified will be immediately referred to the Centre for Health Protection under the Department of Health for follow-up."

The spokesman urged all individuals who were doubtful about their own health conditions to undergo the testing for the protection of themselves and others so that members of the public could fight the epidemic together.

Issued at HKT 19:01

Public hospitals daily update on COVID-19 cases

****

The following is issued on behalf of the Hospital Authority:

As at 9am today (November 4), nine COVID-19 confirmed patients were discharged from hospital in the last 24 hours. So far, a total of 5 118 patients with confirmed or probable infection have been discharged.

At present, there are 619 negative pressure rooms in public hospitals with 1 097 negative pressure beds activated. A total of 92 confirmed patients are currently hospitalised in 20 public hospitals, among which eight patients are in critical condition, three are in serious condition and the remaining 81 patients are in stable condition. In addition, a 70-year-old male patient (case number: 4433) confirmed with COVID-19 infection passed away in Tuen Mun Hospital at 7.12am today. Including this patient, 105 COVID-19 patients have passed away in public hospitals so far.

The Hospital Authority will maintain close contact with the Centre for Health Protection to monitor the latest developments and to inform the public and healthcare workers on the latest information in a timely manner.

Details of the above-mentioned patients are as follows:

Patient condition	Case numbers
Discharged	4383, 5143, 5245, 5248, 5262, 5265, 5298, 5326, 5345
Critical	1989, 3496, 4706, 4833, 4937, 5110, 5185, 5273
Serious	4101, 4788, 5151

Issued at HKT 19:05

November 5[36]

CHP investigates seven additional confirmed cases of COVID-19

****

[36] https://www.info.gov.hk/gia/general/202011/05.htm

The Centre for Health Protection (CHP) of the Department of Health has announced that as of 0.00am, November 5, the CHP was investigating seven additional confirmed cases of coronavirus disease 2019 (COVID-19), taking the number of cases to 5 356 in Hong Kong so far (comprising 5 355 confirmed cases and one probable case).

Among the newly reported cases announced, six had a travel history during the incubation period.

The CHP's epidemiological investigations and relevant contact tracing on the confirmed cases are ongoing. For case details and contact tracing information, please see the Annex or the list of buildings with confirmed cases of COVID-19 in the past 14 days and the latest local situation of COVID-19 available on the website "COVID-19 Thematic Website" (www.coronavirus.gov.hk).

Meanwhile, starting today, the collection hours for deep throat saliva samples for COVID-19 testing in the 13 designated chest clinics or social hygiene/dermatological clinics under the DH have been extended to 9am to 1pm and 2pm to 3pm from Monday to Friday, and remain as 9am to 11am on Saturdays, Sundays and public holidays. Locations of clinics are available on www.chp.gov.hk/files/pdf/list_of_collection_points_en.pdf.

A spokesman for the CHP said, "During the CHP's epidemiological investigations and relevant contact tracing on the confirmed cases, we will compile and upload (www.chp.gov.hk/files/pdf/building_list_eng.pdf) a list of buildings that confirmed patients had visited from two days before the onset of symptoms. Given that cases of local infection continue to occur from time to time, members of the public are urged to seek medical attention immediately if they believe that they had visited the same place at an identical time with a confirmed patient and feel unwell subsequently. If they remain asymptomatic but are concerned that they have been infected, they can also visit the Hospital Authority's designated general out-patient clinics (www.ha.org.hk/haho/ho/covid-19/GOPC_extend_EN.pdf) to obtain specimen collection packs and collect deep throat saliva specimens for free COVID-19 testing."

In view of the severe epidemic situation, the CHP called on members of the public to avoid going out, having social contact and dining out. They should put on a surgical mask and maintain stringent hand hygiene when they need to go out. The CHP strongly urged the elderly to stay home as far as possible and avoid going out. They should consider asking their family and friends to help with everyday tasks such as shopping for basic necessities.

The spokesman said, "Given that the situation of COVID-19 infection remains severe and that there is a continuous increase in the number of cases reported around the world, members of the public are strongly urged to avoid all non-essential travel outside Hong Kong.

"The CHP also strongly urges the public to maintain at all times strict personal and environmental hygiene, which is key to personal protection against infection and prevention of the spread of the disease in the community. On a personal level, members of the public should wear a surgical mask when having respiratory symptoms, taking public transport or staying in crowded places. They should also perform hand hygiene frequently, especially before touching the mouth, nose or eyes.

"As for household environmental hygiene, members of the public are advised to maintain drainage pipes properly, regularly pour water into drain outlets (U-traps) and cover all floor drain outlets when they are not in use. After using the toilet, they should put the toilet lid down before flushing to avoid spreading germs."

Moreover, the Government has launched the website "COVID-19 Thematic Website" (www.coronavirus.gov.hk) for announcing the latest updates on various news on COVID-19 infection and health advice to help the public understand the latest updates. Members of the public may also gain access to information via the COVID-19 WhatsApp Helpline launched by the Office of the Government Chief Information Officer. Simply by saving 9617 1823 in their phone contacts or clicking the link wa.me/85296171823?text=hi, they will be able to obtain information on COVID-19 as well as the "StayHomeSafe" mobile app and wristband via WhatsApp.

Issued at HKT 17:10

Public hospitals daily update on COVID-19 cases

****

The following is issued on behalf of the Hospital Authority:

As at 9am today (November 5), eight COVID-19 confirmed patients were discharged from hospital in the last 24 hours. So far, a total of 5 126 patients with confirmed or probable infection have been discharged.

At present, there are 619 negative pressure rooms in public hospitals with 1 097 negative pressure beds activated. A total of 87 confirmed patients are currently hospitalised in 20 public hospitals, among which eight patients are in critical condition, three are in serious condition and the remaining 76 patients are in stable condition.

The Hospital Authority will maintain close contact with the Centre for Health Protection to monitor the latest developments and to inform the public and healthcare workers on the latest information in a timely manner.

Details of the above-mentioned patients are as follows:

Patient condition	Case numbers
Discharged	4778, 4844, 5263, 5264, 5272, 5292, 5312, 5314

Critical	1989, 3496, 4706, 4833, 4937, 5110, 5185, 5273
Serious	4101, 4788, 5151

Issued at HKT 17:35

Princess Margaret Hospital announces passing away of COVID-19 patient

****

The following is issued on behalf of the Hospital Authority:

The spokesperson for the Princess Margaret Hospital (PMH) announced that a patient confirmed with COVID-19 passed away today (November 5).

A 78-year-old male patient (case number: 3585) with chronic illness was admitted to Caritas Medical Centre on August 2 after being tested positive for COVID-19. The patient was subsequently transferred to PMH for treatment on August 4. His condition continued to deteriorate and he eventually succumbed at 4.26pm today.

The hospital was saddened about the passing away of the patient and would offer necessary assistance to his family.

Including the above case, 106 COVID-19 confirmed patients have passed away in public hospitals so far.

Issued at HKT 20:35

November 6[37]

CHP investigates six additional confirmed cases of COVID-19

****

The Centre for Health Protection (CHP) of the Department of Health has announced that as of 0.00am, November 6, the CHP was investigating six additional confirmed cases of coronavirus

[37] https://www.info.gov.hk/gia/general/202011/06.htm

disease 2019 (COVID-19), taking the number of cases to 5 362 in Hong Kong so far (comprising 5 361 confirmed cases and one probable case).

All the newly reported cases announced had a travel history during the incubation period.

The CHP's epidemiological investigations and relevant contact tracing on the confirmed cases are ongoing. For case details and contact tracing information, please see the Annex or the list of buildings with confirmed cases of COVID-19 in the past 14 days and the latest local situation of COVID-19 available on the website "COVID-19 Thematic Website" (www.coronavirus.gov.hk).

A spokesman for the CHP said, "During the CHP's epidemiological investigations and relevant contact tracing on the confirmed cases, we will compile and upload (www.chp.gov.hk/files/pdf/building_list_eng.pdf) a list of buildings that confirmed patients had visited from two days before the onset of symptoms. Given that cases of local infection continue to occur from time to time, members of the public are urged to seek medical attention immediately if they believe that they had visited the same place at an identical time with a confirmed patient and feel unwell subsequently. If they remain asymptomatic but are concerned that they have been infected, they can also visit the Hospital Authority's designated general out-patient clinics (www.ha.org.hk/haho/ho/covid-19/GOPC_extend_EN.pdf) to obtain specimen collection packs and collect deep throat saliva specimens for free COVID-19 testing."

In view of the severe epidemic situation, the CHP called on members of the public to avoid going out, having social contact and dining out. They should put on a surgical mask and maintain stringent hand hygiene when they need to go out. The CHP strongly urged the elderly to stay home as far as possible and avoid going out. They should consider asking their family and friends to help with everyday tasks such as shopping for basic necessities.

The spokesman said, "Given that the situation of COVID-19 infection remains severe and that there is a continuous increase in the number of cases reported around the world, members of the public are strongly urged to avoid all non-essential travel outside Hong Kong.

"The CHP also strongly urges the public to maintain at all times strict personal and environmental hygiene, which is key to personal protection against infection and prevention of the spread of the disease in the community. On a personal level, members of the public should wear a surgical mask when having respiratory symptoms, taking public transport or staying in crowded places. They should also perform hand hygiene frequently, especially before touching the mouth, nose or eyes.

"As for household environmental hygiene, members of the public are advised to maintain drainage pipes properly, regularly pour water into drain outlets (U-traps) and cover all floor drain outlets when they are not in use. After using the toilet, they should put the toilet lid down before flushing to avoid spreading germs."

Moreover, the Government has launched the website "COVID-19 Thematic Website" (www.coronavirus.gov.hk) for announcing the latest updates on various news on COVID-19 infection and health advice to help the public understand the latest updates. Members of the public may also gain access to information via the COVID-19 WhatsApp Helpline launched by the Office of the Government Chief Information Officer. Simply by saving 9617 1823 in their phone contacts or clicking the link wa.me/85296171823?text=hi, they will be able to obtain information on COVID-19 as well as the "StayHomeSafe" mobile app and wristband via WhatsApp.

Issued at HKT 14:00

Public hospitals daily update on COVID-19 cases

****

The following is issued on behalf of the Hospital Authority:

As at 9am today (November 6), four COVID-19 confirmed patients were discharged from hospital in the last 24 hours. Including a patient (case number: 5350) discharged on November 4, a total of 5 131 patients with confirmed or probable infection have been discharged so far.

At present, there are 619 negative pressure rooms in public hospitals with 1 097 negative pressure beds activated. A total of 88 confirmed patients are currently hospitalised in 20 public hospitals, among which eight patients are in critical condition, four are in serious condition and the remaining 76 patients are in stable condition.

The Hospital Authority will maintain close contact with the Centre for Health Protection to monitor the latest developments and to inform the public and healthcare workers on the latest information in a timely manner.

Details of the above-mentioned patients are as follows:

Patient condition	Case numbers
Discharged	5290, 5293, 5344, 5350, 5355
Critical	1989, 3496, 4706, 4833, 4937, 5110, 5185, 5273
Serious	4101, 4788, 5151, 5282

Issued at HKT 16:18

November 7[38]

CHP investigates three additional confirmed cases of COVID-19

****

The Centre for Health Protection (CHP) of the Department of Health has announced that as of 0.00am, November 7, the CHP was investigating three additional confirmed cases of coronavirus disease 2019 (COVID-19), taking the number of cases to 5 365 in Hong Kong so far (comprising 5 364 confirmed cases and one probable case).

Among the newly reported cases announced, two had a travel history during the incubation period.

The CHP's epidemiological investigations and relevant contact tracing on the confirmed cases are ongoing. For case details and contact tracing information, please see the Annex or the list of buildings with confirmed cases of COVID-19 in the past 14 days and the latest local situation of COVID-19 available on the website "COVID-19 Thematic Website" (www.coronavirus.gov.hk).

A spokesman for the CHP said, "During the CHP's epidemiological investigations and relevant contact tracing on the confirmed cases, we will compile and upload (www.chp.gov.hk/files/pdf/building_list_eng.pdf) a list of buildings that confirmed patients had visited from two days before the onset of symptoms. Given that cases of local infection continue to occur from time to time, members of the public are urged to seek medical attention immediately if they believe that they had visited the same place at an identical time with a confirmed patient and feel unwell subsequently. If they remain asymptomatic but are concerned that they have been infected, they can also visit the Hospital Authority's designated general out-patient clinics (www.ha.org.hk/haho/ho/covid-19/GOPC_extend_EN.pdf) to obtain specimen collection packs and collect deep throat saliva specimens for free COVID-19 testing."

In view of the severe epidemic situation, the CHP called on members of the public to avoid going out, having social contact and dining out. They should put on a surgical mask and maintain stringent hand hygiene when they need to go out. The CHP strongly urged the elderly to stay home as far as possible and avoid going out. They should consider asking their family and friends to help with everyday tasks such as shopping for basic necessities.

The spokesman said, "Given that the situation of COVID-19 infection remains severe and that there is a continuous increase in the number of cases reported around the world, members of the public are strongly urged to avoid all non-essential travel outside Hong Kong.

"The CHP also strongly urges the public to maintain at all times strict personal and environmental hygiene, which is key to personal protection against infection and prevention of the spread of the disease in the community. On a personal level, members of the public should wear a surgical mask when having respiratory symptoms, taking public transport or staying in

[38] https://www.info.gov.hk/gia/general/202011/07.htm

crowded places. They should also perform hand hygiene frequently, especially before touching the mouth, nose or eyes.

"As for household environmental hygiene, members of the public are advised to maintain drainage pipes properly, regularly pour water into drain outlets (U-traps) and cover all floor drain outlets when they are not in use. After using the toilet, they should put the toilet lid down before flushing to avoid spreading germs."

Moreover, the Government has launched the website "COVID-19 Thematic Website" (www.coronavirus.gov.hk) for announcing the latest updates on various news on COVID-19 infection and health advice to help the public understand the latest updates. Members of the public may also gain access to information via the COVID-19 WhatsApp Helpline launched by the Office of the Government Chief Information Officer. Simply by saving 9617 1823 in their phone contacts or clicking the link wa.me/85296171823?text=hi, they will be able to obtain information on COVID-19 as well as the "StayHomeSafe" mobile app and wristband via WhatsApp.

Issued at HKT 17:17

Public hospitals daily update on COVID-19 cases
****

The following is issued on behalf of the Hospital Authority:

As at 9am today (November 7), seven COVID-19 confirmed patients were discharged from hospital in the last 24 hours. Including a patient (case number: 5358) discharged on November 5, a total of 5 139 patients with confirmed or probable infection have been discharged so far.

At present, there are 613 negative pressure rooms in public hospitals with 1 090 negative pressure beds activated. A total of 86 confirmed patients are currently hospitalised in 20 public hospitals, among which seven patients are in critical condition, five are in serious condition and the remaining 74 patients are in stable condition.

The Hospital Authority will maintain close contact with the Centre for Health Protection to monitor the latest developments and to inform the public and healthcare workers on the latest information in a timely manner.

Details of the above-mentioned patients are as follows:

Patient condition	Case numbers

Discharged	3420, 5180, 5286, 5288, 5295, 5296, 5299, 5358
Critical	1989, 3496, 4706, 4833, 4937, 5110, 5185
Serious	4101, 4788, 5151, 5273, 5282

Issued at HKT 17:30

November 8[39]

Mobile van to distribute and collect virus testing specimen bottles in Tai Po from this afternoon (with photos/video)

****

In view of the recent development of the COVID-19 epidemic and based on risk assessment, the Government will arrange a testing agency, Prenetics Limited, to distribute and collect deep throat saliva specimen bottles by mobile van in Tai Po for three consecutive days starting this afternoon (November 8), with a view to facilitating and encouraging residents of the district or individuals who perceive themselves as having a higher risk of exposure to undergo free COVID-19 testing.

The testing agency's mobile van will be parked near to the taxi station in front of Hang Seng Bank at 41 Kwong Fuk Road from 1.30 pm to 6 pm today. Members of the public may collect and return the specimen bottles free of charge. The mobile van will operate from 10 am to 5 pm between November 9 and November 10.

A government spokesman said, "The testing agency will distribute specimen bottles to members of the public for deep throat saliva samples and then collect these samples at the same spot for testing. Positive cases identified will be immediately referred to the Centre for Health Protection under the Department of Health for follow-up."

The spokesman urged all individuals who are doubtful about their own health conditions to undergo the testing for the protection of themselves and others and to fight the epidemic together.

---

[39] https://www.info.gov.hk/gia/general/202011/08.htm

Ends/Sunday, November 8, 2020

Issued at HKT 12:53

CHP investigates 10 additional confirmed cases of COVID-19

****

The Centre for Health Protection (CHP) of the Department of Health has announced that as of 0.00am, November 8, the CHP was investigating 10 additional confirmed cases of coronavirus disease 2019 (COVID-19), taking the number of cases to 5 375 in Hong Kong so far (comprising 5 374 confirmed cases and one probable case).

Among the newly reported cases announced, seven had a travel history during the incubation period. The remaining three cases were local cases with unknown sources.

The first case with unknown sources involves a 38-year-old woman (case 5 372) who had developed fever on October 19. The patient consulted a private doctor on November 5 and submitted a deep throat saliva sample on the following day. She works at Champion Tower on Garden Road in Central and last went to work on October 16.

The second case with unknown sources involves a 42-year-old woman (case 5 373). The patient sought medical attention at Pok Oi Hospital on November 5 and submitted a deep throat saliva sample on the following day. Her husband was a confirmed case earlier.

The third case with unknown sources involves a 50-year-old man (case 5 375) who had developed cough on October 28. The patient sought medical attention at Hong Kong Baptist Hospital on November 4 and submitted a deep throat saliva sample on the following day. He works at Everbright Centre on Gloucester Road in Wan Chai and last went to work on November 6.

The CHP's epidemiological investigations and relevant contact tracing on the confirmed cases are ongoing. For case details and contact tracing information, please see the Annex or the list of buildings with confirmed cases of COVID-19 in the past 14 days and the latest local situation of COVID-19 available on the website "COVID-19 Thematic Website" (www.coronavirus.gov.hk).

A spokesman for the CHP said, "During the CHP's epidemiological investigations and relevant contact tracing on the confirmed cases, we will compile and upload (www.chp.gov.hk/files/pdf/building_list_eng.pdf) a list of buildings that confirmed patients had visited from two days before the onset of symptoms. Given that cases of local infection continue to occur from time to time, members of the public are urged to seek medical attention immediately if they believe that they had visited the same place at an identical time with a confirmed patient and feel unwell subsequently. If they remain asymptomatic but are concerned that they have been infected, they can also visit the Hospital Authority's designated general out-patient clinics (www.ha.org.hk/haho/ho/covid-19/GOPC_extend_EN.pdf) to obtain specimen collection packs and collect deep throat saliva specimens for free COVID-19 testing."

In view of the severe epidemic situation, the CHP called on members of the public to avoid going out, having social contact and dining out. They should put on a surgical mask and maintain stringent hand hygiene when they need to go out. The CHP strongly urged the elderly to stay home as far as possible and avoid going out. They should consider asking their family and friends to help with everyday tasks such as shopping for basic necessities.

The spokesman said, "Given that the situation of COVID-19 infection remains severe and that there is a continuous increase in the number of cases reported around the world, members of the public are strongly urged to avoid all non-essential travel outside Hong Kong.

"The CHP also strongly urges the public to maintain at all times strict personal and environmental hygiene, which is key to personal protection against infection and prevention of the spread of the disease in the community. On a personal level, members of the public should wear a surgical mask when having respiratory symptoms, taking public transport or staying in crowded places. They should also perform hand hygiene frequently, especially before touching the mouth, nose or eyes.

"As for household environmental hygiene, members of the public are advised to maintain drainage pipes properly, regularly pour water into drain outlets (U-traps) and cover all floor drain outlets when they are not in use. After using the toilet, they should put the toilet lid down before flushing to avoid spreading germs."

Moreover, the Government has launched the website "COVID-19 Thematic Website" (www.coronavirus.gov.hk) for announcing the latest updates on various news on COVID-19 infection and health advice to help the public understand the latest updates. Members of the public may also gain access to information via the COVID-19 WhatsApp Helpline launched by the Office of the Government Chief Information Officer. Simply by saving 9617 1823 in their phone contacts or clicking the link wa.me/85296171823?text=hi, they will be able to obtain information on COVID-19 as well as the "StayHomeSafe" mobile app and wristband via WhatsApp.

Issued at HKT 14:00

Public hospitals daily update on COVID-19 cases

****

The following is issued on behalf of the Hospital Authority:

As at 9am today (November 8), five COVID-19 confirmed patients were discharged from hospital in the last 24 hours. So far, a total of 5 144 patients with confirmed or probable infection have been discharged.

At present, there are 613 negative pressure rooms in public hospitals with 1 090 negative pressure beds activated. A total of 84 confirmed patients are currently hospitalised in 20 public hospitals, among which seven patients are in critical condition, four are in serious condition and the remaining 73 patients are in stable condition.

The Hospital Authority will maintain close contact with the Centre for Health Protection to monitor the latest developments and to inform the public and healthcare workers on the latest information in a timely manner.

Details of the above-mentioned patients are as follows:

Patient condition	Case numbers
Discharged	4101, 5278, 5323, 5346, 5359
Critical	1989, 3496, 4706, 4833, 4937, 5110, 5185
Serious	4788, 5151, 5273, 5282

Issued at HKT 17:00

LCSD steps up patrols at public beaches to ensure users comply with anti-epidemic requirements

****

The Leisure and Cultural Services Department (LCSD) reopened all gazetted beaches under its management on November 3. The department has also stepped up patrols to call on users to comply with regulations on the limit of the number of people in group gatherings and the mask-wearing requirement.

The LCSD appeals to beach users to comply with the Prevention and Control of Disease (Prohibition on Group Gathering) Regulation (Cap 599G). The number of people in group gatherings should not be more than that as stipulated by the law. Members of the public should wear masks at all times when being present in any public place in accordance with the Prevention and Control of Disease (Wearing of Mask) Regulation (Cap 599I).

LCSD staff in collaboration with the Police yesterday and today (November 7 and 8), during patrols of public beaches, gave out verbal advice more than 800 times. The spokesman appealed to members of the public to exercise self-discipline in order to reduce the chances of spreading the virus in the community. The LCSD has stepped up cleaning work at the reopened beach facilities. Barbecue sites within gazetted beaches will continue to be closed. The LCSD also calls on members of the public to observe water safety. People should swim at the beaches only when lifeguard services are available. Please do not enter the water when the red flag is hoisted.

Issued at HKT 18:34

Mobile specimen collection stations to be set up in Tai Po from tomorrow

****

In view of a number of confirmed COVID-19 cases relating to residents in Tai Po recently, in order to identify cases in the community as early as possible to help cut the transmission chains, the Government will arrange a testing agency to provide free specimen collection and testing services through mobile specimen collection stations in Tai Po for three consecutive days starting tomorrow (November 9), with a view to facilitating and encouraging residents of the district or individuals who perceive themselves as having a higher risk of exposure to undergo free COVID-19 testing.

The testing agency (Hong Kong Molecular Pathology Diagnostic Centre Limited) will set up mobile stations at the following three locations: volleyball court next to Kwong Wai House of Kwong Fuk Estate; open space outside Fu Shin Community Hall; open space between the Pai Lau and the Pavilion of Wai Tau Tsuen. The mobile stations will operate from 10am to 5pm between November 9 and November 11. Members of the public may visit the mobile stations direct for on-site registration and specimen collections.

A government spokesman said, "The testing agency will provide specimen collection services by combined nasal and throat swab and testing services free of charge. If any specimen tested shows a positive COVID-19 result, the specimen will be referred to the Public Health Laboratory Services Branch of the Department of Health (DH) for a confirmatory test. Confirmed cases will be followed up and announced by the Centre for Health Protection of the DH."

At the same time, the mobile van run by testing agency (Prenetics Limited) will be parked near to the taxi station in front of Hang Seng Bank at 41 Kwong Fuk Road from 10am to 5pm on November 9 and 10 and will continue to distribute and collect deep throat saliva specimen bottles.

The spokesman urged all individuals who are doubtful about their own health conditions to undergo the testing for the protection of themselves and others and to fight the epidemic together.

Issued at HKT 23:58

November 9[40]

CHP investigates six additional confirmed cases of COVID-19

****

The Centre for Health Protection (CHP) of the Department of Health has announced that as of 0.00am, November 9, the CHP was investigating six additional confirmed cases of coronavirus disease 2019 (COVID-19), taking the number of cases to 5 381 in Hong Kong so far (comprising 5 380 confirmed cases and one probable case).

All the newly reported cases announced had a travel history during the incubation period.

The CHP's epidemiological investigations and relevant contact tracing on the confirmed cases are ongoing. For case details and contact tracing information, please see the Annex or the list of buildings with confirmed cases of COVID-19 in the past 14 days and the latest local situation of COVID-19 available on the website "COVID-19 Thematic Website" (www.coronavirus.gov.hk).

A spokesman for the CHP said, "During the CHP's epidemiological investigations and relevant contact tracing on the confirmed cases, we will compile and upload (www.chp.gov.hk/files/pdf/building_list_eng.pdf) a list of buildings that confirmed patients had visited from two days before the onset of symptoms. Given that cases of local infection continue to occur from time to time, members of the public are urged to seek medical attention immediately if they believe that they had visited the same place at an identical time with a confirmed patient and feel unwell subsequently. If they remain asymptomatic but are concerned that they have been infected, they can also visit the Hospital Authority's designated general out-patient clinics (www.ha.org.hk/haho/ho/covid-19/GOPC_extend_EN.pdf) to obtain specimen collection packs and collect deep throat saliva specimens for free COVID-19 testing."

In view of the severe epidemic situation, the CHP called on members of the public to avoid going out, having social contact and dining out. They should put on a surgical mask and maintain stringent hand hygiene when they need to go out. The CHP strongly urged the elderly to stay home as far as possible and avoid going out. They should consider asking their family and friends to help with everyday tasks such as shopping for basic necessities.

The spokesman said, "Given that the situation of COVID-19 infection remains severe and that there is a continuous increase in the number of cases reported around the world, members of the public are strongly urged to avoid all non-essential travel outside Hong Kong.

"The CHP also strongly urges the public to maintain at all times strict personal and environmental hygiene, which is key to personal protection against infection and prevention of

[40] https://www.info.gov.hk/gia/general/202011/09.htm

the spread of the disease in the community. On a personal level, members of the public should wear a surgical mask when having respiratory symptoms, taking public transport or staying in crowded places. They should also perform hand hygiene frequently, especially before touching the mouth, nose or eyes.

"As for household environmental hygiene, members of the public are advised to maintain drainage pipes properly, regularly pour water into drain outlets (U-traps) and cover all floor drain outlets when they are not in use. After using the toilet, they should put the toilet lid down before flushing to avoid spreading germs."

Moreover, the Government has launched the website "COVID-19 Thematic Website" (www.coronavirus.gov.hk) for announcing the latest updates on various news on COVID-19 infection and health advice to help the public understand the latest updates. Members of the public may also gain access to information via the COVID-19 WhatsApp Helpline launched by the Office of the Government Chief Information Officer. Simply by saving 9617 1823 in their phone contacts or clicking the link wa.me/85296171823?text=hi, they will be able to obtain information on COVID-19 as well as the "StayHomeSafe" mobile app and wristband via WhatsApp.

Issued at HKT 14:00

Government to provide medical consultation to HA's chronic disease patients living in Guangdong under COVID-19 epidemic

****

The Hong Kong Special Administrative Region Government announced the launch of the Special Support Scheme for chronic disease patients of the Hospital Authority (HA) residing in Guangdong Province starting from tomorrow (November 10). The Special Support Scheme aims to provide those patients with subsidised medical consultation under the COVID-19 epidemic.

Under the compulsory quarantine measures currently in force, some Hong Kong residents residing in Guangdong Province are unable to travel back and forth between Hong Kong and the Mainland for scheduled medical consultations at the outpatient clinics under the HA as they had done so previously. To ensure that the health conditions of these patients can be effectively monitored and taken care of in a continued and co-ordinated manner, the Government has appointed the University of Hong Kong-Shenzhen Hospital (HKU-SZH) to take up subsidised follow-up consultations for patients with scheduled appointments at designated Specialist Outpatient Clinics (SOPC) or General Outpatient Clinics (GOPC) under the HA.

The Special Support Scheme covers the majority of SOPC and GOPC services, namely anaesthesiology (pain clinic only); cardiothoracic surgery; clinical oncology; ear, nose and throat; eye; gynecology; medicine; neurosurgery; obstetrics; orthopaedics and traumatology; paediatrics, and surgery. Episodic illnesses, inpatient or day inpatient, and Accident and Emergency Departments services are not included.

HA patients with follow-up appointments at the HA's SOPCs or GOPCs between February 17, 2020, and July 31, 2021, may submit applications to the HKU-SZH along with the required supporting documents. Upon patients' consent, the HA will assist the HKU-SZH to verify the identity of the patients with their privacy fully protected during the process. Moreover, to ensure that appropriate treatments are provided for, patients may register for the Electronic Health Record Sharing System (eHRSS) through the HKU-SZH and make a data access request to the Electronic Health Record Office with authorisation for the HKU-SZH to receive copies of the medical records on their behalf. The medical records will be used by relevant healthcare staff in providing appropriate healthcare services.

Eligible patients under the Scheme are required to co-pay RMB100 as a consultation fee per each designated outpatient service at the HKU-SZH (except for specified persons whose medical fees would be waived upon verification by the HA). The rest of the medical fees are subsidised under the Special Support Scheme subject to a cap of RMB2,000 per patient.

The Special Support Scheme will be open for application at the HKU-SZH starting from tomorrow. Eligible persons may receive medical consultations at the HKU-SZH before July 31, 2021, or until the lapse of the quarantine requirement in both Hong Kong and the Mainland (whichever is earlier). The HKU-SZH will accord priority in arranging consultations for patients whose medical appointments are overdue. The Scheme aims to provide an alternative choice for medical services to the patients who are staying in Guangdong Province and unable to return to Hong Kong due to the epidemic situation. It is up to the patients to decide whether to join the Scheme. Such decisions will not affect their appointments previously made with the HA for follow-up medical services.

Details of the Scheme are available at the HA's website (www.ha.org.hk/goto/sss/en) or the HKU-SZH's website (www.hku-szh.org/en/index.html). For enquiries, please call the HA (tel: 2300 7070) between 9am and 6pm from Mondays to Fridays, excluding weekends and public holidays, or the HKU-SZH (tel: (+86) 0755-86913101) from 8am to 12.30pm and 2pm to 5.30pm on Mondays to Fridays, excluding weekends and public holidays.

Issued at HKT 15:21

HA enhances COVID-19 test service in Tai Po District

****

The following is issued on behalf of the Hospital Authority.

The Hospital Authority (HA) made the following announcement today (November 9) on enhancing the COVID-19 test service in Tai Po District to tie in with the Government's actions:

In view of the recent COVID-19 infection cases from an unknown source reported in Tai Po District, the HA has reminded healthcare workers of the general out-patient clinics (GOPCs) and the Accident and Emergency (A&E) Department in the district to stay vigilant and to arrange viral tests for patients where necessary.

Starting from today (November 9), the HA has enhanced the specimen collection pack distribution service in GOPCs in Tai Po District for three consecutive days by increasing the number of specimen collection packs to be distributed in the Tai Po Jockey Club GOPC and Wong Siu Ching Family Medicine Centre. Staff members will closely monitor the situation to co-ordinate the distribution of collection packs and collection of specimens. Members of the public presenting with symptoms should seek consultation at the A&E Department or GOPCs for test arrangements.

Following the Government's enhanced community testing service in the district, the HA would closely work with the Centre for Health Protection to provide medical services for confirmed patients who require hospitalisation.

Issued at HKT 17:15

Public hospitals daily update on COVID-19 cases
****

The following is issued on behalf of the Hospital Authority:

As at 9am today (November 9), one COVID-19 confirmed patient was discharged from hospital in the last 24 hours. Including a patient (case number: 5372) discharged on November 7, a total of 5 146 patients with confirmed or probable infection have been discharged so far.

At present, there are 613 negative pressure rooms in public hospitals with 1 090 negative pressure beds activated. A total of 92 confirmed patients are currently hospitalised in 20 public hospitals, among which seven patients are in critical condition, four are in serious condition and the remaining 81 patients are in stable condition.

The Hospital Authority will maintain close contact with the Centre for Health Protection to monitor the latest developments and to inform the public and healthcare workers on the latest information in a timely manner.

Details of the above-mentioned patients are as follows:

Patient condition	Case numbers

Discharged	5284, 5372
Critical	1989, 3496, 4706, 4833, 4937, 5110, 5185
Serious	4788, 5151, 5273, 5282

Issued at HKT 18:03

Woman sentenced for breaching compulsory quarantine order

****

A 53-year-old woman was sentenced to immediate imprisonment for 14 days by the West Kowloon Magistrates' Courts today (November 9) for violating the Compulsory Quarantine of Certain Persons Arriving at Hong Kong Regulation (Cap 599C) (the Regulation).

The woman was earlier issued a compulsory quarantine order stating that she must conduct quarantine at a hotel for 14 days. Before the expiry of the quarantine order, she left the place of quarantine to handle issues relating to her identity card at the office of the Immigration Department on October 6 without reasonable excuse nor permission given by an authorised officer. She was charged with contravening Sections 8(1) and 8(5) of the Regulation and was sentenced by the West Kowloon Magistrates' Courts today to immediate imprisonment for 14 days.

Pursuant to the Regulation, starting from February 8, save for exempted persons, all persons who have stayed in the Mainland, Macao or Taiwan in the 14 days preceding arrival in Hong Kong, regardless of their nationality or travel documents, will be subject to compulsory quarantine for 14 days. Moreover, pursuant to the Compulsory Quarantine of Persons Arriving at Hong Kong from Foreign Places Regulation (Cap 599E), starting from March 19, all persons arriving from countries or territories outside China would also be subject to compulsory quarantine for 14 days. Breaching a quarantine order is a criminal offence and offenders are subject to a maximum fine of $25,000 and imprisonment for six months.

A spokesman for the Department of Health said the sentence sends a clear message to the community that breaching a compulsory quarantine order is a criminal offence that the Government will not tolerate, and solemnly reminded the public to comply with the Regulation. As of today, a total of 64 persons have been convicted by the courts for breaching compulsory quarantine orders and have received sentences including immediate imprisonment for up to three months or a fine of $15,000. The spokesman reiterated that resolute actions will be taken against anyone who has breached the relevant regulations.

Issued at HKT 18:40

November 10[41]

CHP investigates nine additional confirmed cases of COVID-19

****

The Centre for Health Protection (CHP) of the Department of Health has announced that as of 0.00am, November 10, the CHP was investigating nine additional confirmed cases of coronavirus disease 2019 (COVID-19), taking the number of cases to 5 390 in Hong Kong so far (comprising 5 389 confirmed cases and one probable case).

Among the newly reported cases announced, four had a travel history during the incubation period. Three cases were epidemiologically linked with an imported case and two cases were epidemiologically linked with a local case

The CHP's epidemiological investigations and relevant contact tracing on the confirmed cases are ongoing. For case details and contact tracing information, please see the Annex or the list of buildings with confirmed cases of COVID-19 in the past 14 days and the latest local situation of COVID-19 available on the website "COVID-19 Thematic Website" (www.coronavirus.gov.hk).

A spokesman for the CHP said, "During the CHP's epidemiological investigations and relevant contact tracing on the confirmed cases, we will compile and upload (www.chp.gov.hk/files/pdf/building_list_eng.pdf) a list of buildings that confirmed patients had visited from two days before the onset of symptoms. Given that cases of local infection continue to occur from time to time, members of the public are urged to seek medical attention immediately if they believe that they had visited the same place at an identical time with a confirmed patient and feel unwell subsequently. If they remain asymptomatic but are concerned that they have been infected, they can also visit the Hospital Authority's designated general out-patient clinics (www.ha.org.hk/haho/ho/covid-19/GOPC_extend_EN.pdf) to obtain specimen collection packs and collect deep throat saliva specimens for free COVID-19 testing."

In view of the severe epidemic situation, the CHP called on members of the public to avoid going out, having social contact and dining out. They should put on a surgical mask and maintain stringent hand hygiene when they need to go out. The CHP strongly urged the elderly to stay home as far as possible and avoid going out. They should consider asking their family and friends to help with everyday tasks such as shopping for basic necessities.

The spokesman said, "Given that the situation of COVID-19 infection remains severe and that there is a continuous increase in the number of cases reported around the world, members of the public are strongly urged to avoid all non-essential travel outside Hong Kong.

[41] https://www.info.gov.hk/gia/general/202011/10.htm

"The CHP also strongly urges the public to maintain at all times strict personal and environmental hygiene, which is key to personal protection against infection and prevention of the spread of the disease in the community. On a personal level, members of the public should wear a surgical mask when having respiratory symptoms, taking public transport or staying in crowded places. They should also perform hand hygiene frequently, especially before touching the mouth, nose or eyes.

"As for household environmental hygiene, members of the public are advised to maintain drainage pipes properly, regularly pour water into drain outlets (U-traps) and cover all floor drain outlets when they are not in use. After using the toilet, they should put the toilet lid down before flushing to avoid spreading germs."

Moreover, the Government has launched the website "COVID-19 Thematic Website" (www.coronavirus.gov.hk) for announcing the latest updates on various news on COVID-19 infection and health advice to help the public understand the latest updates. Members of the public may also gain access to information via the COVID-19 WhatsApp Helpline launched by the Office of the Government Chief Information Officer. Simply by saving 9617 1823 in their phone contacts or clicking the link wa.me/85296171823?text=hi, they will be able to obtain information on COVID-19 as well as the "StayHomeSafe" mobile app and wristband via WhatsApp.

Issued at HKT 14:35

Public hospitals daily update on COVID-19 cases and YCH deceased patient

****

The following is issued on behalf of the Hospital Authority:

As at 9am today (November 10), seven COVID-19 confirmed patients were discharged from hospital in the last 24 hours. So far, a total of 5 153 patients with confirmed or probable infection have been discharged.

At present, there are 613 negative pressure rooms in public hospitals with 1 090 negative pressure beds activated. A total of 90 confirmed patients are currently hospitalised in 20 public hospitals, among which six patients are in critical condition, three are in serious condition and the remaining 81 patients are in stable condition.

Besides, an 88-year-old male patient (case number: 4937) confirmed with COVID-19 passed away in Yan Chai Hospital at 9.15pm last night. Including this patient, 107 COVID-19 patients have passed away in public hospitals so far.

The Hospital Authority will maintain close contact with the Centre for Health Protection to

monitor the latest developments and to inform the public and healthcare workers on the latest information in a timely manner.

Details of the above-mentioned patients are as follows:

Patient condition	Case numbers
Discharged	5218, 5305, 5318, 5339, 5357, 5364, 5378
Critical	1989, 3496, 4706, 4833, 5110, 5185
Serious	4788, 5151, 5282

Issued at HKT 16:20

November 11[42]

Designated flights under HK-Singapore Air Travel Bubble to launch November 22
****

The Governments of Hong Kong and Singapore today (November 11) announced the detailed arrangements of the bilateral Air Travel Bubble (ATB), with designated flights to be launched on November 22, taking a significant step forward in resuming cross-border air travel between the two places in an orderly manner

The Secretary for Commerce and Economic Development, Mr Edward Yau, said, "This is the very first ATB for Hong Kong. It matters not only for cross-border travel between the two places, but also reflects the Government's hope to progressively restore the city's economic activities amid the long-drawn battle against COVID-19.

"Hong Kong and Singapore are similar in terms of epidemic control. Both are regional aviation hubs and international cities, enjoying strong trade, investment, finance, tourism and people-to-people ties. The revival of cross-border air travel between the two places is of utmost importance. We hope that aviation, tourism, hotel, retail and catering businesses can benefit from it, thereby enabling Hong Kong's economy to recover gradually," he said

[42] https://www.info.gov.hk/gia/general/202011/11.htm

Under the ATB arrangement, travellers between the two places will not be subject to any quarantine arrangements upon arrival, nor restrictions to their travel purposes or itineraries on the condition that they comply with a set of anti-epidemic protocols.

There are stringent measures in place to safeguard public health under the arrangement, including mutually recognised COVID-19 tests, designated flights for ATB passengers as well as a scalable mechanism to adjust the ATB arrangement having regard to the epidemic situation. All measures are meant to resume cross-border air travel in a safe and progressive manner.

On COVID-19 testing, the ATB travellers must have tested negative in mutually recognised tests taken within 72 hours before their departure. They must also have no travel history to any places other than Singapore or Hong Kong in the last 14 days prior to their departure. The ATB travellers must travel on designated flights to minimise risks. The number of designated flights arriving at Hong Kong will increase progressively, from one flight per day in the first 15 days to two flights per day thereafter depending on the actual implementation. Each designated flight can carry a maximum of 200 ATB travellers. All ATB travellers must undertake COVID-19 tests again via a designated lane at the airport upon arrival at Hong Kong, and then wait at a restricted area of the airport until the receipt of negative test results so that they may leave the airport and start their itineraries.

In addition, the scalable mechanism put in place under the ATB arrangement allows the scale of the ATB to be instantly and flexibly adjusted depending on the epidemic situation of both places and travellers' demands. In short, if the seven-day moving average of the daily number of unlinked local COVID-19 cases is more than five for either Singapore or Hong Kong, the ATB arrangement will be suspended for two weeks. If the relevant figure reported on the last day of the suspension period does not exceed the specified threshold of five, the ATB arrangement can resume. Details of the ATB arrangement are set out in the Annex.

Mr Yau said that not only will the implementation of the ATB arrangement facilitate resumption of air travel between Hong Kong and Singapore, but will also help enable Hong Kong's discussions with places, with epidemic situations controlled, on resuming cross-border travel in an orderly manner.

To dovetail with the above development, the Government announced that the application deadline for the Travel Agents Incentive Scheme will be extended to March 31, 2021, to allow more travel agents to make full use of the scheme through inbound and outbound tours.

Issued at HKT 10:33

Launch of "LeaveHomeSafe" COVID-19 exposure notification mobile app

****

The Government announced today (November 11) the launch of the "LeaveHomeSafe" COVID-19 exposure notification mobile app. Tapping technology to combat the pandemic, the app aims to encourage the public to keep a more precise record of their whereabouts, minimising the risk of further transmission of the virus and protect Hong Kong together. The "LeaveHomeSafe " mobile app will be available for public download from November 16.

There are currently over 6 000 public and private venues that have pledged support for the scheme. The mobile app can also be used directly in over 18 000 taxis. The Government has been actively engaging with trades and businesses, and would welcome more sectors to participate in the scheme and contribute to the epidemic prevention and control work in Hong Kong.

Development of the "LeaveHomeSafe" mobile app is led by the Office of the Government Chief Information Officer. Characterised by voluntary participation and recording visits at users' discretion, it is a digital tool to record accurately the date and time for checking into and leaving different venues. The app is easy to use and can be downloaded for free. App users can check into venues by scanning the venue QR code to log their arrival time and clicking the "Leave" button in the app to mark their departure. Relevant data will then be kept in the app inside the user's mobile phone.

Passengers and taxi drivers can use the app to scan the registration mark located inside the taxi door and click the "Leave" button in the app upon arrival to record their journey.

If a confirmed case is later discovered at a participating venue, the app will notify users who have visited the same venue as the COVID-19 confirmed case at around the same time together with health advice to enhance their vigilance.

The "LeaveHomeSafe" mobile app upholds the principle of protecting personal data privacy, and user registration is not required. The app will not use positioning services or any other data of the users' mobile phones. Venue check-in data will be encrypted and saved on users' devices only. Such data will not be uploaded to the Government or any other systems. Check-in data will be kept in users' mobile phones for 31 days and will then be erased automatically.

The Centre for Health Protection will also release information on premises visited by COVID-19 confirmed cases in the form of open data, regardless of whether those confirmed cases are users of the "LeaveHomeSafe" mobile app or not. The app will send notifications to users who visited the same venues at around the same time as the confirmed cases.

Participating public venues include government office buildings, sports centres, swimming pools, libraries, markets, cooked food markets, community halls/centres, building lobbies and shopping centres of public housing estates, hospitals, clinics, post offices, public works and construction sites. Other participating venues from various sectors and businesses include restaurants, bars or pubs, karaoke establishments, clubs, fitness centres and banks. Venue QR codes will be posted at the participating locations for the public to scan via the app.

The "LeaveHomeSafe" mobile app supports iOS, Android and Huawei mobile devices and will be available for public download from November 16. More details are available on the "LeaveHomeSafe" website (www.leavehomesafe.gov.hk).

Issued at HKT 13:50

LCQ14: COVID-19 Online Dispute Resolution Scheme

****

Following is a question by the Hon Yung Hoi-yan and a written reply by the Secretary for Justice, Ms Teresa Cheng, SC, in the Legislative Council today (November 11):

Question:

The COVID-19 Online Dispute Resolution (ODR) Scheme, established under the Anti-epidemic Fund by the Government, was launched on June 29 this year. Under the Scheme, an arbitration and mediation institution has been appointed to provide speedy ODR services to micro, small and medium-sized enterprises as well as members of the public. The following conditions are to be met for disputes to be admitted under the Scheme: (i) the dispute is related to the Coronavirus Disease 2019 (COVID-19), (ii) the claim amount does not exceed $500,000, and (iii) either one of the parties involved in the dispute is a Hong Kong resident or company. The parties involved are required to pay $200 each as registration fee, while the fees for the mediators and arbitrators will be paid by the Government. In this connection, will the Government inform this Council:

(1) whether it knows the number of cases received so far under the Scheme, with a tabulated breakdown by (i) the group to which the claim amount belongs (each group spanning $100,000), (ii) the type of dispute, and (iii) whether or not either one of the parties involved is a resident or company from (a) the Mainland or (b) an overseas country/region; of the public expenditure incurred so far on the Scheme;

(2) whether it knows, among those cases mentioned in (1), the respective total numbers of cases (a) admitted and (b) rejected; among the cases admitted, the respective numbers of those in which the parties involved (i) are negotiating, (ii) are receiving mediation, (iii) have reached a settlement, (iv) are undergoing arbitration, and (v) have obtained an arbitral award, in respect of their disputes; regarding those cases in which a settlement has been reached, the major types of disputes involved, the average overall processing time for such cases, and the range of the claim amounts agreed to by the parties involved;

(3) whether it knows the respective numbers of arbitrators and mediators participating in the Scheme, with a breakdown by the professional qualifications they possess; whether they are required to undergo any special training and examination before participating in the Scheme; if so, of the details of such training and the passing rate of such examination;

(4) whether it knows the respective to-date numbers and percentages of arbitrators and mediators who have provided services under the Scheme; and

(5) whether it has reviewed, in respect of the Scheme, the response received since its launch, its cost effectiveness and whether its objectives have been achieved; if it has reviewed, of the outcome, and the Government's follow-up measures; if it has not reviewed, the reasons for that?

Reply:

President,

It is a global trend to develop and use online dispute resolution (ODR) services to provide a reliable and efficient platform to facilitate alternative dispute resolution (ADR). In light of the pandemic's impact on the economy and in anticipation of an upsurge of disputes arising from or relating to the pandemic, the Government announced on April 8, 2020 the establishment of the COVID-19 Online Dispute Resolution Scheme (Scheme) under the second round of the Anti-epidemic Fund to provide speedy and cost effective ODR services to the general public and businesses, in particular micro, small and medium-sized enterprises. The Scheme starts from negotiation and mediation so as to prevent entrenched views on the conflicts, thereby helping to foster harmony in society. It also provides an ADR mechanism which may help relieve the Court's caseload in civil claims.

On May 18, 2020, the Department of Justice (DoJ) and eBRAM International Online Dispute Resolution Centre Limited (eBRAM Centre) entered into a Memorandum of Understanding (MoU) on the Scheme to govern and monitor the use of the relevant funding. A funding support totalling $70 million was provided, including (i) $50 million covering the cost of the first 12 months of platform development and initial set-up (including staff), as well as the operation cost in the first year; and (ii) $20 million covering the fees of mediators and arbitrators for an estimate of 2,000 cases in the first year. After the platform has been established and in operation for one year, eBRAM Centre may continue to make use of the platform for other purposes, for example for serving the Asia-Pacific Economic Cooperation (APEC) economies after eBRAM Centre is listed under the APEC Collaborative Framework for ODR. eBRAM Centre may also adapt and make necessary modifications to the platform to handle other cases beyond the Scheme.

The Scheme was launched on June 29, 2020

In relation to the Hon Yung Hoi-yan's questions, the DoJ replies as follows:

(1) to (4) According to the MoU entered into by eBRAM Centre and the Government in May 2020, eBRAM Centre is required to regularly report to the Government on the progress of the Scheme. As the Scheme was launched only less than half a year ago, eBRAM Centre is still in the process of compiling the relevant statistics. It plans to report the latest progress of the Scheme, including the relevant statistics and details, to the Legislative Council Panel on Administration of Justice and Legal Services later this year

According to the preliminary information provided by eBRAM Centre, since the launch of the Scheme, over 150 mediators and arbitrators have been enlisted in the Scheme and the training provided by eBRAM Centre to them has also been completed. The arbitrators and mediators enlisted in the Scheme come from different sectors, while those from the legal sector account for the majority. All of the participants are selected from the lists of arbitrators and mediators maintained by the Hong Kong International Arbitration Centre, Hong Kong Bar Association and the Law Society of Hong Kong, and are professionals who have passed the assessment and possess sufficient experience in arbitration and mediation. Before their eligibility to participate in the Scheme is confirmed, participants must first complete the training course provided by eBRAM Centre. The content of the training course includes understanding of the eBRAM Rules for the Scheme, the arbitration and mediation process and operational guidelines of the online platform, as well as recent developments of ODR etc. The training course was conducted online and was delivered by senior arbitrators, mediators of the sector and prominent academics in the field of ODR. All of the arbitrators and mediators enlisted in the Scheme had passed the training course provided by eBRAM Centre eventually.

(5) As afore-mentioned, the Scheme aims to provide the general public and businesses that are involved in disputes arising from or in relation to the pandemic with a speedy and cost-effective means to resolve such disputes by deploying ODR. The Scheme also provides the benefits of job creation and job advancement for the legal and dispute resolution sectors including mediators, arbitrators and their pupils. At the same time, the DoJ hopes to, through the Scheme, facilitate the development of Hong Kong's ODR services and enhance Hong Kong's LawTech capability.

The Scheme was launched less than half a year ago and is still at its initial stage. We are delighted that the Scheme received very positive response from the general public. The Scheme has also successfully aroused the interest of relevant stakeholders as the number of inquiries and applications received by eBRAM Centre have been on the rise. The DoJ will continue to work closely with eBRAM Centre to jointly promote the Scheme.

eBRAM Centre has been proactively promoting the Scheme locally, to the Mainland and globally through various means and channels, including actively participating in various types of webinars (for example the China International Fair for Trade in Services 2020's Mainland-Hong Kong Services Industry Forum 2020, In-House Community e-Congress Japan 2020 and In-

House Community e-Congress Hong Kong 2020). Furthermore, eBRAM Centre also promoted the Scheme through interviews with different media and with various chambers of commerce in Hong Kong. Currently, eBRAM Centre has reached consensus with relevant local organisations and bodies to jointly further promote the Scheme.

Moreover, the Scheme has helped advance the relevant skills and capabilities of mediators and arbitrators, as well as facilitated the development of an ODR platform by eBRAM Centre, which signifies an important milestone for Hong Kong's ODR services development. The DoJ will continue to monitor the progress of the Scheme and conduct timely review of its effectiveness.

Issued at HKT 14:25

LCQ3: Coping with the Coronavirus Disease 2019
****

Following is a question by Ir Dr the Hon Lo Wai-kwok and a reply by the Secretary for Food and Health, Professor Sophia Chan, in the Legislative Council today (November 11):

Question:

Last month, the Secretary for Commerce and Economic Development indicated that, in order to facilitate the movement of people between Hong Kong and other parts of the world, the Government was studying the introduction of a rapid nucleic acid test for Coronavirus Disease 2019 (COVID-19) at the airport. In this connection, will the Government inform this Council:

(1) of the details of the relevant study, including the progress made so far and the implementation timetable; whether it will study the provision of rapid test services at all boundary control points; if so, of the details; if not, the reasons for that;

(2) as the World Health Organization (WHO) announced in September this year that affordable antigen rapid test kits, which were to be priced at a maximum of about HK$40 per unit and could provide results in 15 to 30 minutes, would be made available for low and middle-income countries, whether the Government has gained an understanding from WHO of the suitability of using such test kits in Hong Kong and discussed with it the procurement arrangements; if so, of the details; if not, the reasons for that; and

(3) whether it will allocate additional resources to promote the collaboration between local universities and research institutions in the research and development of rapid test kits, vaccines and drugs for COVID-19; if so, of the details; if not, the reasons for that?

Reply:

President,

The Government's priority at the moment is to incorporate disease prevention and control and infection management into the new normal of the day-to-day operation of society with an aim to minimising new cases as far as possible. Adhering to the principle of "preventing the importation of cases and the spreading of the virus in the community", on one hand, we have strictly implemented epidemic control measures at various boundary control points, including testing and quarantine for inbound travelers to suppress any chance that the virus might enter the community. On the other hand, we have continued to implement various prevention and control measures, including monitoring and surveillance, targeted group testing, social distancing measures, etc., in accordance with the principle of "early identification, early isolation and early treatment of the infected" to prevent the spread of the virus in the community

The Government has been implementing suitable cross-boundary control measures having regard to the epidemic situation to prevent importation of COVID-19 cases. Although we have now restricted the entry of foreigners who are non-Hong Kong residents, there are still local residents who continue to return to Hong Kong from abroad, and quite a number of them are returning from places with severe epidemic situations. The continued risk of importation of the virus and infected patients has created considerable strain on disease prevention and control in Hong Kong. As the epidemic is still rampant across the globe, Hong Kong will need to continue to strictly implement entry testing and quarantine arrangements for some time. At the same time, we must allow limited cross-boundary people flow having regard to actual needs with the implementation of risk control measures.

In consultation with the Innovation and Technology Bureau, our reply to the various parts of the question raised by Ir Dr the Hon Lo Wai-kwok is as follows:

(1) At present, all persons arriving at the Hong Kong International Airport (HKIA) are required to undertake testing for COVID-19. Currently, the arrival testing is based on a nucleic acid test using the reverse transcription polymerase chain reaction (RT-PCR) technique, which normally takes a few hours. With the exception of a few exempted persons (e.g. Government officials and consular corps), the majority of persons entering Hong Kong must wait for the test results before leaving the airport (i.e. the "test-and-hold" arrangement).

As it is necessary to continue the arrival testing arrangement to prevent the importation of virus, and with an increase in the number of travellers who need to undertake testing under various entry facilitating measures such as "travel bubbles", the Government has been closely monitoring the development of various COVID-19 testing technologies. The goal is to adopt faster and reliable testing technologies where appropriate, in order to ensure prevention of importation of cases with controllable risks while facilitating travellers as far as practicable.

After a preliminary assessment conducted by the Department of Health (DH), a trial run of a nucleic acid test using reverse transcription loop-mediated isothermal amplification (RT-LAMP) technique began at HKIA on October 28. The trial run was conducted in parallel with the RT-PCR nucleic acid test, which is the highest standard currently used by the DH to examine the sensitivity and reliability of the RT-LAMP technique. During the trial, passengers were still required to wait for a negative RT-PCR test result before proceeding to compulsory quarantine. The trial run was expected to last for two weeks, and may be extended subject to the amount of data gathered during the trial period. We will study the data collected from the trial, and assess the efficacy of the testing technique and the feasibility for applying it to different uses, including testing for arriving passengers.

As regards the identification of rapid test technologies, the Government and the Airport Authority Hong Kong are open to any testing technologies that have the potential in achieving a level of sensitivity and specificity suitable for boundary screening purposes.

(2) On nucleic acid tests, laboratories in Hong Kong are using the nucleic acid test which is adopted as the reference method. Although the World Health Organization (WHO) considered that antigen tests could expand the scope of testing, particularly in countries that do not have extensive laboratory facilities or trained health workers to implement molecular (polymerase-chain reaction) tests, the WHO guidance published on September 11 reiterated that antigen tests are only valuable in areas where community transmission is widespread and where nucleic acid testing is either unavailable or where test results are significantly delayed. The Government will closely monitor the latest development of the technology concerned.

(3) In order to combat the epidemic, since April 2020, the Health and Medical Research Fund (HMRF) administered by the Food and Health Bureau has approved a total funding of $47 million to support four local universities to conduct 11 studies relating to the testing methods, vaccines and antivirals of COVID-19. The HMRF will suitably allocate additional resources to support research in these areas in order to complement the Government's work in combating the epidemic.

On the other hand, through the Innovation and Technology Fund (ITF), the Innovation and Technology Commission (ITC) has provided funding support for local Research and Development (R&D) centres, universities, other designated local public research institutes and private companies to conduct R&D projects. From 2017-18 to 2019-20, the ITF has funded 35 public health-related R&D projects, involving funding of about $75.4 million.

Besides, the ITC launched a special call for projects under the Public Sector Trial Scheme in March this year to support product development and application of technologies for the prevention and control of the epidemic. In August this year, the ITF also supported in-principle a COVID-19 related project on the development of technology for vaccine production.

Thank you, President.

Issued at HKT 15:10

Four community testing centres to commence service this Sunday

****

Four community testing centres set up by the Government on Hong Kong Island and in Kowloon, New Territories East and New Territories West will commence service at 8am on November 15 (Sunday).

The four community testing centres will be located at Quarry Bay Community Hall in Eastern District, Henry G Leong Yaumatei Community Centre, Lek Yuen Community Hall in Sha Tin and Yuen Long Town East Community Hall respectively. The community testing centres will mainly provide self-paid testing services for the public at a more affordable price to serve general community or private purposes such as certification for travelling or work. The price of testing services will be capped at $240, with payment to be made in accordance with the arrangement of testing contractors. The Government will also, as and when necessary (such as in situations with higher risks of community transmission), conduct testing for target groups, specified persons or other members of the public at the testing centres for public health reasons on a needs basis, and separate announcements will be made at that time. The four testing centres will operate for an initial period of three months, which may be extended for another three months depending on the situation.

A Government spokesman said, "Through the provision of venues by the Government and competitive tendering, the price of self-paid testing services at the community testing centres has been substantially reduced to $240. The community testing centres also enable the Government to meet unexpected testing demand in a more efficient and flexible manner, with a view to strengthening disease prevention and control in Hong Kong."

The community testing centres will provide specimen collection services (using combined nasal and throat swabs) and COVID-19 testing services for all asymptomatic individuals (excluding children under 6 years old and people not suitable for testing) holding valid Hong Kong identity cards, Hong Kong birth certificates or other valid identity documents (including Hong Kong residents and non-Hong Kong residents). The centres will be open daily from 8am to 1.30pm and from 2.30pm to 8pm. Deep cleaning and disinfection will be conducted when they close in the afternoon and at night.

Booking and walk-in services will be available. Bookings can only be made by holders of a Hong Kong identity card or a Hong Kong birth certificate. With the launch of the 24-hour booking system (www.communitytest.gov.hk) today (November 11), members of the public only need to provide simple personal information (including their name, Hong Kong identity card or Hong Kong birth certificate number and phone number) to select the testing centre and time slot. They may also visit the testing centres direct for on-site registration and testing. Participants with a negative result will receive a test report for a COVID-19 nucleic acid test within 24 hours. Those who test positive as confirmed by the Department of Health (DH) will receive calls from the DH to arrange for isolation and treatment in public hospitals in accordance with established procedures.

For enquiries, please call the following hotlines of the community testing centres:

Quarry Bay Community Hall, Eastern District (Prenetics)	3008 8325
Henry G Leong Yaumatei Community Centre (Kingmed Diagnostics (Hong Kong) Limited)	9869 3603
Lek Yuen Community Hall, Sha Tin (Hong Kong Molecular Pathology Diagnostic Centre Limited)	2986 1272 2986 1270
Yuen Long Town East Community Hall (BGI)	2818 9690

Issued at HKT 16:54

Government announces "Return2hk - Travel Scheme for Hong Kong Residents returning from Guangdong Province or Macao without being subject to quarantine under the Compulsory Quarantine of Certain Persons Arriving at Hong Kong Regulation (Cap. 599C)"

****

The Government today (November 11) announced the introduction of "Return2hk – Travel Scheme for Hong Kong Residents returning from Guangdong Province or Macao without being subject to quarantine under the Compulsory Quarantine of Certain Persons Arriving at Hong Kong Regulation (Cap. 599C)" (Return2hk Scheme). Starting from November 23 (Monday), Hong Kong residents who, upon fulfilment of the conditions specified under sections 12(2) and 12A of the Regulation, including not having been to places other than Hong Kong, Guangdong Province or Macao in the past 14 days, could be exempted from the 14-day compulsory quarantine requirement when they return to Hong Kong under the Return2hk Scheme.

To ensure that Hong Kong residents who are currently in Guangdong Province or Macao would be returning to Hong Kong in a gradual and orderly manner to avoid increased public health risks at overcrowded ports, a quota arrangement will be put in place to control the number of cross-boundary travellers during the initial stage of the implementation of the Return2hk Scheme. A daily quota of 3 000 has been set for the Shenzhen Bay Port, while that for the Hong Kong-Zhuhai-Macao Bridge (HZMB) Hong Kong Port is 2 000.

Hong Kong residents who wish to return to Hong Kong under the Return2hk Scheme should apply for a quota using the online booking system. The online booking system will be open every Wednesday at 9am until Friday at 6pm to accept quota applications for the seven-day period of the following week (i.e. Monday to Sunday). The first batch of quotas will be opened for booking from November 18 to November 21. Successful quota applicants who also fulfil other specified conditions would be exempted from the 14-day compulsory quarantine requirement when they return to Hong Kong from Guangdong Province or Macao on November 23 at the earliest.

Any Hong Kong residents who are 18 or above may apply for a quota through the Return2hk Scheme booking system during the above-mentioned opening hours of the system. When making an application, the applicant is required to provide his/her Hong Kong Identity Card number, and to specify the date and the boundary control point (i.e. the Shenzhen Bay Port or the HZMB Hong Kong Port) to be used for the return. In the same application, he/she may also apply for the quota for three accompanying Hong Kong residents at most. Applications for Hong Kong residents who are under 18 should be made on their behalf by their parents or guardians, and the number of their Hong Kong Identity Card or other personal identity document(s) (e.g. HKSAR passport, HKSAR re-entry permit, birth certificate, other passports) should be provided. Quotas are administered on a first-come-first-served basis.

The Government spokesman reminded Hong Kong residents who have successfully applied for a quota to allow sufficient time for taking a COVID-19 (RT-PCR) nucleic acid test at one of the medical institutions mutually recognised by the Governments of Hong Kong and Guangdong, and, Hong Kong and Macao, such that he/she can present the proof of a valid negative nucleic acid test result upon arrival in Hong Kong. The sample should be taken within three days prior to, or on the day of the person's entry into Hong Kong. The list of recognised medical or testing institutions in Guangdong Province is available at www.coronavirus.gov.hk/pdf/List_of_recognised_laboratories_GD.pdf; whereas the list of recognised medical or testing institutions in Macao is available at www.coronavirus.gov.hk/pdf/List_of_recognised_laboratories_MO.pdf.

Hong Kong residents with a quota must return to Hong Kong on the date and at the boundary control point as specified in the booking, and they should present their Hong Kong Identity Card or other identification documents and the confirmation of a successful booking (i.e. a printout of the booking confirmation page). Before arriving at the boundary control point, they should transmit a valid negative COVID-19 nucleic acid test result to the electronic health declaration system of the Department of Health through "Yuekang code" (粵康碼) or "Macao health code" (澳康碼), and fill in all other required information for completing the health declaration. A

"Green" QR code will be issued to those who have fulfilled all the specified conditions, with which they would be exempted from the 14-day compulsory quarantine requirement upon their return to Hong Kong.

"A dedicated channel will be set up at both the Shenzhen Bay Port and HZMB Hong Kong Port for the use of travellers with a 'Green' QR code. We strongly advise Hong Kong residents with a quota to complete the code conversion process to obtain a 'Green' QR code within 24 hours before their return trip to Hong Kong to expedite the clearance process," said the Government spokesman.

"If a traveler receives a QR code of a different colour (e.g. a 'Pink' QR code) after transmitting a valid negative COVID-19 nucleic acid test result to the electronic health declaration system of the Department of Health through 'Yuekang code' (粵康碼) or 'Macao health code' (澳康碼), it means that he/she has yet to fulfil all the specified conditions, and may thus be subject to 14-day compulsory quarantine requirement upon entry into Hong Kong."

The Government spokesman noted that Hong Kong residents who can fulfil all the specified conditions and are returning to Hong Kong under the Return2hk Scheme should still exercise self-monitoring of their health conditions for at least 14 days after their entry into Hong Kong. They should observe the points listed in the "Health-monitoring Checklist for Inbound Travellers". If they feel unwell, they should seek medical advice promptly and reveal their travel history to medical practitioners. If there is any concern about their symptoms, they may make a request to their doctors for taking a relevant virus test

The spokesman also reminded Hong Kong residents who are returning to Hong Kong under the Return2hk Scheme that they would still be subject to the prevailing quarantine arrangements of Guangdong Province or Macao (e.g. 14-day compulsory quarantine) when they subsequently leave Hong Kong for the two places, unless exemption has been granted for them separately. They should take note of the latest quarantine arrangements of Guangdong Province and Macao, and make necessary preparations.

Details of the Return2hk Scheme are available at the "COVID-19 Thematic Website" (return2hk.gov.hk or 回港易.政府.香港). Members of the public may also call the hotline of the Return2hk Scheme at 3142 2330 if they have any enquiries.

Issued at HKT 17:59

Public hospitals daily update on COVID-19 cases

****

The following is issued on behalf of the Hospital Authority:

As at 9am today (November 11), six COVID-19 confirmed patients were discharged from hospital in the last 24 hours. So far, a total of 5 159 patients with confirmed or probable infection have been discharged.

At present, there are 613 negative pressure rooms in public hospitals with 1 090 negative pressure beds activated. A total of 93 confirmed patients are currently hospitalised in 20 public hospitals, among which six patients are in critical condition, three are in serious condition and the remaining 84 patients are in stable condition.

The Hospital Authority will maintain close contact with the Centre for Health Protection to monitor the latest developments and to inform the public and healthcare workers on the latest information in a timely manner.

Details of the above-mentioned patients are as follows:

Patient condition	Case numbers
Discharged	4225, 5307, 5361, 5367, 5370, 5380
Critical	1989, 3496, 4706, 4833, 5110, 5185
Serious	4788, 5151, 5282

Ends/Wednesday, November 11, 2020
Issued at HKT 18:15

Government extends social distancing measures under Prevention and Control of Disease Ordinance

****

The Government will gazette directions and specifications under the Prevention and Control of Disease (Requirements and Directions) (Business and Premises) Regulation (Cap. 599F), the Prevention and Control of Disease (Prohibition on Group Gathering) Regulation (Cap. 599G) and the Prevention and Control of Disease (Wearing of Mask) Regulation (Cap. 599I) today (November 11) to maintain the social distancing measures currently in place. These measures will take effect at 0.00am on November 13 for a period of seven days till November 19.

A spokesman for the Food and Health Bureau said, "While the third wave of the local epidemic has been subsiding after reaching the peak in late July, new confirmed cases with unknown sources of infection have still been identified over the past week, indicating the existence of silent transmission chains in the community. In addition, it is worrying that the number of locally acquired cases has shown an increasing trend in recent days and that we are seeing small cluster outbreaks in the community as a result of, inter alia, anti-epidemic fatigue, frequent social activities and delay in taking tests. Meanwhile, the global epidemic situation has continued to worsen, with the number of new confirmed cases hitting a record high of some 600 000 cases daily. The past 14 days have seen over 60 imported cases involving new sources of infection in areas such as Europe, America and Africa, in addition to those involving very high-risk places. While we have strengthened the testing and quarantine requirements for arrivals, imported cases would continue to pose discernible public health risks to Hong Kong.

"Having regard to the development of the epidemic situation, we have relaxed the various social distancing measures under a refined and sophisticated approach in a gradual and orderly manner over the past two months or so. The relaxation includes that under the latest round of measures which took effect since October 30, further extending the hours when dine-in services are allowed in catering business premises and relaxing the number of persons allowed to be seated together at one table therein, as well as raising the total number of people allowed in catering business premises and some scheduled premises, etc. While our intention is to allow members of the public to further resume social and economic activities as far as practicable under the new normal, with the relaxation of social distancing measures, members of the public appeared to become less alert in combating the epidemic. Amongst others, there was even a new cluster relating to a staycation at a local hotel identified in early November. As the number of locally acquired cases has shown signs of a rebound in recent days, there is no room for us to further relax the social distancing measures currently in place at this stage."

Taking into account the latest public health risk assessment, starting from this Friday (November 13), the Government will maintain all existing requirements and restrictions applicable to catering business premises and scheduled premises. The Government will continue to closely monitor the development of the epidemic situation and make adjustments to the social distancing measures in a timely manner upon considering and striking a balance among factors such as public health, economic impact and social acceptance.

The spokesman added, "As we have stressed time and again, co-operation and self-discipline of members of the public are the keys to the effectiveness of social distancing measures in preventing the spread of the disease in the community. In particular, we would like to remind members of the public to avoid mask-off group activities, which will pose significant risk of spreading the virus. In light of the staycation-related local cases identified in recent days, while such gatherings in private places may not contravene the social distancing measures, they should be avoided as far as possible from a public health perspective. If cases involving congregations in hotels or other private places continue to be identified, we do not rule out the need to explore amending relevant regulations under the Prevention and Control of Disease Regulations (Cap. 599) to regulate the said activities and premises. Again, we would like to call for the public's concerted efforts in fighting the epidemic. While resuming social and economic activities, members of the public should continue to stay vigilant in maintaining personal hygiene, and complying with anti-epidemic measures and social distancing, with a view to putting the epidemic under control as soon as possible. If the epidemic situation shows signs of a rebound and there is another large-scale outbreak in the community, the Government will have no choice but to significantly tighten anti-epidemic measures. As the rebound of the epidemic situation may bring about early the fourth wave of the local epidemic, which would likely coincide with the peak of the winter influenza season, such tightening of anti-epidemic measures may need to be pursued within a shorter period of time and to a larger extent as compared with that of the previous wave."

Details of the aforementioned social distancing measures which are to be effective during the seven-day period from November 13 to 19, 2020, are as follows:

(I) Catering business and scheduled premises

(1) The requirements and restrictions applicable to catering business and scheduled premises (see Annex 1 for details) will be maintained during the seven-day period from November 13 to 19, 2020. Amongst others, facilities involving higher health risks such as steam and sauna facilities and ball pits will continue to be prohibited from opening.

Persons responsible for carrying on catering businesses and managers of scheduled premises that contravene the statutory requirements under Cap. 599F would have committed a criminal offence. Offenders are subject to a maximum fine of $50,000 and imprisonment for six months.

(II) Group gatherings

(2) Unless exempted, the prohibition on group gatherings of more than four persons in public places will continue during the seven-day period from November 13 to 19, 2020.

Any person who participates in a prohibited group gathering; organises a prohibited group gathering; owns, controls or operates the place of such a gathering; and knowingly allows the taking place of such gathering commits an offence under Cap. 599G. Offenders are liable to a maximum fine of $25,000 and imprisonment for six months. Persons who participate in a prohibited group gathering may discharge liability for the offence by paying a fixed penalty of $2,000.

(III) Mask-wearing requirement

(3) The mandatory mask-wearing requirement will be extended for a period of seven days from November 13 to 19, 2020. During the aforementioned period, a person must wear a mask all the

time when the person is boarding or on board a public transport carrier, is entering or present in an MTR paid area, or is entering or present in a specified public place (i.e. all public places, save for outdoor public places in country parks and special areas as defined in section 2 of the Country Parks Ordinance (Cap. 208)).

Under Cap. 599I, if a person does not wear a mask in accordance with the requirement, an authorised person may deny that person from boarding a public transport carrier or entering the area concerned, as well as require that person to wear a mask and disembark from the carrier or leave the said area. A person in contravention of the relevant provision commits an offence and the maximum penalty is a fine at level 2 ($5,000). In addition, authorised public officers may issue fixed penalty notices to persons who do not wear a mask in accordance with the requirement and such persons may discharge liability for the offence by paying a fixed penalty of $2,000.

Issued at HKT 18:34

CHP investigates 18 additional confirmed cases of COVID-19
****

The Centre for Health Protection (CHP) of the Department of Health has announced that as of 0.00am, November 11, the CHP was investigating 18 additional confirmed cases of coronavirus disease 2019 (COVID-19), taking the number of cases to 5 408 in Hong Kong so far (comprising 5 407 confirmed cases and one probable case).

Among the newly reported cases announced, 15 had a travel history during the incubation period.

The CHP's epidemiological investigations and relevant contact tracing on the confirmed cases are ongoing. For case details and contact tracing information, please see the Annex or the list of buildings with confirmed cases of COVID-19 in the past 14 days and the latest local situation of COVID-19 available on the website "COVID-19 Thematic Website" (www.coronavirus.gov.hk).

In view of the latest epidemic developments in the Mainland, starting tomorrow (November 12), inbound travellers who have been to Shanghai and Tianjin in the past 14 days arriving via land boundary control points will be provided with specimen collection containers. They are required to collect their deep throat saliva samples by themselves in accordance with the instructions and return the samples for conducting COVID-19 testing. The arrangement of distributing specimen collection containers to inbound travellers who have been to Shandong Province and Xinjiang in the past 14 days arriving via land boundary control points, which has come into effect earlier, remains unchanged.

A spokesman for the CHP said, "During the CHP's epidemiological investigations and relevant contact tracing on the confirmed cases, we will compile and upload (www.chp.gov.hk/files/pdf/building_list_eng.pdf) a list of buildings that confirmed patients had visited from two days before the onset of symptoms. Given that cases of local infection continue to occur from time to time, members of the public are urged to seek medical attention immediately if they believe that they had visited the same place at an identical time with a confirmed patient and feel unwell subsequently. If they remain asymptomatic but are concerned that they have been infected, they can also visit the Hospital Authority's designated general out-patient clinics (www.ha.org.hk/haho/ho/covid-19/GOPC_extend_EN.pdf) to obtain specimen collection packs and collect deep throat saliva specimens for free COVID-19 testing."

In view of the severe epidemic situation, the CHP called on members of the public to avoid going out, having social contact and dining out. They should put on a surgical mask and maintain stringent hand hygiene when they need to go out. The CHP strongly urged the elderly to stay home as far as possible and avoid going out. They should consider asking their family and friends to help with everyday tasks such as shopping for basic necessities.

The spokesman said, "Given that the situation of COVID-19 infection remains severe and that there is a continuous increase in the number of cases reported around the world, members of the public are strongly urged to avoid all non-essential travel outside Hong Kong.

"The CHP also strongly urges the public to maintain at all times strict personal and environmental hygiene, which is key to personal protection against infection and prevention of the spread of the disease in the community. On a personal level, members of the public should wear a surgical mask when having respiratory symptoms, taking public transport or staying in crowded places. They should also perform hand hygiene frequently, especially before touching the mouth, nose or eyes.

"As for household environmental hygiene, members of the public are advised to maintain drainage pipes properly, regularly pour water into drain outlets (U-traps) and cover all floor drain outlets when they are not in use. After using the toilet, they should put the toilet lid down before flushing to avoid spreading germs."

Moreover, the Government has launched the website "COVID-19 Thematic Website" (www.coronavirus.gov.hk) for announcing the latest updates on various news on COVID-19 infection and health advice to help the public understand the latest updates. Members of the public may also gain access to information via the COVID-19 WhatsApp Helpline launched by the Office of the Government Chief Information Officer. Simply by saving 9617 1823 in their phone contacts or clicking the link wa.me/85296171823?text=hi, they will be able to obtain information on COVID-19 as well as the "StayHomeSafe" mobile app and wristband via WhatsApp.

Issued at HKT 19:00

Two persons sentenced for breaching compulsory quarantine order

****

Two persons were sentenced by magistrates' courts today (November 11) for violating the Compulsory Quarantine of Certain Persons Arriving at Hong Kong Regulation (Cap 599C) and the Compulsory Quarantine of Persons Arriving at Hong Kong from Foreign Places Regulation (Cap 599E) respectively.

The first case involved a man aged 33, who was earlier issued a compulsory quarantine order stating that he must conduct quarantine at home for 14 days. Before the expiry of the quarantine order, he left the place of quarantine on March 23 and 24 without reasonable excuse nor permission given by an authorised officer. He was charged with two counts of contravening Sections 8(1) and 8(5) of the Compulsory Quarantine of Persons Arriving at Hong Kong from Foreign Places Regulation (Cap 599E) and was sentenced by the Eastern Magistrates' Courts today to a fine of $15,000 for each of the two charges.

The second case involved a woman aged 46. Before the expiry of the quarantine order, she left the place of quarantine on October 3 and 4 without reasonable excuse nor permission given by an authorised officer. She was charged with two counts of contravening Sections 8(1) and 8(5) of the Compulsory Quarantine of Certain Persons Arriving at Hong Kong Regulation (Cap 599C) and was sentenced by the Kwun Tong Magistrates' Courts today to immediate imprisonment for a total of 14 days for the two charges.

Pursuant to the Compulsory Quarantine of Certain Persons Arriving at Hong Kong Regulation (Cap 599C) starting from February 8, save for exempted persons, all persons who have stayed in the Mainland, Macao or Taiwan in the 14 days preceding arrival in Hong Kong, regardless of their nationality or travel documents, will be subject to compulsory quarantine for 14 days. Moreover, pursuant to the Compulsory Quarantine of Persons Arriving at Hong Kong from Foreign Places Regulation (Cap 599E), starting from March 19, all persons arriving from countries or territories outside China would also be subject to compulsory quarantine for 14 days. Breaching a quarantine order is a criminal offence and offenders are subject to a maximum fine of $25,000 and imprisonment for six months.

A spokesman for the Department of Health said the sentence sends a clear message to the community that breaching a compulsory quarantine order is a criminal offence that the Government will not tolerate, and solemnly reminded the public to comply with the Regulation. As of today, a total of 66 persons have been convicted by the courts for breaching compulsory quarantine orders and have received sentences including immediate imprisonment for up to three months or a fine of $15,000. The spokesman reiterated that resolute actions will be taken against anyone who has breached the relevant regulations.

Issued at HKT 19:15

Transport Department to continue to arrange free COVID-19 testing for taxi drivers

****

In order to identify cases in the community as early as possible to help cut the transmission chains, and in light of a few taxi drivers being preliminary tested positive for COVID-19, the Transport Department (TD) announced today (November 11) that starting from tomorrow (November 12) until November 18, another round of testing service will be provided for taxi drivers.

Making reference to the previous rounds of testing service, the TD will set up four temporary testing kit distribution/collection centres. The location, opening dates and hours of the temporary testing kit distribution/collection centres are at Annex 1. The testing is free of charge. Taxi drivers can visit any one of the specific temporary distribution centres to collect the testing kit upon presenting their valid taxi driver identity plate. Drivers are required to register their personal information at the Government website (www.tgptest.gov.hk), and should self-collect their deep throat saliva specimen and return it to any one of the temporary collection centre on the same day. The testing agency will deliver the specimens collected to the laboratory for testing. As no personal information will be indicated on the specimen bottles, the testing agency will only have records of the barcode number of the specimen bottles and will not collect personal information. Drivers will be notified by the Government of the negative test result by SMS through mobile phone, while cases with positive test results will be referred to the Centre for Health Protection of the Department of Health for follow-up.

Taxi drivers can collect the "Anti-epidemic Tag for Taxi Drivers" from the relevant taxi trade organisations with the SMS indicating the negative test result and display the tag at a prominent position inside the taxi compartment to enable passengers' checking. The list of taxi trade organisations distributing the "Anti-epidemic Tag for Taxi Drivers" is at Annex 2.

The TD strongly appeals to taxi drivers to undergo the testing for the protection of themselves and others and to fight the epidemic together. For details of the testing service and the collection of the "Anti-epidemic Tag for Taxi Drivers", please visit the website of the TD (www.td.gov.hk).

Issued at HKT 19:50

November 12[43]

Public hospitals daily update on COVID-19 cases

****

The following is issued on behalf of the Hospital Authority:

---

[43] https://www.info.gov.hk/gia/general/202011/12.htm

As at 9am today (November 12), 11 COVID-19 confirmed patients were discharged from hospital in the last 24 hours. So far, a total of 5 170 patients with confirmed or probable infection have been discharged.

At present, there are 613 negative pressure rooms in public hospitals with 1 090 negative pressure beds activated. A total of 100 confirmed patients are currently hospitalised in 20 public hospitals, among which six patients are in critical condition, two are in serious condition and the remaining 92 patients are in stable condition.

The Hospital Authority will maintain close contact with the Centre for Health Protection to monitor the latest developments and to inform the public and healthcare workers on the latest information in a timely manner.

Details of the above-mentioned patients are as follows:

Patient condition	Case numbers
Discharged	4187, 4788, 5317, 5319, 5320, 5324, 5331, 5336, 5353, 5354, 5393
Critical	1989, 3496, 4706, 4833, 5110, 5185
Serious	5151, 5282

Issued at HKT 17:35

CHP investigates 23 additional confirmed cases of COVID-19

****

The Centre for Health Protection (CHP) of the Department of Health has announced that as of 0.00am, November 12, the CHP was investigating 23 additional confirmed cases of coronavirus disease 2019 (COVID-19), taking the number of cases to 5 431 in Hong Kong so far (comprising 5 430 confirmed cases and one probable case).

Among the newly reported cases announced, 16 had a travel history during the incubation period.

The CHP's epidemiological investigations and relevant contact tracing on the confirmed cases are ongoing. For case details and contact tracing information, please see the Annex or the list of buildings with confirmed cases of COVID-19 in the past 14 days and the latest local situation of COVID-19 available on the website "COVID-19 Thematic Website" (www.coronavirus.gov.hk).

A spokesman for the CHP said, "During the CHP's epidemiological investigations and relevant contact tracing on the confirmed cases, we will compile and upload (www.chp.gov.hk/files/pdf/building_list_eng.pdf) a list of buildings that confirmed patients had visited from two days before the onset of symptoms. Given that cases of local infection continue to occur from time to time, members of the public are urged to seek medical attention immediately if they believe that they had visited the same place at an identical time with a confirmed patient and feel unwell subsequently. If they remain asymptomatic but are concerned that they have been infected, they can also visit the Hospital Authority's designated general out-patient clinics (www.ha.org.hk/haho/ho/covid-19/GOPC_extend_EN.pdf) to obtain specimen collection packs and collect deep throat saliva specimens for free COVID-19 testing."

In view of the severe epidemic situation, the CHP called on members of the public to avoid going out, having social contact and dining out. They should put on a surgical mask and maintain stringent hand hygiene when they need to go out. The CHP strongly urged the elderly to stay home as far as possible and avoid going out. They should consider asking their family and friends to help with everyday tasks such as shopping for basic necessities

The spokesman said, "Given that the situation of COVID-19 infection remains severe and that there is a continuous increase in the number of cases reported around the world, members of the public are strongly urged to avoid all non-essential travel outside Hong Kong.

"The CHP also strongly urges the public to maintain at all times strict personal and environmental hygiene, which is key to personal protection against infection and prevention of the spread of the disease in the community. On a personal level, members of the public should wear a surgical mask when having respiratory symptoms, taking public transport or staying in crowded places. They should also perform hand hygiene frequently, especially before touching the mouth, nose or eyes.

"As for household environmental hygiene, members of the public are advised to maintain drainage pipes properly, regularly pour water into drain outlets (U-traps) and cover all floor drain outlets when they are not in use. After using the toilet, they should put the toilet lid down before flushing to avoid spreading germs."

Moreover, the Government has launched the website "COVID-19 Thematic Website" (www.coronavirus.gov.hk) for announcing the latest updates on various news on COVID-19 infection and health advice to help the public understand the latest updates. Members of the public may also gain access to information via the COVID-19 WhatsApp Helpline launched by the Office of the Government Chief Information Officer. Simply by saving 9617 1823 in their phone contacts or clicking the link wa.me/85296171823?text=hi, they will be able to obtain information on COVID-19 as well as the "StayHomeSafe" mobile app and wristband via WhatsApp.

Issued at HKT 18:00

Man sentenced for breaching compulsory quarantine order

****

A 67-year-old man was sentenced by the West Kowloon Magistrates' Courts today (November 12) to six days' imprisonment, suspended for 12 months, for violating the Compulsory Quarantine of Certain Persons Arriving at Hong Kong Regulation (Cap. 599C) (the Regulation).

The man was earlier issued a compulsory quarantine order stating that he must conduct quarantine at home for 14 days. Before the expiry of the quarantine order, he left the place of quarantine without reasonable excuse nor permission given by an authorised officer and was stopped by an immigration officer at the Shenzhen Bay Control Point on September 23. He was charged with contravening Sections 8(4) and 8(5) of the Regulation and was sentenced by the West Kowloon Magistrates' Courts today to six days' imprisonment, suspended for 12 months.

Pursuant to the Regulation, starting from February 8, save for exempted persons, all persons who have stayed in the Mainland, Macao or Taiwan in the 14 days preceding arrival in Hong Kong, regardless of their nationality or travel documents, will be subject to compulsory quarantine for 14 days. Moreover, pursuant to the Compulsory Quarantine of Persons Arriving at Hong Kong from Foreign Places Regulation (Cap. 599E), starting from March 19, all persons arriving from countries or territories outside China would also be subject to compulsory quarantine for 14 days. Breaching a quarantine order is a criminal offence and offenders are subject to a maximum fine of $25,000 and imprisonment for six months.

A spokesman for the Department of Health said the sentence sends a clear message to the community that breaching a compulsory quarantine order is a criminal offence that the Government will not tolerate, and solemnly reminded the public to comply with the Regulation. As of today, a total of 67 persons have been convicted by the courts for breaching compulsory quarantine orders and have received sentences including immediate imprisonment for up to three months or a fine of $15,000. The spokesman reiterated that resolute actions will be taken against anyone who has breached the relevant regulations.

Issued at HKT 18:30

November 13[44]

[44] https://www.info.gov.hk/gia/general/202011/13.htm

CHP investigates six additional confirmed cases of COVID-19

****

The Centre for Health Protection (CHP) of the Department of Health has announced that as of 0.00am, November 13, the CHP was investigating six additional confirmed cases of coronavirus disease 2019 (COVID-19), taking the number of cases to 5 437 in Hong Kong so far (comprising 5 436 confirmed cases and one probable case).

Among the newly reported cases announced, two had a travel history during the incubation period, two were local cases with unknown sources while the other two were epidemiologically linked with a local case.

The first case with unknown sources involves a 56-year-old man (case 5 432) who had developed fever, cough, runny nose and sore throat on November 7. The patient sought medical attention at a private clinic on November 9 and submitted a deep throat saliva sample on the following day. He works at Li Ping Medical Library in Prince of Wales Hospital and last went to work on November 9.

The second case with unknown sources involves a 65-year-old man (case 5 433) who had developed fever, cough and runny nose on November 9. The patient sought medical attention at Yau Ma Tei Jockey Club General Out-patient Clinic on November 10 and submitted a deep throat saliva sample on the following day. He is a retiree.

The CHP's epidemiological investigations and relevant contact tracing on the confirmed cases are ongoing. For case details and contact tracing information, please see the Annex or the list of buildings with confirmed cases of COVID-19 in the past 14 days and the latest local situation of COVID-19 available on the website "COVID-19 Thematic Website" (www.coronavirus.gov.hk).

A spokesman for the CHP said, "During the CHP's epidemiological investigations and relevant contact tracing on the confirmed cases, we will compile and upload (www.chp.gov.hk/files/pdf/building_list_eng.pdf) a list of buildings that confirmed patients had visited from two days before the onset of symptoms. Given that cases of local infection continue to occur from time to time, members of the public are urged to seek medical attention immediately if they believe that they had visited the same place at an identical time with a confirmed patient and feel unwell subsequently. If they remain asymptomatic but are concerned that they have been infected, they can also visit the Hospital Authority's designated general out-patient clinics (www.ha.org.hk/haho/ho/covid-19/GOPC_extend_EN.pdf) to obtain specimen collection packs and collect deep throat saliva specimens for free COVID-19 testing."

In view of the severe epidemic situation, the CHP called on members of the public to avoid going out, having social contact and dining out. They should put on a surgical mask and maintain

stringent hand hygiene when they need to go out. The CHP strongly urged the elderly to stay home as far as possible and avoid going out. They should consider asking their family and friends to help with everyday tasks such as shopping for basic necessities.

The spokesman said, "Given that the situation of COVID-19 infection remains severe and that there is a continuous increase in the number of cases reported around the world, members of the public are strongly urged to avoid all non-essential travel outside Hong Kong.

"The CHP also strongly urges the public to maintain at all times strict personal and environmental hygiene, which is key to personal protection against infection and prevention of the spread of the disease in the community. On a personal level, members of the public should wear a surgical mask when having respiratory symptoms, taking public transport or staying in crowded places. They should also perform hand hygiene frequently, especially before touching the mouth, nose or eyes.

"As for household environmental hygiene, members of the public are advised to maintain drainage pipes properly, regularly pour water into drain outlets (U-traps) and cover all floor drain outlets when they are not in use. After using the toilet, they should put the toilet lid down before flushing to avoid spreading germs."

Moreover, the Government has launched the website "COVID-19 Thematic Website" (www.coronavirus.gov.hk) for announcing the latest updates on various news on COVID-19 infection and health advice to help the public understand the latest updates. Members of the public may also gain access to information via the COVID-19 WhatsApp Helpline launched by the Office of the Government Chief Information Officer. Simply by saving 9617 1823 in their phone contacts or clicking the link wa.me/85296171823?text=hi, they will be able to obtain information on COVID-19 as well as the "StayHomeSafe" mobile app and wristband via WhatsApp.

Issued at HKT 14:00

Public hospitals daily update on COVID-19 cases

****

The following is issued on behalf of the Hospital Authority:

As at 9am today (November 13), seven COVID-19 confirmed patients were discharged from hospital in the last 24 hours. So far, a total of 5 177 patients with confirmed or probable infection have been discharged.

At present, there are 613 negative pressure rooms in public hospitals with 1 090 negative pressure beds activated. A total of 116 confirmed patients are currently hospitalised in 20 public hospitals, among which six patients are in critical condition, one is in serious condition and the remaining 109 patients are in stable condition.

The Hospital Authority will maintain close contact with the Centre for Health Protection to monitor the latest developments and to inform the public and healthcare workers on the latest information in a timely manner.

Details of the above-mentioned patients are as follows:

Patient condition	Case numbers
Discharged	5332, 5338, 5373, 5405, 5408, 5410, 5423
Critical	1989, 3496, 4706, 4833, 5110, 5185
Serious	5151

Issued at HKT 17:43

S for IT attends briefing sessions on "LeaveHomeSafe" mobile app

****

The Secretary for Innovation and Technology, Mr Alfred Sit, today (November 13) attended two briefing sessions for representatives from the wholesale and retail sectors and the beauty and massage industries to actively solicit their support for the "LeaveHomeSafe" mobile app and encouraged more businesses to join the scheme and fight the virus together.

Mr Sit said, "Under the new normal, we need concerted efforts from various sectors to fight the virus so that people will feel comfortable going out and the economy can regain its momentum. There are currently over 6 000 public and private venues that have pledged support for the scheme. The app can also be used directly in over 18 000 taxis. We will continue to get the message across and engage various sectors and businesses such as retail, shopping malls and property management to fight the virus together."

The Government has been actively inviting various industries to participate in the scheme. The Office of the Government Chief Information Officer (OGCIO) has organised a number of briefing sessions in collaboration with relevant government departments to introduce the scheme to trade organisations from restaurants, bars or pubs, karaoke establishments, clubs, taxis, fitness centres, banks, cinemas and social welfare institutions. Interested organisations or institutions should contact the OGCIO through the designated email address (leavehomesafe@ogcio.gov.hk).

The "LeaveHomeSafe" mobile app is a digital tool that brings convenience and can assist the public in recording the date and time for checking into and leaving different venues, and encouraging them to keep a more precise record of their whereabouts to minimise the risk of further transmission of the virus. Downloading the app does not require user registration. When checking into participating venues, app users can scan the venue QR code to log their arrival time and click the "Leave" button in the app to mark their departure. Relevant data will then be kept in the app inside the user's mobile phone and will be erased automatically after 31 days. If a confirmed case is later discovered at a participating venue, the app will notify users who have visited the same venue as the COVID-19 confirmed case at around the same time together with health advice to enhance their vigilance.

The "LeaveHomeSafe" mobile app will be available for public download from next Monday (November 16). For details, please refer to the "LeaveHomeSafe" website (www.leavehomesafe.gov.hk).

Issued at HKT 17:59

November 14[45]

S for IT speaks on LeaveHomeSafe mobile app

****

Following is the transcript of remarks by the Secretary for Innovation and Technology, Mr Alfred Sit, at a media session after attending a radio programme today (November 14):

Reporter: Mr Sit, how do you convince the public that no data will be stored in government and also do you have a target on how many downloads?

Secretary for Innovation and Technology: We understand very well that our people have concern on data privacy, so we have put much emphasis on developing this app. We have three steps in protecting data privacy. First, the app is voluntary participation, people can download the app at their own discretion. When they go to some premises, it is also up to them, at their own discretion to scan the QR code or not. Also, all the data are contained in their own phones, there is no central system to control or store the movement or the visiting data of our people. So three

[45] https://www.info.gov.hk/gia/general/202011/14.htm

steps, voluntary download, voluntary scanning QR code and also all the data is contained in their own phones. There is no central system to record all the data, and for all the data contained in their phones, they are going to be erased automatically in 31 days.

Reporter: Any target about download?

Secretary for Innovation and Technology: We don't set any target because it is all voluntary arrangement, and we are looking forward to people's support, but we don't set any target.

Issued at HKT 12:13

CHP investigates eight additional confirmed cases of COVID-19
****

The Centre for Health Protection (CHP) of the Department of Health has announced that as of 0.00am, November 14, the CHP was investigating eight additional confirmed cases of coronavirus disease 2019 (COVID-19), taking the number of cases to 5 445 in Hong Kong so far (comprising 5 444 confirmed cases and one probable case).

Among the newly reported cases announced, five had a travel history during the incubation period.

The CHP's epidemiological investigations and relevant contact tracing on the confirmed cases are ongoing. For case details and contact tracing information, please see the Annex or the list of buildings with confirmed cases of COVID-19 in the past 14 days and the latest local situation of COVID-19 available on the website "COVID-19 Thematic Website" (www.coronavirus.gov.hk).

A spokesman for the CHP said, "During the CHP's epidemiological investigations and relevant contact tracing on the confirmed cases, we will compile and upload (www.chp.gov.hk/files/pdf/building_list_eng.pdf) a list of buildings that confirmed patients had visited from two days before the onset of symptoms. Given that cases of local infection continue to occur from time to time, members of the public are urged to seek medical attention immediately if they believe that they had visited the same place at an identical time with a confirmed patient and feel unwell subsequently. If they remain asymptomatic but are concerned that they have been infected, they can also visit the Hospital Authority's designated general out-patient clinics (www.ha.org.hk/haho/ho/covid-19/GOPC_extend_EN.pdf) to obtain specimen collection packs and collect deep throat saliva specimens for free COVID-19 testing.

In view of the severe epidemic situation, the CHP called on members of the public to avoid going out, having social contact and dining out. They should put on a surgical mask and maintain stringent hand hygiene when they need to go out. The CHP strongly urged the elderly to stay home as far as possible and avoid going out. They should consider asking their family and friends to help with everyday tasks such as shopping for basic necessities.

The spokesman said, "Given that the situation of COVID-19 infection remains severe and that there is a continuous increase in the number of cases reported around the world, members of the public are strongly urged to avoid all non-essential travel outside Hong Kong.

"The CHP also strongly urges the public to maintain at all times strict personal and environmental hygiene, which is key to personal protection against infection and prevention of the spread of the disease in the community. On a personal level, members of the public should wear a surgical mask when having respiratory symptoms, taking public transport or staying in crowded places. They should also perform hand hygiene frequently, especially before touching the mouth, nose or eyes.

"As for household environmental hygiene, members of the public are advised to maintain drainage pipes properly, regularly pour water into drain outlets (U-traps) and cover all floor drain outlets when they are not in use. After using the toilet, they should put the toilet lid down before flushing to avoid spreading germs."

Moreover, the Government has launched the website "COVID-19 Thematic Website" (www.coronavirus.gov.hk) for announcing the latest updates on various news on COVID-19 infection and health advice to help the public understand the latest updates. Members of the public may also gain access to information via the COVID-19 WhatsApp Helpline launched by the Office of the Government Chief Information Officer. Simply by saving 9617 1823 in their phone contacts or clicking the link wa.me/85296171823?text=hi, they will be able to obtain information on COVID-19 as well as the "StayHomeSafe" mobile app and wristband via WhatsApp.

Issued at HKT 17:45

Public hospitals daily update on COVID-19 cases
****

The following is issued on behalf of the Hospital Authority:

As at 9am today (November 14), nine COVID-19 confirmed patients were discharged from hospital in the last 24 hours. Including a patient (case number: 5434) discharged on November 12, a total of 5 187 patients with confirmed or probable infection have been discharged so far.

At present, there are 613 negative pressure rooms in public hospitals with 1 090 negative pressure beds activated. A total of 112 confirmed patients are currently hospitalised in 20 public hospitals, among which six patients are in critical condition, two are in serious condition and the remaining 104 patients are in stable condition.

The Hospital Authority will maintain close contact with the Centre for Health Protection to monitor the latest developments and to inform the public and healthcare workers on the latest information in a timely manner.

Details of the above-mentioned patients are as follows:

Patient condition	Case numbers
Discharged	4205, 5159, 5267, 5330, 5337, 5341, 5394, 5401, 5419, 5434
Critical	1989, 3496, 4706, 4833, 5110, 5185
Serious	5151, 5273

Issued at HKT 18:50

Government tightens social distancing measures

****

In view of the development of COVID-19 in Hong Kong, the Government announced today (November 14) that social distancing measures will be tightened.

A spokesman for the Food and Health Bureau said, "With the relaxation of social distancing measures, members of the public appeared to become less alert in combating the epidemic, and we have seen anti-epidemic fatigue in the community with an increase in mask-off social gatherings. At the same time, the global epidemic situation has continued to worsen, and there are signs of rebound in local confirmed cases with unknown source of infection recently. The fourth wave of outbreak could be triggered at any moment."

"The Government has to adopt a 'preventing the importation of cases and the spreading of the virus in the community' infection control strategy to curb the epidemic. On prevention of importation of cases, we have extensively tightened testing and quarantine requirements for inbound travellers and exempted persons since July. The Secretary for Food and Health also announced further tightening measures on November 13 and today."

"At the same time, the Government needs to prevent spreading of the virus in the community by swiftly tightening infection control measures, targeting at risks brought about by mask-off gathering activities in particular. In view of the latest public health risk assessment, in particular the higher risks brought about by staycation as shown in recent cases, we consider it necessary to tighten social distancing measures under the Prevention and Control of Disease (Requirements and Directions) (Business and Premises) Regulation (Cap. 599F), targeting at mask-off gathering activities, including gatherings in hotels (the so-called staycation). We will also tighten the visiting arrangement for confinees under hotel quarantine, with a view to stopping the transmission of virus by imported cases in the community."

The latest details of requirements and restrictions are as follows:

(I) Catering premises and scheduled premises (details at Annex 1)

(1) From 12.00am to 4.59am daily, save for specific premises (details at Annex 2), a person responsible for carrying on a catering business must cease selling or supplying food or drink for consumption on the premises of the business; and close any premises, or part of the premises, on which food or drink is sold or supplied by the business for consumption on the premises. The premises concerned may still sell or supply food and/or drink for takeaway services and deliveries. A person responsible for carrying on a catering business is also required to put up a notice at the entrance to the catering premises to remind customers that food or drink should not be consumed in areas adjacent to the catering premises;

(2) No more than two persons may be seated together at one table within bars or pubs as well as clubs or nightclubs; no more than four persons may be seated together at one table within other catering business premises;

(3) Members of public must only consume food or drink at the table (but not any other places) within catering business premises. In other words, a person must not consume food or drink and must wear a mask when he or she is away from the table (such as toasting at weddings);

(4) The total number of people allowed in catering business premises (including bars or pubs), clubs or nightclubs, and swimming pools will be capped at 50 per cent of the normal seating capacity/maximum capacity of the respective premises;

(5) Members of the public must wear masks when doing exercise in indoor sports premises and public skating rinks, except when there is a distance of at least 1.5 metres or effective partition(s), or when doing certain exercises involving little physical contact;

(6) Other requirements and restrictions on catering business and scheduled premises will be maintained. Amongst others, facilities involving higher health risks such as steam and sauna facilities and ball pits will continue to be prohibited from opening; and

(7) The Government will explore to incorporate hotels /guesthouses into the list of scheduled

premises, and requirements will be imposed to this newly added scheduled premises, including:

- limiting the number of guests in each guestroom to four persons (except people living in the same household);
- requiring all guests visiting guestrooms to register their personal particulars with the hotel/guesthouse operator;
- conducting body temperature screening on a person before the person is allowed to enter the hotel/guesthouse;
- conducting cleaning and disinfection of facilities and accessories before the use of the next customer;
- providing hand sanitisers at the hotel/guesthouse for any person therein;
- ensuring the guestrooms for hotel confinees and non-confinees must be separated in different floors; and
- hotel operators must take effective measures to prevent hotel confinees from leaving their guestrooms.

The Government has gazetted the directions and specification under Cap. 599F to implement the above measures in (1) to (6). The above measures will take effect from November 16 for a period of 11 days till November 26, 2020. The Government has also started preparing for the legislative amendment work related to the above new requirements set out in (7).

Persons responsible for carrying on catering businesses and managers of scheduled premises that contravene the statutory requirements under Cap. 599F would have committed a criminal offence. Offenders are subject to a maximum fine of $50,000 and imprisonment for six months.

(II) Tightening the visiting arrangement for persons under quarantine in hotels

(8) The Department of Health (DH) will shortly disallow visitors for any person under compulsory quarantine in hotels during the quarantine period. If confinees have the need to replenish goods or food, their friends, family members or hotel staff can place them outside the guestrooms for the confinees to pick up without face-to-face contact. If a person under compulsory hotel quarantine requires the company of a carer, with the prior permission from DH, the carer also has to be quarantined in the hotel till the end of the quarantine period. The above measures will take effect from November 18, 2020.

The Government strongly appeals to the confinees to follow the quarantine requirement strictly in order to protect the health of their own selves and others. The measure is of utmost importance to prevent the spreading of COVID-19 in the community. Breaking Quarantine Orders is a criminal offence and offenders are subject to a maximum imprisonment of six months and a fine of $25,000.

(III) Group gatherings

(9) Unless exempted, the prohibition on group gatherings of more than four persons in public places will continue during the 11-day period from November 16 to 26, 2020.

Any person who participates in a prohibited group gathering; organises a prohibited group gathering; owns, controls or operates the place of such a gathering; and knowingly allows the taking place of such gathering commits an offence under the Prevention and Control of Disease (Prohibition on Group Gathering) Regulation (Cap. 599G). Offenders are liable to a maximum fine of $25,000 and imprisonment for six months. Persons who participate in a prohibited group gathering may discharge liability for the offence by paying a fixed penalty of $2,000.

(IV) Mask-wearing requirement

(10) The mandatory mask-wearing requirement under the Prevention and Control of Disease (Wearing of Mask) Regulation (Cap. 599I) will be extended for a period of eleven days from November 16 to November 26, 2020. During the aforementioned period, a person must wear a mask all the time when the person is boarding or on board a public transport carrier, is entering or present in an MTR paid area, or is entering or present in a specified public place (i.e. all public places, save for outdoor public places in country parks and special areas as defined in section 2 of the Country Parks Ordinance (Cap. 208).

Under Cap. 599I, if a person does not wear a mask in accordance with the requirement, an authorised person may deny that person from boarding a public transport carrier or entering the area concerned, as well as require that person to wear a mask and disembark from the carrier or leave the said area. A person in contravention of the relevant provision commits an offence and the maximum penalty is a fine at level 2 ($5,000). In addition, authorised public officers may issue fixed penalty notices to persons who do not wear a mask in accordance with the requirement and such persons may discharge liability for the offence by paying a fixed penalty of $2,000.

The spokesman said, "The Government will review the various measures in place from time to time in accordance with the development of the epidemic situation, and make suitable adjustments taking into account all relevant factors."

Issued at HKT 20:05

Prevention and Control of Disease (Compulsory Testing for Certain Persons) Regulation gazetted

****

The Government has published the Prevention and Control of Disease (Compulsory Testing for Certain Persons) Regulation (Cap. 599J) in the Gazette today (November 14), which provides the legal framework for the Government to require certain categories of persons to undergo COVID-19 testing, and for specified medical practitioners to require symptomatic patients to undergo COVID-19 testing. The Regulation will commence at 0.00am on November 15

Strengthening COVID-19 testing is an integral part of the epidemic control strategy, which can help to slow down the transmission of the virus by early identification, early isolation and early treatment. The Government has been urging all individuals who are in doubt about their own health conditions, or individuals with infection risks (such as individuals who visited places with epidemic outbreaks or contacted confirmed cases) to undergo testing for early identification of infected persons.

To further strengthen testing, the Regulation provides a legal framework for the Government to specify by compulsory testing notice published in the Gazette, a category or description of persons who are required to undergo a test for COVID-19, taking into account the epidemic development. Examples include persons who live or work in specified premises with outbreak of cases, persons of a particular occupation, or persons who are close to completion of the compulsory 14-day quarantine upon their arrival at Hong Kong. The Secretary for Food and Health (SFH) will publish the relevant notices when necessary taking into account the epidemic development and the testing participation rate.

In addition, the Regulation allows SFH to specify by notice published in the Gazette a period of not more than 14 days, during which a specified medical practitioner can require a person whom he clinically suspects has contracted COVID-19 to undergo testing by written direction issued to that person.

Those who are subject to compulsory testing may either choose the testing service provided by the Department of Health (DH) or a qualified private laboratory in accordance with the existing mechanism. To facilitate members of the public to undergo testing, we will further streamline the logistical arrangements for the distribution and collection of specimen bottles by the DH and Hospital Authority. The Government will also facilitate private medical practitioners to order COVID-19 testing for patients

Any person who fails to comply with the testing notice or testing direction commits an offence and may be fined a fixed penalty of $2,000. The person would also be issued with a compulsory testing order requiring him/her to undergo testing within a specified timeframe. Failure to comply with the order is an offence and the offender would be liable to a fine at level 4 ($25,000) and to imprisonment for six months.

The Regulation is made in accordance with the Prevention and Control of Disease Ordinance (Cap. 599). Section 8 of the Ordinance empowers the Chief Executive in Council to make public health emergency regulation for the purposes of preventing, combating or alleviating the effects of a public health emergency and protecting public health.

The Government has launched the website "COVID-19 Thematic Website" (www.coronavirus.gov.hk) for announcing the latest updates on various news on COVID-19 infection and health advice to help the public understand the latest updates. Members of the public may also gain access to information via the COVID-19 WhatsApp Helpline launched by the Office of the Government Chief Information Officer. Simply by saving 9617 1823 in their phone contacts or clicking the link wa.me/85296171823?text=hi, they will be able to obtain information on COVID-19 as well as the "StayHomeSafe" mobile app and wristband via WhatsApp.

Issued at HKT 20:10

November 15[46]

Transport Department to provide additional temporary testing kit distribution/collection centres
****

To further encourage taxi drivers to participate in the COVID-19 testing, the Transport Department (TD) announced today (November 15) that starting from tomorrow (November 16), seven additional temporary testing kit distribution/collection centres will be set up to provide free COVID-19 testing for taxi drivers.

From November 16 to 18, the total number of temporary testing kit distribution/collection centres will be increased from four to 11. The location, opening dates and hours of the temporary testing kit distribution/collection centres are at Annex 1.

The arrangement of the additional temporary testing kit distribution/collection centres is the same as the existing centres. The testing is free of charge. Taxi drivers can visit any one of the specific temporary distribution centres to collect the testing kit upon presenting their valid taxi driver identity plate. Drivers are required to register their personal information at the Government website (www.tgptest.gov.hk), and should self-collect their deep throat saliva specimen and return it to any one of the temporary collection centre on the same day. The testing agency will deliver the specimens collected to the laboratory for testing. As no personal information will be indicated on the specimen bottles, the testing agency will only have records of the barcode number of the specimen bottles and will not collect personal information. Drivers will be notified by the Government of the negative test result by SMS through mobile phone, while cases with positive test results will be referred to the Centre for Health Protection of the Department of Health for follow-up.

[46] https://www.info.gov.hk/gia/general/202011/15.htm

Taxi drivers can collect the "Anti-epidemic Tag for Taxi Drivers" from the relevant taxi trade organisations with the SMS indicating the negative test result and display the tag at a prominent position inside the taxi compartment to enable passengers' checking.

The TD strongly appeals to taxi drivers to undergo the testing for the protection of themselves and others and to fight the epidemic together. For details of the testing service and the collection of the "Anti-epidemic Tag for Taxi Drivers", please visit the website of the TD (www.td.gov.hk).

Issued at HKT 10:00

FEHD steps up inspections and reminds catering business operators and public to continue complying with anti-epidemic regulations

****

The Food and Environmental Hygiene Department (FEHD) stepped up inspections at catering premises (including eateries and cooked food centres) in Tai Po District, Mong Kok District and Wong Tai Sin District and reminded the catering business operators to strictly comply with the requirements under the Prevention and Control of Disease (Requirements and Directions) (Business and Premises) Regulation (Cap. 599F) (the Regulation), and the public to comply with the various restrictions in relation to group gatherings and mask-wearing under the anti-epidemic regulations and directions when patronising catering premises.

FEHD officers yesterday (November 14) conducted inspections in Tai Po District and Mong Kok District, and conducted joint operations with the Police in Tsz Wan Shan. During the operations, a total of 102 catering premises (including 50 eateries and 52 cooked food stalls) were inspected. Twenty-five verbal warnings were given. Procedures on prosecution were initiated against four catering business operators for breaching the Regulation, mainly violating the requirements on the distance between tables or partition serving as effective buffer and the requirement on mask-wearing; and also against two catering business operators for breaching the Food Business Regulation (Cap. 132X) in terms of illegal extension of the business areas of their catering premises. In addition, fixed penalty notices were issued against two persons for breaching the regulation on mask-wearing.

A spokesman for the FEHD said, "According to the prevailing directions issued by the Secretary for Food and Health in relation to catering business under the Regulation, catering business operators have to strictly comply with a series of requirements and restrictions, including, no more than six persons may be at one table in catering premises; the total number of customers allowed in catering premises must not exceed 75 per cent of the normal seating capacity; a mask must be worn within the premises except when the person is consuming food or drink; tables must be arranged in a way to ensure there is a distance of at least 1.5m or some form of partition which could serve as effective buffer between one table and another table; body temperature screening must be conducted before the person is allowed to enter the catering premises; and hand sanitisers must be provided, etc."

The spokesman supplemented, "According to the latest directions issued by the Secretary for Food and Health in relation to catering business under the Regulation that apply to the period from November 16 to 26 (see Gazette Notice published on November 14), the updated requirements and restrictions include: no more than two persons may be at one table for a bar/pub or night establishment/nightclub while no more than four persons may be at one table for other catering premises; the total number of customers allowed in catering premises must not exceed 50 per cent of the normal seating capacity; a mask must be worn within the premises except when the person is consuming food or drink at a table therein."

As a warm reminder, the spokesman said, "Communal seating areas adjoining cooked food stalls in a public market are public places. The public must comply with the Prevention and Control of Disease (Prohibition in Group Gathering) Regulation (Cap. 599G) that prohibits group gatherings of more than four persons in public places."

The spokesman stressed that for catering premises across the territory (including eateries and cooked food centres), the FEHD will continue to step up inspections and, as needed, conduct joint operations with the Police, to ensure that catering business operators and the public strictly comply with relevant regulations. Enforcement actions will be taken against offenders so as to minimise the risk of transmission of COVID-19 in food premises. If catering business operators contravene the Regulation, they are liable to a maximum fine of $50,000 and imprisonment for six months. Persons who violate the group gathering restriction of the Prevention and Control of Disease (Prohibition in Group Gathering) Regulation (Cap. 599G) are subject to a fixed penalty of $2,000.

The spokesman appealed to catering business operators to comply with relevant regulations on prevention and control of disease in a concerted and persistent manner, with a view to keeping their staff, customers and the public safe. Members of the public also have to comply with the related regulations and directions on group gatherings at catering premises.

Issued at HKT 13:48

CHP investigates 14 additional confirmed cases of COVID-19

****

The Centre for Health Protection (CHP) of the Department of Health has announced that as of 0.00am, November 15, the CHP was investigating 14 additional confirmed cases of coronavirus disease 2019 (COVID-19), taking the number of cases to 5 459 in Hong Kong so far (comprising 5 458 confirmed cases and one probable case).

Among the newly reported cases announced, nine had a travel history during the incubation period, one was local case with unknown sources while the other four were epidemiologically linked with a local case.

The case with unknown sources involves a 49-year-old man (case 5 446) who had developed fever on November 6. The patient consulted a private doctor on November 12 and submitted a deep throat saliva sample on the same day. He last went to work on November 9 at 25 Shan Kwong Road in Happy Valley.

The CHP's epidemiological investigations and relevant contact tracing on the confirmed cases are ongoing. For case details and contact tracing information, please see the Annex or the list of buildings with confirmed cases of COVID-19 in the past 14 days and the latest local situation of COVID-19 available on the website "COVID-19 Thematic Website" (www.coronavirus.gov.hk).

A spokesman for the CHP said, "During the CHP's epidemiological investigations and relevant contact tracing on the confirmed cases, we will compile and upload (www.chp.gov.hk/files/pdf/building_list_eng.pdf) a list of buildings that confirmed patients had visited from two days before the onset of symptoms. Given that cases of local infection continue to occur from time to time, members of the public are urged to seek medical attention immediately if they believe that they had visited the same place at an identical time with a confirmed patient and feel unwell subsequently. If they remain asymptomatic but are concerned that they have been infected, they can also visit the Hospital Authority's designated general out-patient clinics (www.ha.org.hk/haho/ho/covid-19/GOPC_extend_EN.pdf) to obtain specimen collection packs and collect deep throat saliva specimens for free COVID-19 testing."

In view of the severe epidemic situation, the CHP called on members of the public to avoid going out, having social contact and dining out. They should put on a surgical mask and maintain stringent hand hygiene when they need to go out. The CHP strongly urged the elderly to stay home as far as possible and avoid going out. They should consider asking their family and friends to help with everyday tasks such as shopping for basic necessities.

The spokesman said, "Given that the situation of COVID-19 infection remains severe and that there is a continuous increase in the number of cases reported around the world, members of the public are strongly urged to avoid all non-essential travel outside Hong Kong.

"The CHP also strongly urges the public to maintain at all times strict personal and environmental hygiene, which is key to personal protection against infection and prevention of the spread of the disease in the community. On a personal level, members of the public should wear a surgical mask when having respiratory symptoms, taking public transport or staying in crowded places. They should also perform hand hygiene frequently, especially before touching the mouth, nose or eyes.

"As for household environmental hygiene, members of the public are advised to maintain drainage pipes properly, regularly pour water into drain outlets (U-traps) and cover all floor drain outlets when they are not in use. After using the toilet, they should put the toilet lid down before flushing to avoid spreading germs."

Moreover, the Government has launched the website "COVID-19 Thematic Website" (www.coronavirus.gov.hk) for announcing the latest updates on various news on COVID-19 infection and health advice to help the public understand the latest updates. Members of the public may also gain access to information via the COVID-19 WhatsApp Helpline launched by the Office of the Government Chief Information Officer. Simply by saving 9617 1823 in their phone contacts or clicking the link wa.me/85296171823?text=hi, they will be able to obtain information on COVID-19 as well as the "StayHomeSafe" mobile app and wristband via WhatsApp.

Issued at HKT 14:00

Public hospitals daily update on COVID-19 cases

****

The following is issued on behalf of the Hospital Authority:

As at 9am today (November 15), seven COVID-19 confirmed patients were discharged from hospital in the last 24 hours. So far, a total of 5 194 patients with confirmed or probable infection have been discharged.

At present, there are 613 negative pressure rooms in public hospitals with 1 090 negative pressure beds activated. A total of 113 confirmed patients are currently hospitalised in 20 public hospitals, among which seven patients are in critical condition, two are in serious condition and the remaining 104 patients are in stable condition.

The Hospital Authority will maintain close contact with the Centre for Health Protection to monitor the latest developments and to inform the public and healthcare workers on the latest information in a timely manner.

Details of the above-mentioned patients are as follows:

Patient condition	Case numbers
Discharged	5308, 5334, 5369, 5395, 5411, 5413, 5414
Critical	1989, 3496, 4706, 4833, 5110, 5185, 5409
Serious	5151, 5273

Issued at HKT 17:06

November 16[47]

Mobile specimen collection stations in Tai Po cease operation
****

The mobile specimen collection stations in Tai Po set up by the Government provided specimen collection services by combined nasal and throat swab and COVID-19 testing services for 736 people on November 15, and their operation ended at 8pm. Together with the distribution and collection services of deep throat saliva specimen bottles provided by mobile van earlier, the mobile specimen collection stations have provided free COVID-19 testing services for a total of more than 12 590 people.

As at 10pm on November 15, a total of 7 598 specimens collected under the mobile specimen collection stations arrangement had been tested. If any specimen tested shows a positive COVID-19 result, the specimen will be referred to the Public Health Laboratory Services Branch of the Department of Health (DH) for a confirmatory test. Confirmed cases will be followed up and announced by the Centre for Health Protection of the DH.

In view of a number of confirmed COVID-19 cases relating to residents in Tai Po in early November, in order to identify cases in the community as early as possible to help cut the transmission chains, the Government arranged testing agencies to Tai Po to provide free distribution and collection services of deep throat saliva specimen bottles by mobile van from November 8, and provide free specimen collection and testing services through mobile specimen collection stations from November 9, with a view to facilitating and encouraging residents of the district or individuals who perceive themselves as having a higher risk of exposure to undergo free COVID-19 testing.

A Government spokesman said, "The Government will continue to closely monitor the situation. In the eventuality of a sudden outbreak in certain groups, the Government may arrange for urgent cluster testing in the community testing centres or through mobile facilities for the relevant locations or premises with confirmed cases based on a need and risk assessment in order to identify the infected persons and cut the transmission chains as soon as possible."

While the mobile specimen collection stations have ceased operation, members of the public can still receive free COVID-19 tests by collecting deep throat saliva specimen collection packs at the 46 general outpatient clinics of the Hospital Authority.

[47] https://www.info.gov.hk/gia/general/202011/16.htm

The spokesman appealed to all members of the public who have doubts about their health condition to undergo testing to protect oneself and others and to fight the virus together.

Issued at HKT 1:05

Four community testing centres commence service

****

Four community testing centres set up by the Government on Hong Kong Island and in Kowloon, New Territories East and New Territories West commenced service on November 15. The centres provided self-paid COVID-19 testing services for general community or private purposes at a more affordable price for more than 2 380 people on November 15.

The four community testing centres are located at Quarry Bay Community Hall in Eastern District, Henry G Leong Yaumatei Community Centre, Lek Yuen Community Hall in Sha Tin and Yuen Long Town East Community Hall respectively. The price of the relevant service is capped at $240. The community testing centres provide specimen collection services (using combined nasal and throat swabs) and COVID-19 testing services for all asymptomatic individuals (excluding children under 6 years old and people not suitable for testing) holding valid Hong Kong identity cards, Hong Kong birth certificates or other valid identity documents (including Hong Kong residents and non-Hong Kong residents). The testing centres open daily from 8am to 1.30pm and from 2.30pm to 8pm. Deep cleaning and disinfection will be conducted when they close in the afternoon and at night.

A Government spokesman said, "To reduce the waiting time at the testing centres, members of the public holding a Hong Kong identity card or a Hong Kong birth certificate are encouraged to make use of the 24-hour booking system (www.communitytest.gov.hk). Members of the public only need to provide simple personal information (including their name, Hong Kong identity card or Hong Kong birth certificate number and phone number) to select the testing centre and time slot."

For enquiries, please call the following hotlines of the community testing centres:

Quarry Bay Community Hall, Eastern District (Prenetics)	3008 8325
Henry G Leong Yaumatei Community Centre (Kingmed Diagnostics (Hong Kong) Limited)	9869 3603
Lek Yuen Community Hall, Sha Tin (Hong Kong Molecular Pathology Diagnostic Centre Limited)	2986 1272 2986 1270

Yuen Long Town East Community Hall (BGI)	2818 9690

The Government spokesman reminded that those who have undergone COVID-19 testing in Hong Kong with negative test results would still be subject to the prevailing quarantine arrangements of the Mainland/Guangdong Province or Macao (e.g. 14-day compulsory quarantine) when they visit the two places, unless exemption has been granted for them separately. They should take note of the latest quarantine arrangement of the Mainland/Guangdong Province and Macao, and make necessary preparations.

Issued at HKT 1:09

CHP investigates eight additional confirmed cases of COVID-19

****

The Centre for Health Protection (CHP) of the Department of Health has announced that as of 0.00am, November 16, the CHP was investigating eight additional confirmed cases of coronavirus disease 2019 (COVID-19), taking the number of cases to 5 467 in Hong Kong so far (comprising 5 466 confirmed cases and one probable case).

All the newly reported cases announced had a travel history during the incubation period.

The CHP's epidemiological investigations and relevant contact tracing on the confirmed cases are ongoing. For case details and contact tracing information, please see the Annex or the list of buildings with confirmed cases of COVID-19 in the past 14 days and the latest local situation of COVID-19 available on the website "COVID-19 Thematic Website" (www.coronavirus.gov.hk).

A spokesman for the CHP said, "During the CHP's epidemiological investigations and relevant contact tracing on the confirmed cases, we will compile and upload (www.chp.gov.hk/files/pdf/building_list_eng.pdf) a list of buildings that confirmed patients had visited from two days before the onset of symptoms. Given that cases of local infection continue to occur from time to time, members of the public are urged to seek medical attention immediately if they believe that they had visited the same place at an identical time with a confirmed patient and feel unwell subsequently. If they remain asymptomatic but are concerned that they have been infected, they can also visit the Hospital Authority's designated general out-patient clinics (www.ha.org.hk/haho/ho/covid-19/GOPC_extend_EN.pdf) to obtain specimen collection packs and collect deep throat saliva specimens for free COVID-19 testing."

In view of the severe epidemic situation, the CHP called on members of the public to avoid going out, having social contact and dining out. They should put on a surgical mask and maintain

stringent hand hygiene when they need to go out. The CHP strongly urged the elderly to stay home as far as possible and avoid going out. They should consider asking their family and friends to help with everyday tasks such as shopping for basic necessities.

The spokesman said, "Given that the situation of COVID-19 infection remains severe and that there is a continuous increase in the number of cases reported around the world, members of the public are strongly urged to avoid all non-essential travel outside Hong Kong.

"The CHP also strongly urges the public to maintain at all times strict personal and environmental hygiene, which is key to personal protection against infection and prevention of the spread of the disease in the community. On a personal level, members of the public should wear a surgical mask when having respiratory symptoms, taking public transport or staying in crowded places. They should also perform hand hygiene frequently, especially before touching the mouth, nose or eyes.

"As for household environmental hygiene, members of the public are advised to maintain drainage pipes properly, regularly pour water into drain outlets (U-traps) and cover all floor drain outlets when they are not in use. After using the toilet, they should put the toilet lid down before flushing to avoid spreading germs."

Moreover, the Government has launched the website "COVID-19 Thematic Website" (www.coronavirus.gov.hk) for announcing the latest updates on various news on COVID-19 infection and health advice to help the public understand the latest updates. Members of the public may also gain access to information via the COVID-19 WhatsApp Helpline launched by the Office of the Government Chief Information Officer. Simply by saving 9617 1823 in their phone contacts or clicking the link wa.me/85296171823?text=hi, they will be able to obtain information on COVID-19 as well as the "StayHomeSafe" mobile app and wristband via WhatsApp.

Issued at HKT 14:00

Public hospitals daily update on COVID-19 cases

****

The following is issued on behalf of the Hospital Authority:

As at 9am today (November 16), three COVID-19 confirmed patients were discharged from hospital in the last 24 hours. Including a patient (case number: 5454) discharged on November 14, a total of 5 198 patients with confirmed or probable infection have been discharged so far.

At present, there are 595 negative pressure rooms in public hospitals with 1 078 negative pressure beds activated. A total of 123 confirmed patients are currently hospitalised in 20 public hospitals, among which seven patients are in critical condition, two are in serious condition and the remaining 114 patients are in stable condition.

The Hospital Authority will maintain close contact with the Centre for Health Protection to monitor the latest developments and to inform the public and healthcare workers on the latest information in a timely manner.

Details of the above-mentioned patients are as follows:

Patient condition	Case numbers
Discharged	5387, 5396, 5428, 5454
Critical	1989, 3496, 4706, 4833, 5110, 5185, 5409
Serious	5151, 5273

Issued at HKT 16:40

FEHD continues to arrange free COVID-19 testing services for targeted groups

****

The Food and Environmental Hygiene Department (FEHD) announced today (November 16) that it will continue to arrange voluntary free COVID-19 testing services for targeted groups. In view of the detection of the virus on packaging materials of frozen commodities in the Mainland and other places in recent days, the FEHD is extending the testing services to cover practitioners of cold stores to safeguard public health. Registration is not required and the testing agency (Prenetics Limited) will contact the operators of all licensed cold stores as soon as possible to arrange testing services for their staff starting from November 18.

A spokesman for the FEHD said, "To broaden surveillance at the community level, and incorporate disease prevention and infection control into the new normal of the daily operation of society, the Government will integrate and regularise the Targeted Group Testing Scheme (TGTS) as part of its sentinel surveillance. The TGTS will become part of the surveillance and early-warning system. By facilitating contact tracing and epidemiological investigations, it will be conducive to 'early identification, early isolation and early treatment', and can provide reference data for the overall assessment of the epidemic situation."

The FEHD currently has been arranging testing every week for those working in the Sheung Shui Slaughterhouse, and will continue to provide voluntary free virus testing services for high-exposure groups, including catering premises staff (licensed general restaurants, licensed light refreshment restaurants, licensed marine restaurants, licensed factory canteens, school canteens, staff canteens, bars and pubs), staff and personnel working in FEHD markets, hawker licensees and registered assistants.

Under the scheme, the testing agency will be responsible for the provision of one-stop services covering specimen taking and testing. The testing agency will deliver specimen bottles to the premises for collecting deep throat saliva samples, and then collect the samples in the subsequent one to two days for testing. The person-in-charge of the premises should return all unused specimen bottles to the testing agency on the day of the sample collection. Cases with preliminary positive results will be relayed to the Centre for Health Protection of the Department of Health for follow-up.

The FEHD strongly appeals to the groups concerned to actively participate in the testing scheme, and continue to comply with the directions made under the Prevention and Control of Disease (Requirements and Directions) (Business and Premises) Regulation (Cap. 599F), and to maintain personal and environmental hygiene continuously with a view to ensuring cleanliness of the premises and food safety.

For details of the testing programme, please call the hotline of the testing agency at 3008 8319 or visit the FEHD website (www.fehd.gov.hk).

Issued at HKT 16:53

OGCIO explains access right issues on "LeaveHomeSafe" COVID-19 exposure notification mobile app

****

The "LeaveHomeSafe" COVID-19 exposure notification mobile app was officially launched today (November 16). With regard to some media reports on the access rights of the mobile app, including access to photos and media, files and storage space, modification or deletion of content, and access to Wi-Fi network and network permissions, the Office of the Government Chief Information Officer (OGCIO) gave the following response:

The "LeaveHomeSafe" mobile app assists the public in recording the date and time for checking into and leaving different venues by scanning the venue QR code or the registration mark located at the inside of the taxi door. The app requires the camera function of the mobile phone to scan the venue QR code and the taxi registration mark. After scanning, relevant check-in data, including the venue name and address, taxi registration mark, date, arrival and departure time, will all be stored in the storage space of the mobile phone. The app therefore requires permission to access the camera and storage space of the mobile phone.

In addition, cloud-based Optical Character Recognition (OCR) technology is used to enable scanning of the taxi registration mark. Text images captured by the camera will be converted to text files for storage. The mobile app will then delete relevant images instantly and user's check-in data will also be erased automatically after 31 days. The mobile app thus requires access permissions to mobile network, Wi-Fi network (to conserve data usage), media and files in order to protect user's privacy.

The Centre for Health Protection (CHP) has been releasing information on premises visited by COVID-19 confirmed cases in the form of open data. The "LeaveHomeSafe" mobile app needs to run in the background, and use the network function to download the data from CHP for comparing with user's venue check-in data regularly in the mobile phone, in order to notify any user who has visited the same venue as the COVID-19 confirmed case at around the same time automatically. Hence, the mobile app requires network access, Wi-Fi access and relevant permissions in allowing the app to run in the background and send notifications when needed. Moreover, the "LeaveHomeSafe" mobile app would perform checking (with access permission to the "retrieve running apps" under "device & app history") in order to ensure previous task of data download has been completed, and retrieval of the correct version of data.

The spokesman for the OGCIO stressed that the Government understands public concerns over privacy, and therefore uphold the principle of protecting personal data privacy when designing the "LeaveHomeSafe" mobile app. The program designs of the app on Android and iOS are the same. The app only needs the least amount of access permissions to enable smooth operation and it has also passed relevant code reviews of Google and Apple. The spokesman reiterated that the Government recognises public concerns over the access permissions that the "LeaveHomeSafe" mobile app uses and will continue to explain to the public in this regard, and also invite more members of the public to use the app so as to minimise the risk of virus transmission.

Issued at HKT 23:50

November 17[48]

Public hospitals daily update on COVID-19 cases

****

The following is issued on behalf of the Hospital Authority:

As at 9am today (November 17), 14 COVID-19 confirmed patients were discharged from hospital in the last 24 hours. So far, a total of 5 212 patients with confirmed or probable infection have been discharged.

---

[48] https://www.info.gov.hk/gia/general/202011/17.htm

At present, there are 594 negative pressure rooms in public hospitals with 1 077 negative pressure beds activated. A total of 117 confirmed patients are currently hospitalised in 19 public hospitals, among which seven patients are in critical condition, two are in serious condition and the remaining 108 patients are in stable condition.

The Hospital Authority will maintain close contact with the Centre for Health Protection to monitor the latest developments and to inform the public and healthcare workers on the latest information in a timely manner.

Details of the above-mentioned patients are as follows:

Patient condition	Case numbers
Discharged	5333, 5342, 5347, 5349, 5362, 5365, 5375, 5416, 5417, 5418, 5420, 5429, 5442, 5467
Critical	1989, 3496, 4706, 4833, 5110, 5185, 5409
Serious	5151, 5273

Issued at HKT 17:20

CHP investigates four additional confirmed cases of COVID-19

****

The Centre for Health Protection (CHP) of the Department of Health has announced that as of 0.00am, November 17, the CHP was investigating four additional confirmed cases of coronavirus disease 2019 (COVID-19), taking the number of cases to 5 471 in Hong Kong so far (comprising 5 470 confirmed cases and one probable case).

Among the newly reported cases announced, three had a travel history during the incubation period.

A total of 130 cases were recorded in the past 14 days (from November 3 to 16), including 33 local cases (in which 18 have unknown sources).

The CHP's epidemiological investigations and relevant contact tracing on the confirmed cases are ongoing. For case details and contact tracing information, please see the Annex or the list of buildings with confirmed cases of COVID-19 in the past 14 days and the latest local situation of COVID-19 available on the website "COVID-19 Thematic Website" (www.coronavirus.gov.hk).

A spokesman for the CHP said, "During the CHP's epidemiological investigations and relevant contact tracing on the confirmed cases, we will compile and upload (www.chp.gov.hk/files/pdf/building_list_eng.pdf) a list of buildings that confirmed patients had visited from two days before the onset of symptoms. Given that cases of local infection continue to occur from time to time, members of the public are urged to seek medical attention immediately if they believe that they had visited the same place at an identical time with a confirmed patient and feel unwell subsequently. If they remain asymptomatic but are concerned that they have been infected, they can also visit the Hospital Authority's designated general out-patient clinics (www.ha.org.hk/haho/ho/covid-19/GOPC_extend_EN.pdf) to obtain specimen collection packs and collect deep throat saliva specimens for free COVID-19 testing."

In view of the severe epidemic situation, the CHP called on members of the public to avoid going out, having social contact and dining out. They should put on a surgical mask and maintain stringent hand hygiene when they need to go out. The CHP strongly urged the elderly to stay home as far as possible and avoid going out. They should consider asking their family and friends to help with everyday tasks such as shopping for basic necessities.

The spokesman said, "Given that the situation of COVID-19 infection remains severe and that there is a continuous increase in the number of cases reported around the world, members of the public are strongly urged to avoid all non-essential travel outside Hong Kong.

"The CHP also strongly urges the public to maintain at all times strict personal and environmental hygiene, which is key to personal protection against infection and prevention of the spread of the disease in the community. On a personal level, members of the public should wear a surgical mask when having respiratory symptoms, taking public transport or staying in crowded places. They should also perform hand hygiene frequently, especially before touching the mouth, nose or eyes.

"As for household environmental hygiene, members of the public are advised to maintain drainage pipes properly, regularly pour water into drain outlets (U-traps) and cover all floor drain outlets when they are not in use. After using the toilet, they should put the toilet lid down before flushing to avoid spreading germs."

Moreover, the Government has launched the website "COVID-19 Thematic Website" (www.coronavirus.gov.hk) for announcing the latest updates on various news on COVID-19 infection and health advice to help the public understand the latest updates. Members of the public may also gain access to information via the COVID-19 WhatsApp Helpline launched by the Office of the Government Chief Information Officer. Simply by saving 9617 1823 in their phone contacts or clicking the link wa.me/85296171823?text=hi, they will be able to obtain information on COVID-19 as well as the "StayHomeSafe" mobile app and wristband via WhatsApp.

Issued at HKT 17:32

"Return2hk - Travel Scheme for Hong Kong Residents returning from Guangdong Province or Macao without being subject to quarantine under the Compulsory Quarantine of Certain Persons Arriving at Hong Kong Regulation (Cap. 599C)" to open for application tomorrow

****

"Return2hk - Travel Scheme for Hong Kong Residents returning from Guangdong Province or Macao without being subject to quarantine under the Compulsory Quarantine of Certain Persons Arriving at Hong Kong Regulation (Cap. 599C)" (Return2hk Scheme) will be open for application from tomorrow (November 18). Hong Kong residents who are currently in Guangdong Province or Macao will be exempted from the 14-day compulsory quarantine requirement when they return to Hong Kong under the Return2hk Scheme upon fulfilment of all the conditions specified under sections 12 and 12A of the Regulation.

Quota applications

The first batch of quotas under the Return2hk Scheme will be open for application from 9am tomorrow until 6pm on November 20 (Friday) for bookings to return to Hong Kong between November 23 (Monday) and November 29 (Sunday). Hong Kong residents who wish to return to Hong Kong under the Return2hk Scheme should apply under a quota using the online booking system (www.quotabooking.gov.hk). A daily quota of 3 000 has been set for Shenzhen Bay Port, while that for the Hong Kong-Zhuhai-Macao Bridge (HZMB) Hong Kong Port is 2 000.

Quota allocation will be administered on a first-come, first-served basis. The online booking system will be open each Wednesday at 9am and run until 6pm on Friday to accept quota applications for the seven-day period of the following week (i.e. Monday to Sunday).

Eligibility

Any Hong Kong resident aged 18 or above who is currently in Guangdong Province or Macao may apply under a quota through the Return2hk Scheme booking system during the above-mentioned opening hours of the system. When making an application, the applicant is required to provide his/her Hong Kong identity card number, and to specify the date and the boundary control point (i.e. Shenzhen Bay Port or the HZMB Hong Kong Port) to be used for the return. In the same application, he/she may also apply under the quota for three accompanying Hong Kong residents at most. Applications for Hong Kong residents who are under 18 should be made on their behalf by their parents or guardians, and the number of their Hong Kong identity card or other personal identity document(s) (e.g. Hong Kong Special Administrative Region (HKSAR) passport, HKSAR re-entry permit, birth certificate or other passports) should be provided.

A Government spokesman stressed that Hong Kong residents who can fulfil all the specified conditions and are returning to Hong Kong under the Return2hk Scheme should still exercise self-monitoring of their health conditions for at least 14 days after their entry into Hong Kong. They should observe the points listed in the "Health-monitoring Checklist for Inbound

Travellers". If they feel unwell, they should seek medical advice promptly and reveal their travel history to medical practitioners.

Details about the Return2hk Scheme, including those relating to nucleic acid testing, documents to be provided, health code conversion and more, are available at the "COVID-19 Thematic Website" (return2hk.gov.hk or 回港易.政府.香港). Members of the public may also call the hotline of the Return2hk Scheme at 3142 2330 if they have any enquiries.

Issued at HKT 18:17

Man sentenced for breaching compulsory quarantine order

****

A 76-year-old man was sentenced to immediate imprisonment for 14 days by the Tuen Mun Magistrates' Courts today (November 17) for violating the Compulsory Quarantine of Certain Persons Arriving at Hong Kong Regulation (Cap 599C) (the Regulation).

The man was issued a compulsory quarantine order when he entered Hong Kong on November 2, stating that he must conduct quarantine at home for 14 days. He did not enter the place of quarantine without reasonable excuse nor permission given by an authorised officer and tried to leave Hong Kong on the same day. He was stopped by an immigration officer at the Shenzhen Bay Control Point. He was charged with contravening sections 8(4) and 8(5) of the Regulation and was sentenced by the Tuen Mun Magistrates' Courts today to immediate imprisonment for 14 days.

Pursuant to the Regulation, starting from February 8, save for exempted persons, all persons who have stayed in the Mainland, Macao or Taiwan in the 14 days preceding arrival in Hong Kong, regardless of their nationality or travel documents, will be subject to compulsory quarantine for 14 days. Moreover, pursuant to the Compulsory Quarantine of Persons Arriving at Hong Kong from Foreign Places Regulation (Cap 599E), starting from March 19, all persons arriving from countries or territories outside China would also be subject to compulsory quarantine for 14 days. Breaching a quarantine order is a criminal offence and offenders are subject to a maximum fine of $25,000 and imprisonment for six months.

A spokesman for the Department of Health said the sentence sends a clear message to the community that breaching a compulsory quarantine order is a criminal offence that the Government will not tolerate, and solemnly reminded the public to comply with the Regulation. As of today, a total of 68 persons have been convicted by the courts for breaching compulsory quarantine orders and have received sentences including immediate imprisonment for up to three months or a fine of $15,000. The spokesman reiterated that resolute actions will be taken against anyone who has breached the relevant regulations.

Issued at HKT 18:35

Government announces further tightening of testing and isolation arrangement for consular and diplomatic officers exempted from compulsory quarantine

****

The Government today (November 17) announced that the testing and isolation arrangements for consular and diplomatic officers who are exempted from quarantine requirement upon arriving Hong Kong will be tightened with effect from tomorrow (November 18).

A Government spokesman pointed out that in view of the development and severity of the global epidemic situation, based on the prevention and risk assessment, the Government decided to tighten the epidemic control measures on inbound travellers comprehensively. With effect from November 18 (Wednesday), the Government will tighten the testing and isolation arrangement for consular and diplomatic officers who are exempted from quarantine arrangement upon arriving Hong Kong, particularly those who have visited very high risk places (i.e. the specified very high-risk places gazetted under the Prevention and Control of Disease (Regulation of Cross-boundary Conveyances and Travellers) Regulation (Cap.599H)), with details as follows:

Consular and diplomatic officers who have visited very high risk places during the 14 days prior to arrival in Hong Kong:

• They must possess a negative result of SARS-CoV-2 nucleic acid test done at an ISO15189-accredited laboratory or a laboratory recognised by the Government where the laboratory is located with the specimen collected within 48 hours prior to boarding the flight to Hong Kong;

• They must take a post-arrival SARS-CoV-2 nucleic acid test at the Department of Health's (DH) Temporary Specimen Collection Centre (TSCC) and wait for the results there or any other location as designated by DH upon arrival at Hong Kong International Airport (HKIA);

• Except Consul Generals or representatives in HKSAR at equivalent level, all other consular and diplomatic officers must be subject to self-isolation for 14 days at an accommodation arranged by respective organisations;

• Specimen bottles will be distributed to the consular and diplomatic officers upon arrival. They must collect and return their deep throat saliva sample at Day-12 upon their arrival in accordance with the instructions for SARS-CoV-2 nucleic acid test again; and

• Respective organisations must arrange point-to-point transportation for the consular and diplomatic officers. The use of public transport is prohibited.

Consular and diplomatic officers who have not visited very high risk places during the 14-day prior to arrival in Hong Kong:

• If they possess a negative result of SARS-CoV-2 nucleic acid test done at an ISO15189-accredited laboratory or a laboratory recognised by the Government where the laboratory is located with the specimen collected within 48 hours prior to boarding the flight to Hong Kong, they are required to take a post-arrival SARS-CoV-2 nucleic acid test at the DH's TSCC before leaving HKIA;

• If they do not possess a negative result of SARS-CoV-2 nucleic acid test done at an ISO15189-accredited laboratory or a laboratory recognised by the Government where the laboratory is located with the specimen collected within 48 hours prior to boarding the flight to Hong Kong, they must take a post-arrival SARS-CoV-2 nucleic acid test at the DH's TSCC and wait for the results there or any other location as designated by DH upon arrival at HKIA;

• Specimen bottles will be distributed to the consular and diplomatic officers upon arrival. They must collect and return their deep throat saliva sample at Day-12 upon their arrival in accordance with the instructions for SARS-CoV-2 nucleic acid test again; and

• Respective organisations must arrange point-to-point transportation for the consular and diplomatic officers. The use of public transport is prohibited.

The spokesman said, "The exemption status and the itineraries of the consular and diplomatic officers carrying out governmental duties are determined by their official capacity and relevant official duties with a view to safeguarding normal operation of the governments. Nevertheless, we consider there is a need to tighten respective exemption arrangement to strengthen the prevention of imported cases as well as avoiding the respective exempted persons' contact with the local community during the exemption period, so as to achieve the strategic goal to 'Controlling the epidemic with precision'."

The spokesman added, "The testing and quarantine arrangement imposed by the Government on incoming passengers was made on the basis of public health risk assessment and has been adjusting rapidly in response to the latest epidemic situation and experts' views. The Government will continue to closely monitor the epidemic situation around the world, and review the quarantine and testing arrangements for all inbound travellers (including exempted persons) entering Hong Kong.

Issued at HKT 21:03

November 18[49]

[49] https://www.info.gov.hk/gia/general/202011/18.htm

CHP investigates nine additional confirmed cases of COVID-19

****

The Centre for Health Protection (CHP) of the Department of Health has announced that as of 0.00am, November 18, the CHP was investigating nine additional confirmed cases of coronavirus disease 2019 (COVID-19), taking the number of cases to 5 480 in Hong Kong so far (comprising 5 479 confirmed cases and one probable case).

Among the newly reported cases announced, six had a travel history during the incubation period, one was local case with unknown sources while the other two were epidemiologically linked with a local case.

The case with unknown sources involves a 76-year-old man (case 5 479) who had developed cough on November 10 and shortness of breath on November 16. The patient sought medical attention at Prince of Wales Hospital on November 16 and was admitted. He is a taxi driver and last went to work on November 16.

A total of 125 cases have been recorded in the past 14 days (November 4 - 17), including 31 local cases of which 18 are from unknown sources.

The CHP's epidemiological investigations and relevant contact tracing on the confirmed cases are ongoing. For case details and contact tracing information, please see the Annex or the list of buildings with confirmed cases of COVID-19 in the past 14 days and the latest local situation of COVID-19 available on the website "COVID-19 Thematic Website" (www.coronavirus.gov.hk).

Starting today, the DH will disallow visitors for any person under compulsory quarantine in hotels during the quarantine period. If confinees have the need to replenish goods or food, their friends, family members or hotel staff can place them outside the guestrooms for the confinees to pick up without face-to-face contact. If a person under compulsory hotel quarantine requires the company of a carer which requires prior permission from DH, the carer also has to be quarantined in the hotel till the end of the quarantine period.

The Government strongly appeals to the confinees to follow the quarantine requirement strictly in order to protect the health of their own selves and others. The measure is of utmost importance to prevent the spreading of COVID-19 in the community. Breaking Quarantine Orders is a criminal offence and offenders are subject to a maximum imprisonment of six months and a fine of $25,000.

A spokesman for the CHP said, "During the CHP's epidemiological investigations and relevant contact tracing on the confirmed cases, we will compile and upload (www.chp.gov.hk/files/pdf/building_list_eng.pdf) a list of buildings that confirmed patients had visited from two days before the onset of symptoms. Given that cases of local infection continue to occur from time to time, members of the public are urged to seek medical attention immediately if they believe that they had visited the same place at an identical time with a confirmed patient and feel unwell subsequently. If they remain asymptomatic but are concerned

that they have been infected, they can also visit the Hospital Authority's designated general out-patient clinics (www.ha.org.hk/haho/ho/covid-19/GOPC_extend_EN.pdf) to obtain specimen collection packs and collect deep throat saliva specimens for free COVID-19 testing."

In view of the severe epidemic situation, the CHP called on members of the public to avoid going out, having social contact and dining out. They should put on a surgical mask and maintain stringent hand hygiene when they need to go out. The CHP strongly urged the elderly to stay home as far as possible and avoid going out. They should consider asking their family and friends to help with everyday tasks such as shopping for basic necessities.

The spokesman said, "Given that the situation of COVID-19 infection remains severe and that there is a continuous increase in the number of cases reported around the world, members of the public are strongly urged to avoid all non-essential travel outside Hong Kong.

"The CHP also strongly urges the public to maintain at all times strict personal and environmental hygiene, which is key to personal protection against infection and prevention of the spread of the disease in the community. On a personal level, members of the public should wear a surgical mask when having respiratory symptoms, taking public transport or staying in crowded places. They should also perform hand hygiene frequently, especially before touching the mouth, nose or eyes.

"As for household environmental hygiene, members of the public are advised to maintain drainage pipes properly, regularly pour water into drain outlets (U-traps) and cover all floor drain outlets when they are not in use. After using the toilet, they should put the toilet lid down before flushing to avoid spreading germs."

Moreover, the Government has launched the website "COVID-19 Thematic Website" (www.coronavirus.gov.hk) for announcing the latest updates on various news on COVID-19 infection and health advice to help the public understand the latest updates. Members of the public may also gain access to information via the COVID-19 WhatsApp Helpline launched by the Office of the Government Chief Information Officer. Simply by saving 9617 1823 in their phone contacts or clicking the link wa.me/85296171823?text=hi, they will be able to obtain information on COVID-19 as well as the "StayHomeSafe" mobile app and wristband via WhatsApp.

Issued at HKT 14:00

Public hospitals daily update on COVID-19 cases

****

The following is issued on behalf of the Hospital Authority:

As at 9am today (November 18), 12 COVID-19 confirmed patients were discharged from hospital in the last 24 hours. So far, a total of 5 224 patients with confirmed or probable infection have been discharged.

At present, there are 594 negative pressure rooms in public hospitals with 1 077 negative pressure beds activated. A total of 109 confirmed patients are currently hospitalised in 19 public hospitals, among which eight patients are in critical condition, two are in serious condition and the remaining 99 patients are in stable condition.

The Hospital Authority will maintain close contact with the Centre for Health Protection to monitor the latest developments and to inform the public and healthcare workers on the latest information in a timely manner.

Details of the above-mentioned patients are as follows:

Patient condition	Case numbers
Discharged	3170, 5271, 5297, 5343, 5348, 5356, 5391, 5430, 5441, 5458, 5461, 5462
Critical	1989, 3496, 4706, 4833, 5110, 5185, 5409,5433
Serious	5151, 5273

Issued at HKT 17:41

S for IT visits Kowloon City to keep abreast of "LeaveHomeSafe" mobile app implementation (

****

The Secretary for Innovation and Technology, Mr Alfred Sit, today (November 18) toured a market, restaurants, a bar and a karaoke establishment in Kowloon City District to keep abreast of the implementation of the "LeaveHomeSafe" mobile app.

Accompanied by the Deputy Director of the Food and Environmental Hygiene Department (FEHD), Miss Diane Wong, Mr Sit started his visit at the To Kwa Wan Market. He toured market stalls to learn more about the FEHD's work in guarding against COVID-19 with the aid of technology and promoting the "LeaveHomeSafe" mobile app. Venue QR codes are put up at market entrances and prominent positions, with posters being displayed alongside with QR codes to allow members of the public to better understand how to download and use the mobile app, and to keep a more precise record of their whereabouts. The FEHD's subsidy scheme for promotion of contactless payment in public markets will provide a one-off subsidy to tenants of public markets to promote the use of contactless payment in market stalls. This will help reduce virus transmission in the markets. He exchanged views with representatives of trade associations, stall tenants and market patrons present on the implementation of the anti-epidemic measures.

Mr Sit then visited different premises in the vicinity, including a karaoke establishment, a local cafe kitchen, a foot massage parlour, a bar, a noodle stall and a Chinese restaurant. He chatted with shop operators and members of the public and listened to their views for further refinements.

Mr Sit said, "We have all along been actively engaging various sectors and enlisting their support for the 'LeaveHomeSafe' mobile app. The response is encouraging and so far we have over 10 000 public and private venues taking part in the scheme. We will continue to step up our efforts to get the message across and invite more sectors, such as restaurant chains, retail outlets and property management businesses to participate. With concerted efforts and the aid of technology, we can encourage the public to develop a habit of keeping a more precise record of their whereabouts which can help fight the virus and get better prepared for guarding against the fourth wave of the pandemic."

There are currently over 10 000 public and private venues participating in the scheme. Among them, 6 000 are public venues, which include government office buildings, sports centres, swimming pools, libraries, markets, cooked food markets, community halls/centres, building lobbies and shopping centres of public housing estates, hospitals, clinics, post offices and terminals. Nearly 4 000 participating venues are privately owned, including banks, restaurants, coffee shops, karaoke establishments, bars and pubs, clubs, hotels, fitness centres, cinemas, malls, shops, and commercial and residential buildings. The "LeaveHomeSafe" mobile app can be used directly in over 18 000 taxis. Interested institutions or organisations should contact the Office of the Government Chief Information Officer direct (Designated email address: leavehomesafe@ogcio.gov.hk).

Issued at HKT 18:29

Woman sentenced for breaching compulsory quarantine order

****

A 19-year-old woman was sentenced to 14 days' imprisonment, suspended for 12 months by the Shatin Magistrates' Courts today (November 18) for violating the Compulsory Quarantine of Certain Persons Arriving at Hong Kong Regulation (Cap. 599C) (the Regulation).

The woman was earlier issued a compulsory quarantine order stating that she must conduct quarantine at home for 14 days. Before the expiry of the quarantine order, she left the place of quarantine twice on May 15 and 16 without reasonable excuse nor permission given by an authorised officer. She was charged with two counts of contravening Sections 8(1) and 8(5) of the Regulation and was sentenced by the Shatin Magistrates' Courts today to 14 days' imprisonment, suspended for 12 months for each of the two charges, which are to run concurrently.

Pursuant to the Regulation, starting from February 8, save for exempted persons, all persons who have stayed in the Mainland, Macao or Taiwan in the 14 days preceding arrival in Hong Kong, regardless of their nationality or travel documents, will be subject to compulsory quarantine for 14 days. Moreover, pursuant to the Compulsory Quarantine of Persons Arriving at Hong Kong from Foreign Places Regulation (Cap. 599E), starting from March 19, all persons arriving from countries or territories outside China would also be subject to compulsory quarantine for 14 days. Breaching a quarantine order is a criminal offence and offenders are subject to a maximum fine of $25,000 and imprisonment for six months.

A spokesman for the Department of Health said the sentence sends a clear message to the community that breaching a compulsory quarantine order is a criminal offence that the Government will not tolerate, and solemnly reminded the public to comply with the Regulation. As of today, a total of 69 persons have been convicted by the courts for breaching compulsory quarantine orders and have received sentences including imprisonment for up to three months or a fine of $15,000. The spokesman reiterated that resolute actions will be taken against anyone who has breached the relevant regulations.

Issued at HKT 18:57

Latest amendments to Prevention and Control of Disease (Requirements and Directions) (Business and Premises) Regulation and Prevention and Control of Disease (Prohibition on Group Gathering) Regulation

****

In view of the development of COVID-19 epidemic situation in Hong Kong, the Government will gazette the amendments to the Prevention and Control of Disease (Requirements and Directions) (Business and Premises) Regulation (Cap. 599F) and the Prevention and Control of Disease (Prohibition on Group Gathering) Regulation (Cap. 599G) today (November 18). The amendments provide the legal framework for the Government to promulgate relevant measures later to restrict group gatherings and strengthen the infection prevention and control in hotels/guesthouses, as well as to enhance the legal power under Cap. 599F and Cap. 599G.

A spokesman for the Food and Health Bureau said, "Since the fourth wave of outbreak could happen at any moment, the Government has to implement preventive measures in a targeted manner to reduce the infectious risks brought by mask-off gatherings."

"As announced by the Secretary for Food and Health on November 14, we notice that there has recently been an increasing trend of 'staycation' activities in hotels/guesthouses. The participants of the relevant gatherings usually did not wear masks, and sometimes there were a considerable number of participants in such gatherings. Since there was a cluster of COVID-19 cases related to this kind of gatherings earlier, the relevant health risks should not be overlooked. Furthermore, as general travellers arriving in Hong Kong from places outside China must be put under compulsory quarantine in hotels for 14 days, we consider it necessary to strengthen measures to reduce cross infection risks between confinees and local guests. The Government will therefore amend the relevant legislations to restrict gatherings and strengthen infection prevention and control measures in hotels/guesthouses, as well as imposing legal responsibility to people who organise or participate in prohibited group gatherings. Compared with the current practice where the hotel/guesthouse operators could only appeal for the self-discipline of customers, this legislative amendment exercise will facilitate the operators to manage infection prevention and control within the premises more effectively."

The latest details of the Regulations are as follows:

(1) Hotels/guesthouses referred under the Hotel and Guesthouse Accommodation Ordinance (Cap. 349) will be incorporated into the list of scheduled premises under Cap. 599F.

(2) The legal power under Cap. 599F and Cap. 599G will be enhanced, which includes expanding the scope of Cap. 599G to prohibit group gatherings at non-public places of scheduled premises regulated under Cap. 599F (for examples places within club-houses). Accordingly, for all the group gatherings in premises regulated under Cap. 599F, the participants must comply with the relevant group gathering requirements and restrictions specified under Cap. 599F in order to be exempted under Cap. 599G. Otherwise, summons can be issued against the participants under Cap. 599G.

(3) The enforcement power of authorised officers under Cap. 599F and Cap. 599G will be aligned, and a defence will be provided to the manager of the scheduled premises if he has taken all reasonable steps to ensure that the group gatherings comply with the requirements.

The relevant legislative amendments will take effect from November 20, 2020. Regarding amendment (1) above, after discussing the details with the hotel/guesthouse industry, the Government will separately gazette the directions under Cap. 599F to set out the details and the effective date of the measures restricting group gatherings and strengthening infection prevention and control in hotels/guesthouses.

Furthermore, the Department of Health (DH) has tightened the requirement to disallow visitors for any person under compulsory quarantine in hotels during the quarantine period starting from today (November 18). If confinees have the need to replenish goods or food, their friends, family members or hotel staff can place them outside the guestrooms for the confinees to pick up without face-to-face contact. If a person under compulsory hotel quarantine requires the company of a carer, with the prior permission from DH, the carer also has to be quarantined in the hotel till the end of the quarantine period. Breaking quarantine orders, including leaving quarantine places without permission or allowing visitors to enter quarantine guestrooms, is a criminal offence and offenders are subject to a maximum imprisonment of six months and a fine of $25,000.

The spokesman said, "The Government will review the various measures in place from time to time in accordance with the development of the epidemic situation, and make suitable adjustments taking into account all relevant factors."

Issued at HKT 21:09

November 19[50]

Special scheme on delivering prescription medications to Hong Kong people in Guangdong and Fujian with urgent need for medications to cease shortly

****

The Hong Kong Special Administrative Region (HKSAR) Government today (November 19) announced that the special scheme to deliver prescription medications to Hong Kong residents who are currently in Guangdong and Fujian Provinces with urgent need for medications (special scheme) will cease after December 23, 2020.

As the HKSAR Government has introduced the Special Support Scheme for Hospital Authority Chronic Disease Patients Living in the Guangdong Province to Sustain Their Medical Consultation since November 10, and announced on November 11 details of the "Return2hk" scheme under which Hong Kong residents, upon fulfilment of specified conditions, will be exempted from the 14-day compulsory quarantine requirement when returning to Hong Kong from Guangdong Province and Macao, Hong Kong residents who are currently in Guangdong Province could seek suitable medical services through various means. In this connection, the Government decided that the special scheme on delivering prescription medications will cease after its last occasion of prescription medications delivery on December 23, 2020.

"The special scheme is a temporary measure which originally aimed to address the issues faced by Hong Kong residents currently living in the Mainland who are unable to attend follow-up medical consultations in Hong Kong and return to the Mainland as usual owing to the mandatory quarantine measures and the prescription medications taken by them may soon be running out. The special scheme has been launched for about nine months since February 24, 2020. Although prescription medications have been delivered to the patients concerned, for the sake of their health, the patients are urged to consult a doctor as soon as possible if they have not attended medical consultations for a long time," the spokesman said.

---

[50] https://www.info.gov.hk/gia/general/202011/19.htm

For enquiries on the special scheme, please call the Social Welfare Department's 24-hour Hotline (Tel: 2343 2255), or the hotline of the Hong Kong Federation of Trade Unions Hong Kong office (Tel: 3652 5833) from 9am to 6pm from Monday to Friday.

Issued at HKT 14:30

Specifications under Prevention and Control of Disease (Regulation of Cross-boundary Conveyances and Travellers) Regulation to be gazetted

****

In view of the global development and severity of the COVID-19 pandemic situation, the Government announced today (November 19) that it will gazette the specifications under the Prevention and Control of Disease (Regulation of Cross-boundary Conveyances and Travellers) Regulation (Cap. 599H) to include Ecuador and Germany as specified places starting from November 28 to more effectively combat the epidemic.

A spokesman for the Food and Health Bureau said, "The global pandemic situation is becoming increasingly severe. The daily number of new cases increased from around 70 000 to 100 000 between late March and mid-May, and further increased to reach a new height of around 660 000 in mid-November. In view of the severe global pandemic situation, Hong Kong cannot afford to drop its guard on entry prevention and control measures."

Travellers who visited very high-risk places

The Government has earlier introduced Cap. 599H to impose testing and quarantine conditions on travellers coming to Hong Kong from very high-risk places to reduce the health risk they may bring to Hong Kong. The Secretary for Food and Health (SFH) has previously published in the Gazette specifications on the relevant measures applicable to 15 specified places (i.e. Bangladesh, Belgium, Ethiopia, France, India, Indonesia, Kazakhstan, Nepal, Pakistan, the Philippines, Russia, South Africa, Turkey, the United Kingdom and the United States of America) and adjusted the relevant conditions having regard to the circumstances on the ground since the implementation of the regulation.

Taking into account the latest public health risk assessment, and the changes and developments of the epidemic situation, the SFH will publish in the Gazette new specifications to maintain the conditions imposed and to include Ecuador and Germany as specified places. The relevant specifications will come into effect on November 28 and remain until further notice.

According to the latest specifications, a traveller who, on the day on which the traveller boarded a civil aviation aircraft that arrives at, or is about to arrive at, Hong Kong (specified aircraft), or during the 14 days before that day, has stayed in one of the aforementioned specified places must provide the following documents:

(1) A test report in English or Chinese issued by a laboratory or healthcare institution bearing the name of the relevant traveller from the aforementioned specified places identical to that in his or her valid travel document to show that:

(a) the relevant traveller from the aforementioned specified places underwent a nucleic acid test for COVID-19, the sample for which was taken from the relevant traveller from the aforementioned specified places within 72 hours before the scheduled time of departure of the specified aircraft;

(b) the test conducted on the sample is a nucleic acid test for COVID-19; and

(c) the result of the test is that the relevant traveller from the aforementioned specified places was tested negative for COVID-19; and

(2) If the relevant report is not in English or Chinese or does not contain all of the above information, a written confirmation in English or Chinese issued by the laboratory or healthcare institution bearing the name of the relevant traveller from the aforementioned specified places identical to that in his or her valid travel document and setting out all of the above information. The said written confirmation should be presented together with the test report; and

(3) Documentary proof in English or Chinese to show that the laboratory or healthcare institution is ISO 15189 accredited or is recognised or approved by the relevant authority of the government of the place in which the laboratory or healthcare institution is located; and

(4) The relevant traveller from the aforementioned specified places has confirmation in English or Chinese of room reservation in a hotel in Hong Kong for not less than 14 days starting on the day of the arrival in Hong Kong of the relevant traveller from the aforementioned specified places.

Travellers who visited any country outside China

The spokesman reminded with effect from November 13, 2020, a traveller who, on the day on which the traveller boarded a specified aircraft, or during the 14 days before that day, has stayed in a specified place outside China (excluding very high-risk areas specified otherwise), must provide confirmation in English or Chinese of room reservation in a hotel in Hong Kong for not less than 14 days starting on the day of the arrival in Hong Kong of the relevant traveller from the rest of the world.

The operator of the specified aircraft should submit to the Department of Health (DH) before the specified aircraft arrives at Hong Kong a document in a form specified by the DH confirming that each relevant traveller from the rest of the world has, before being checked in for the flight to Hong Kong on the aircraft, produced for boarding on the aircraft the above document.

A person who is in transit in Hong Kong, a person exempted by the Chief Secretary for Administration from compulsory quarantine under section 4(1) of either the Compulsory Quarantine of Certain Persons Arriving at Hong Kong Regulation (Cap. 599C) or the Compulsory Quarantine of Persons Arriving at Hong Kong from Foreign Places Regulation (Cap. 599E), and a person who arrives at Hong Kong from Singapore and meets all conditions specified for Singapore as a Category 2 specified foreign place by the SFH under section 12(2) of Cap. 599E will not be affected.

Government continues to strengthen law enforcement

If any condition specified by the SFH is not met in relation to any relevant traveller on the conveyance, each of the operators of the conveyance commits an offence and is liable on conviction to the maximum penalty of a fine at level 5 ($50,000) and imprisonment for six months. If an operator fails to comply with a requirement to provide information, or knowingly or recklessly provides any information that is false or misleading in a material particular, he or she is liable on conviction to the maximum penalty of a fine at level 5 ($50,000) and imprisonment for six months.

As for travellers, if a traveller coming to Hong Kong fails to comply with a requirement to provide information, or knowingly or recklessly provides any information that is false or misleading in a material particular, he or she is liable on conviction to the maximum penalty of a fine at level 3 ($10,000) and imprisonment for six months.

Travellers to Hong Kong should note that they will be mandated to wait for their test results at a designated location after their deep throat saliva samples are collected for conducting testing for COVID-19 at the DH's Temporary Specimen Collection Centre pursuant to the Prevention and Control of Disease Regulation (Cap. 599A). If their test results are negative, they will be allowed to go to the hotel for which they made the reservation to continue the 14-day compulsory quarantine until completion. If their results are positive, the travellers will be transferred to hospital for isolation and treatment.

The Government will continue to monitor closely the situation including the developments of the epidemic situation both globally and locally and changes in the volume of cross-boundary passenger traffic, and will not hesitate to adopt more resolute and severe measures as and when necessary.

Issued at HKT 17:10

HA to install more vending machines for specimen collection pack distribution

****

The following is issued on behalf of the Hospital Authority:

The Hospital Authority (HA) today (November 19) announced that more vending machines will be installed to distribute specimen collection packs, to tie in with the "Enhanced Laboratory Surveillance Programme" of the Centre for Health Protection (CHP) of the Department of Health in order to identify infected cases earlier and minimise the risk of community transmission. Members of the public who perceive themselves to have a higher risk of exposure and experience mild discomfort can undergo COVID-19 testing with greater convenience.

"The HA has earlier piloted the use of vending machines in distributing specimen collection packs in three General Out-patient Clinics (GOPCs). With satisfactory results in the trial run, the HA decided to install another 14 vending machines in selected GOPCs in the coming week starting from tomorrow (November 20), enabling members of public to obtain specimen collection packs. The clinics can then focus manpower on providing patient services," the HA spokesman said.

In addition, to enable the public to obtain specimen collection packs with greater convenience, the HA has been exploring using vending machines in clinics that could not serve as distribution points previously due to site limitations. With due consideration, a vending machine will be installed at North Lantau Community Health Centre, adding the number of GOPCs distributing specimen collection packs to 47. Details of the collection submission times and clinics are provided in the attachment.

"The vending machines will be placed outside the usual service areas of clinics. Members of the public should observe relevant infection control measures and maintain social distancing when obtaining specimen collection packs. The public can contact clinic staff if assistance is required in the process," the spokesman said.

The HA will closely monitor the utilisation of the specimen collection pack vending machines by the public. If space and operation allow, more clinics will install vending machines in the future.

Issued at HKT 17:35

CHP investigates 12 additional confirmed cases of COVID-19

****

The Centre for Health Protection (CHP) of the Department of Health has announced that as of 0.00am, November 19, the CHP was investigating 12 additional confirmed cases of coronavirus disease 2019 (COVID-19), taking the number of cases to 5 492 in Hong Kong so far (comprising 5 491 confirmed cases and one probable case).

Among the newly reported cases announced, eight had a travel history during the incubation period, two were local cases with unknown sources while the other two were epidemiologically linked with a local case and an imported case respectively.

A total of 131 cases have been recorded in the past 14 days (November 5 - 18), including 32 local cases of which 19 are from unknown sources.

The CHP's epidemiological investigations and relevant contact tracing on the confirmed cases are ongoing. For case details and contact tracing information, please see the Annex or the list of buildings with confirmed cases of COVID-19 in the past 14 days and the latest local situation of COVID-19 available on the website "COVID-19 Thematic Website" (www.coronavirus.gov.hk).

A spokesman for the CHP said, "During the CHP's epidemiological investigations and relevant contact tracing on the confirmed cases, we will compile and upload (www.chp.gov.hk/files/pdf/building_list_eng.pdf) a list of buildings that confirmed patients had visited from two days before the onset of symptoms. Given that cases of local infection continue to occur from time to time, members of the public are urged to seek medical attention immediately if they believe that they had visited the same place at an identical time with a confirmed patient and feel unwell subsequently. If they remain asymptomatic but are concerned that they have been infected, they can also visit the Hospital Authority's designated general out-patient clinics (www.ha.org.hk/haho/ho/covid-19/GOPC_extend_EN.pdf) to obtain specimen collection packs and collect deep throat saliva specimens for free COVID-19 testing."

In view of the severe epidemic situation, the CHP called on members of the public to avoid going out, having social contact and dining out. They should put on a surgical mask and maintain stringent hand hygiene when they need to go out. The CHP strongly urged the elderly to stay home as far as possible and avoid going out. They should consider asking their family and friends to help with everyday tasks such as shopping for basic necessities.

The spokesman said, "Given that the situation of COVID-19 infection remains severe and that there is a continuous increase in the number of cases reported around the world, members of the public are strongly urged to avoid all non-essential travel outside Hong Kong.

"The CHP also strongly urges the public to maintain at all times strict personal and environmental hygiene, which is key to personal protection against infection and prevention of the spread of the disease in the community. On a personal level, members of the public should wear a surgical mask when having respiratory symptoms, taking public transport or staying in crowded places. They should also perform hand hygiene frequently, especially before touching the mouth, nose or eyes.

"As for household environmental hygiene, members of the public are advised to maintain drainage pipes properly, regularly pour water into drain outlets (U-traps) and cover all floor drain outlets when they are not in use. After using the toilet, they should put the toilet lid down before flushing to avoid spreading germs."

Moreover, the Government has launched the website "COVID-19 Thematic Website" (www.coronavirus.gov.hk) for announcing the latest updates on various news on COVID-19 infection and health advice to help the public understand the latest updates. Members of the public may also gain access to information via the COVID-19 WhatsApp Helpline launched by the Office of the Government Chief Information Officer. Simply by saving 9617 1823 in their phone contacts or clicking the link wa.me/85296171823?text=hi, they will be able to obtain information on COVID-19 as well as the "StayHomeSafe" mobile app and wristband via WhatsApp.

Issued at HKT 18:05

Public hospitals daily update on COVID-19 cases

****

The following is issued on behalf of the Hospital Authority:

As at 9am today (November 19), nine COVID-19 confirmed patients were discharged from hospital in the last 24 hours. So far, a total of 5 233 patients with confirmed or probable infection have been discharged.

At present, there are 594 negative pressure rooms in public hospitals with 1 077 negative pressure beds activated. A total of 109 confirmed patients are currently hospitalised in 19 public hospitals, among which eight patients are in critical condition, two are in serious condition and the remaining 99 patients are in stable condition.

The Hospital Authority will maintain close contact with the Centre for Health Protection to monitor the latest developments and to inform the public and healthcare workers on the latest information in a timely manner.

Details of the above-mentioned patients are as follows:

Patient condition	Case numbers
Discharged	4861, 5151, 5181, 5322, 5335, 5368, 5376, 5415, 5476

Critical	1989, 3496, 4706, 4833, 5110, 5185, 5409, 5433
Serious	5273, 5439

Issued at HKT 18:38

Reminder for Hong Kong residents with quota under Return2hk Scheme before their return
****

"Return2hk - Travel Scheme for Hong Kong Residents returning from Guangdong Province or Macao without being subject to quarantine under the Compulsory Quarantine of Certain Persons Arriving at Hong Kong Regulation (Cap. 599C)" (Return2hk Scheme) began accepting quota applications yesterday (November 18). Up to 5pm today (November 19), over 10 570 quota applications for the 7-day period of the following week have been received through the online booking system. Of these around 9 240 applications were for returning to Hong Kong through the Shenzhen Bay Port while around 1 330 applications were for returning through the Hong Kong-Zhuhai-Macao Bridge (HZMB) Hong Kong Port.

To ensure that immigration clearance would be smooth at the boundary control points, Hong Kong residents who have successfully reserved a quota should pay attention to the necessary steps to take before returning to Hong Kong and make sure all the specified conditions have been met, including:

- Not having been to places other than Hong Kong, Guangdong Province or Macao in the past 14 days;
- Undergone a COVID-19 (RT-PCR) nucleic acid test at one of the medical institutions mutually recognised by the governments of Hong Kong and Guangdong/Hong Kong and Macao, such that he/she can present the proof of a valid negative nucleic acid test result upon arrival in Hong Kong. The sample should be taken within three days prior to, or on the day of the person's entry into Hong Kong. For example, if a Hong Kong resident takes the test at a recognised medical institution on November 20, the negative test result will be valid until November 23. He/she should therefore return to Hong Kong with the test result on or before November 23, or otherwise he/she will still be subject to 14-day compulsory quarantine. The list of the 39 recognised medical or testing institutions in the Guangdong Province is available at www.coronavirus.gov.hk/pdf/List_of_recognised_laboratories_GD.pdf; whereas the list of the four recognised medical or testing institutions in Macao is available at www.coronavirus.gov.hk/pdf/List_of_recognised_laboratories_MO.pdf.

- Trasmit the valid negative COVID-19 nucleic acid test result to the electronic health declaration system of the Department of Health through "Yuekang code" (粵康碼) or "Macao health code" (澳康碼), and fill in all other required information for completing the health declaration within twenty-four hours before arriving at the boundary control point and obtain a "Green" QR code to be exempted from the 14-day compulsory quarantine requirement upon their return to Hong Kong. If a QR code of a different colour (e.g. a "Pink" QR code) is received after the code conversion process, it means not all the specified conditions have been fulfilled, and the traveller may still be subject to the 14-day compulsory quarantine requirement upon entry into Hong Kong; and

- Return to Hong Kong on the date and at the boundary control point as specified in the booking, and bring along the Hong Kong Identity Card or other identification documents, the confirmation of a successful booking (i.e. a printout of the booking confirmation page) as well as the proof of a valid negative nucleic acid test result (paper or electronic copy are both acceptable).

Re-entry into Guangdong Province or Macao

The Government spokesman specifically reminded that, if returning Hong Kong residents would subsequently enter the Guangdong Province or Macao again, they would still be subject to the prevailing quarantine arrangement of the two places (e.g. 14-day compulsory quarantine), unless exemption has been granted for them separately. They should therefore take note of the latest quarantine arrangements of Guangdong Province and Macao, and make necessary preparations.

Self-monitoring of health conditions after returning Hong Kong

The spokesman stressed that Hong Kong residents who can fulfil all the specified conditions and are returning to Hong Kong under the Return2hk Scheme should still exercise self-monitoring of their health conditions for at least 14 days after their entry into Hong Kong. They should observe the points listed in the "Health-monitoring Checklist for Inbound Travellers". If they feel unwell, they should seek medical advice promptly and reveal their travel history to medical practitioners. They may proactively make a request to their doctor for testing when there is any suspicion.

Details about the Return2hk Scheme are available at the "COVID-19 Thematic Website" (return2hk.gov.hk or 回港易.政府.香港). Members of the public may also call the Return2hk Scheme hotline at 3142 2330 if they have any enquiries.

Issued at HKT 20:53

November 20[51]

Transcript of remarks by SFH at media session

****

Following is the transcript of remarks by the Secretary for Food and Health, Professor Sophia Chan, at a media session this afternoon (November 20) about the latest situation of COVID-19:

Reporter: Professor Chan, several experts have said that the fourth wave has officially started, is it your view that the fourth wave officially started today in Hong Kong, can you confirm that?

Dr Chan, you have just said that the upper respiratory tract outbreaks have been more severe than last year and have been rising more rapidly, can you give us some figures to prove that, to compare this year's figures with last year's to show why it is much more severe and much more rapid?

Professor Chan, why have you suspended junior primary schools when there haven't been one case of COVID-19 found in those upper respiratory tract infected students, but why have you instead not announced any implementation date for hotel staycations and for mandatory testing, when there have been several cases linked to the hotel staycation groups, why are the relevant bureaux still considering that when you have already announced school suspension for junior primary schools? Professor Yuen today also recommended that the border strategy is not "water tight", that's his words. So he suggested that perhaps the quarantine period for travellers from high risk places has to be extended to 21 days, and he also said that perhaps there should be no food served in primary schools. Is that what you will be considering? Would you take up his suggestions and implement in those areas as well?

Finally, can I just get some clarifications from Professor Chan, because we are not quite sure that the dance studios are under the regulation of Cap. 599F. We have seen some cases linked to the Starlight Dance Club. Can you confirm whether dance studios are actually one of those 14 scheduled premises? And if not, why not?

Secretary for Food and Health: Thank you for your questions. First of all, just very quickly to answer your question on Starlight Dance Club. The Home Affairs Bureau is looking into whether

[51] https://www.info.gov.hk/gia/general/202011/20.htm

these kind of dancing studios are considered as party rooms, for example, so we are actively looking into that. But in any case, if there is such a cluster - people are dancing and do not wear masks - it is very high risk, and therefore I would appeal to people to stop all the unnecessary gatherings because the situation is severe now in Hong Kong.

Of course, according to the experts and also the information from the Centre for Health Protection, we have probably entered into a new wave of cases. But of course we are now doing our best, and before this severe situation started, in the past week, we have already tightened many of our measures, including border control measures, quarantine measures, hotel regulation measures, and also some of the social distancing measures. We have also ramped up our testing capacity and set up four community testing centres, and also improved the accessibility of people getting tested, not only the distribution of bottles, but also getting tested in our centres.

We will continue to tighten the measures. If you remember back in September, we have already listed six major areas in preparation for the fourth wave, so that our capacity, and also many of our current measures, can be executed as soon as possible in response to this wave.

Regarding your question about the timing of mandatory testing, the law is already here, and we will be issuing directions for mandatory testing for the three groups that I have earlier listed - those who have symptoms, residential elderly homes staff, and also taxi drivers. On staycation, as I have said earlier, we met with the hotel industry last night and ironed out all the details that we would like the hotel industry to follow. Many of those instructions and measures, some of the hotels are already following or executing. But now that we have the law, we want to be very clear that we will be issuing the directions to the hotels as soon as possible.

We have been in communication with our experts very frequently, all our four experts including Professor Yuen. We will definitely look into his suggestions and will consider the suggestions. The border control measures, Professor Yuen has actually said many times that there is no way for it to be "water tight", and therefore we must do more at different junctures, different points, in terms of border control measures. Before people come into Hong Kong, for example, we require pre-departure tests; also we stop flights if they have more confirmed cases. Most recently we have tightened our testing measures at the airport, everybody has to be tested at the airport. We have also been increasing the number of high risk countries under Cap. 599H, and we have also required returnees from all countries except China to have hotel quarantine rather than home quarantine. We will look into the science and the quarantine period to see how best we can actually be more "water tight" in these measures.

Regarding no food in primary schools, we have made a recommendation to the Education Bureau about mask-off activities. I think it would be the best if students would severely cut down all mask-off activities, including extra-curricular activities and so on.

Issued at HKT 15:30

CHP investigates 26 additional confirmed cases of COVID-19

****

The Centre for Health Protection (CHP) of the Department of Health has announced that as of 0.00am, November 20, the CHP was investigating 26 additional confirmed cases of coronavirus disease 2019 (COVID-19), taking the number of cases to 5 518 in Hong Kong so far (comprising 5 517 confirmed cases and one probable case).

Among the newly reported cases announced, five had a travel history during the incubation period.

A total of 136 cases have been recorded in the past 14 days (November 6 - 19), including 34 local cases of which 20 are from unknown sources.

The CHP's epidemiological investigations and relevant contact tracing on the confirmed cases are ongoing. For case details and contact tracing information, please see the Annex or the list of buildings with confirmed cases of COVID-19 in the past 14 days and the latest local situation of COVID-19 available on the website "COVID-19 Thematic Website" (www.coronavirus.gov.hk).

A spokesman for the CHP said, "During the CHP's epidemiological investigations and relevant contact tracing on the confirmed cases, we will compile and upload (www.chp.gov.hk/files/pdf/building_list_eng.pdf) a list of buildings that confirmed patients had visited from two days before the onset of symptoms. Given that cases of local infection continue to occur from time to time, members of the public are urged to seek medical attention immediately if they believe that they had visited the same place at an identical time with a confirmed patient and feel unwell subsequently. If they remain asymptomatic but are concerned that they have been infected, they can also visit the Hospital Authority's designated general out-patient clinics (www.ha.org.hk/haho/ho/covid-19/GOPC_extend_EN.pdf) to obtain specimen collection packs and collect deep throat saliva specimens for free COVID-19 testing."

In view of the severe epidemic situation, the CHP called on members of the public to avoid going out, having social contact and dining out. They should put on a surgical mask and maintain stringent hand hygiene when they need to go out. The CHP strongly urged the elderly to stay home as far as possible and avoid going out. They should consider asking their family and friends to help with everyday tasks such as shopping for basic necessities.

The spokesman said, "Given that the situation of COVID-19 infection remains severe and that there is a continuous increase in the number of cases reported around the world, members of the public are strongly urged to avoid all non-essential travel outside Hong Kong.

"The CHP also strongly urges the public to maintain at all times strict personal and environmental hygiene, which is key to personal protection against infection and prevention of the spread of the disease in the community. On a personal level, members of the public should wear a surgical mask when having respiratory symptoms, taking public transport or staying in crowded places. They should also perform hand hygiene frequently, especially before touching the mouth, nose or eyes.

"As for household environmental hygiene, members of the public are advised to maintain drainage pipes properly, regularly pour water into drain outlets (U-traps) and cover all floor drain outlets when they are not in use. After using the toilet, they should put the toilet lid down before flushing to avoid spreading germs."

Moreover, the Government has launched the website "COVID-19 Thematic Website" (www.coronavirus.gov.hk) for announcing the latest updates on various news on COVID-19 infection and health advice to help the public understand the latest updates. Members of the public may also gain access to information via the COVID-19 WhatsApp Helpline launched by the Office of the Government Chief Information Officer. Simply by saving 9617 1823 in their phone contacts or clicking the link wa.me/85296171823?text=hi, they will be able to obtain information on COVID-19 as well as the "StayHomeSafe" mobile app and wristband via WhatsApp.

Issued at HKT 18:18

Man sentenced for breaching compulsory quarantine order

****

A 49-year-old man was sentenced to immediate imprisonment for three weeks by the Kowloon City Magistrates' Courts today (November 20) for violating the Compulsory Quarantine of Certain Persons Arriving at Hong Kong Regulation (Cap. 599C) (the Regulation).

The man was earlier issued a compulsory quarantine order stating that he must conduct quarantine at home for 14 days. Before the expiry of the quarantine order, he left the place of quarantine on September 30 without reasonable excuse nor permission given by an authorised officer. He was charged with contravening Sections 8(1) and 8(5) of the Regulation and was sentenced by the Kowloon City Magistrates' Courts today to immediate imprisonment for three weeks.

Pursuant to the Regulation, starting from February 8, save for exempted persons, all persons who have stayed in the Mainland, Macao or Taiwan in the 14 days preceding arrival in Hong Kong, regardless of their nationality or travel documents, will be subject to compulsory quarantine for 14 days. Moreover, pursuant to the Compulsory Quarantine of Persons Arriving at Hong Kong from Foreign Places Regulation (Cap. 599E), starting from March 19, all persons arriving from countries or territories outside China would also be subject to compulsory quarantine for 14 days. Breaching a quarantine order is a criminal offence and offenders are subject to a maximum fine of $25,000 and imprisonment for six months.

A spokesman for the Department of Health said the sentence sends a clear message to the community that breaching a compulsory quarantine order is a criminal offence that the Government will not tolerate, and solemnly reminded the public to comply with the Regulation. As of today, a total of 70 persons have been convicted by the courts for breaching compulsory quarantine orders and have received sentences including immediate imprisonment for up to three months or a fine of $15,000. The spokesman reiterated that resolute actions will be taken against anyone who has breached the relevant regulations.

Issued at HKT 18:25

Public hospitals daily update on COVID-19 cases

****

The following is issued on behalf of the Hospital Authority:

As at 9am today (November 20), six COVID-19 confirmed patients were discharged from hospital in the last 24 hours. So far, a total of 5 239 patients with confirmed or probable infection have been discharged.

At present, there are 577 negative pressure rooms in public hospitals with 1 060 negative pressure beds activated. A total of 115 confirmed patients are currently hospitalised in 19 public hospitals, among which eight patients are in critical condition, two are in serious condition and the remaining 105 patients are in stable condition.

The Hospital Authority will maintain close contact with the Centre for Health Protection to monitor the latest developments and to inform the public and healthcare workers on the latest information in a timely manner.

Details of the above-mentioned patients are as follows:

Patient condition	Case numbers
Discharged	5377, 5385, 5436, 5451, 5471, 5486
Critical	1989, 3496, 4706, 4833, 5110, 5185, 5409, 5433
Serious	5273, 5439

Issued at HKT 18:50

Suspension of face-to-face classes of Primary One to Primary Three

****

In light of the latest situation of the COVID-19 epidemic and the outbreak of upper respiratory tract infections (URTI) in schools, the Government announced today (November 20) that starting from next Monday (November 23), face-to-face classes and all school activities of Primary One to Primary Three of all primary schools (including schools offering non-local curriculum) and primary sections of special schools, would be suspended until December 6 (Sunday).

A spokesman for the Education Bureau (EDB) said, "As for Primary Four to Primary Six of primary schools and all levels of secondary schools (including special schools and schools offering non-local curriculum), schools should strictly observe all the health protection measures when conducting face-to-face classes and school activities, including maintaining appropriate social distances, checking of body temperatures upon entry into school premises, wearing of masks at all times inside the school premises, etc, so as to safeguard the health and well-being of teachers and students. In view of the worsening trend of the epidemic, schools are requested not to arrange activities which require students to take off their masks."

The spokesman continued, "In case of any URTI or confirmed case of COVID-19 being reported, schools must follow the advice of the Centre for Health Protection on suspension of face-to-face classes and related epidemic prevention measures, including suspending the affected classes concerned during specified periods."

In addition, the Government has earlier announced that kindergartens and kindergarten-cum-child care centres would suspend face-to-face classes and all school activities for two weeks starting from November 14 (Saturday) to November 27 (Friday). In view of the latest situation, all kindergartens and kindergarten-cum-child care centres will continue to suspend face-to-face classes and all school activities to December 6 (Sunday).

The EDB will issue letters to inform schools of the related arrangements and measures that schools should implement during this period to sustain students' learning at home through flexible use of various learning modes. During the suspension of face-to-face classes, schools should remain open to take care of those students who have to go back to schools because of the lack of carers at home. Schools should arrange staff to be on duty to handle school affairs, answer parents' enquiries and take care of those students who have returned to schools. Schools should also ensure that the campus environment is clean and hygienic.

Parents should take precautionary measures for influenza and pay close attention to the health conditions of their children. They should avoid bringing their children to crowded places with poor ventilation. Students should maintain a balanced diet, exercise regularly and take adequate rest in order to strengthen their immunity. If students are feeling unwell (even if the symptoms are very mild), they must not return to schools and should seek medical advice promptly to receive appropriate diagnoses and treatments.

The Government will closely monitor the development of the epidemic, maintain close liaison with the school sector and provide timely support to schools.

Issued at HKT 18:57

S for IT solicits catering businesses to support "LeaveHomeSafe" mobile app

****

The Secretary for Innovation and Technology, Mr Alfred Sit, today (November 20) attended a briefing session for representatives from catering businesses to solicit their support for the "LeaveHomeSafe" mobile app and fight the virus together.

Legislative Council member, Mr Tommy Cheung, and representatives of several catering chains also attended the briefing.

Mr Sit said that the "LeaveHomeSafe" mobile app enables users to keep a more precise record of their whereabouts under the new normal, and fight the virus with the aid of technology. Users with risk of exposure to the virus will be notified by the mobile app to enhance their vigilance. If people with exposure risk undergo COVID-19 testing early, the objective of "early identification, early isolation and early treatment" can then be achieved. It will make contact tracing more efficient and minimise the risk of further transmission of the virus, which in turn helps save both livelihoods and the economy.

"Anti-epidemic work is a shared responsibility and everyone has a role to play. We need active participation and co-operation from members of the public and various sectors. I appeal to more catering businesses to join the scheme, display QR codes and posters at prominent positions and make it easy for members of the public to use the 'LeaveHomeSafe' mobile app. It will help drive the message across and make the scheme more effective," he said.

Venue QR code registration function is now available on the "LeaveHomeSafe" website. Venue operators are welcome to apply via the "LeaveHomeSafe" website (www.leavehomesafe.gov.hk/registration/) or contact the Office of the Government Chief Information Officer direct (designated email address: leavehomesafe@ogcio.gov.hk).

There are currently nearly 12 000 public and private venues participating in the scheme. Among them, about 7 000 are public venues while nearly 5 000 are private venues. The "LeaveHomeSafe" mobile app can be used directly in over 18 000 taxis.

Issued at HKT 19:42

November 21[52]

[52] https://www.info.gov.hk/gia/general/202011/21.htm

Government further tightens social distancing measures

****

In view of the development of COVID-19 in Hong Kong, the Government announced today (November 21) that it has gazetted directions and specifications under the Prevention and Control of Disease (Requirements and Directions) (Business and Premises) Regulation (Cap. 599F) to further tighten social distancing measures. The above directions will take effect at 0.00am on November 22.

A spokesman for the Food and Health Bureau said, "The number of confirmed local cases with unknown sources of infection has been on a rising trend recently, indicating the existence of silent transmission chains in the community. The Government announced a series of measures to tighten social distancing on November 14, targeting at restrictions on mask-off gathering activities. In view of the latest public health risk assessment, in particular the higher risks brought about by activities conducted without wearing masks as well as various social activities as shown in recent cases, we are of the view that it is now necessary to further tighten social distancing measures implemented under Cap. 599F."

"We urge the public to stay at home as much as possible, go out less often unless necessary, and avoid dining out and unnecessary social activities (including private gatherings, in particular mask-off activities or group gatherings in indoor premises). At this key moment when the epidemic situation is worsening, the public should fight the epidemic together without letting down one's guard and take every possible step to prevent the virus from continuing to spread in the community. Maintaining good personal and environmental hygiene at all times is key to prevention of infection and the spread of the virus in the community."

The details of the tightening measures are as follows:

(1) Live performance and dancing must not be allowed in any catering premises (including bars or pubs) as well as clubs or nightclubs.

(2) Premises (commonly known as party rooms) that are maintained or intended to be maintained for hire for holding social gatherings must be closed.

The Government has gazetted the directions and specifications under Cap. 599F to implement the above measures (details at Annex 1). The above measures will take effect from November 22 for a period of five days till November 26, 2020. Persons responsible for carrying on catering businesses and managers of scheduled premises that contravene the statutory requirements under Cap. 599F would have committed a criminal offence. Offenders are subject to a maximum fine of $50,000 and imprisonment for six months.

The spokesman added that apart from the above additional social distancing measures, other measures, including requirements on group gatherings and mask wearing as announced on November 14 are still in effect until November 26.

"We will continue to closely monitor the development of the epidemic situation and review the various measures in place from time to time with a view to making suitable adjustments taking into account all relevant factors," said the spokesman.

Issued at HKT 6:00

S for IT speaks on "LeaveHomeSafe" mobile app

****

Following is the transcript of remarks by the Secretary for Innovation and Technology, Mr Alfred Sit, at a media session after attending an event in support of the "LeaveHomeSafe" mobile app today (November 21):

Reporter: Could you explain what are the factors that you would consider to decide what high risk areas would be applied the app first? And then also could you offer more details on the 12 000 public and private places, how many of them are shops and how many of them are other public places, thank you.

Secretary for Innovation and Technology: About the breakdown of those shops or restaurants that they have already used our QR code of the "LeaveHomeSafe" app, I don't have the record in hand with me. But I assure you that we are going to have more shops and restaurants joining the scheme. Up to present, we have altogether 7 000 public venues using the "LeaveHomeSafe" app and about 5 000 are shops and restaurants. Thank you.

Issued at HKT 15:28

Inaugural flights under HK-Singapore Air Travel Bubble deferred for two weeks

****

The Government of the Hong Kong Special Administrative Region (HKSAR) announced today (November 21) that in view of the recent epidemic situation in Hong Kong, the Governments of HKSAR and Singapore have decided to defer the inaugural flights under the Hong Kong-Singapore Air Travel Bubble (ATB) for two weeks.

A Government spokesman said that the epidemic situation in Hong Kong has deteriorated rapidly. The increasing trend of the number of unlinked local cases shows that there is an invisible and continuous transmission chain in the community. It is expected that the epidemic situation in Hong Kong will still remain severe in the near future. If the ATB is to be launched as scheduled tomorrow, chances of making immediate adjustment are high. The deferral of the inaugural flights is a suitable and responsible arrangement to minimise the inconvenience caused to the ATB travellers and reduce the uncertainty in their itineraries.

The Governments of HKSAR and Singapore will continue to closely monitor the epidemic situation of both places, exchange relevant data and statistics, and maintain close communication. The new date of inaugural flights will be announced in early December. Travellers who wish to travel between the two places via the ATB arrangement should watch out for the latest announcement and adjust their itineraries according to their own situation.

To cater for possible fluctuation in the epidemic situation, the ATB has a built-in mechanism whereby the number of designated flights may be increased, decreased or even suspended depending on the situation. If the latest seven-day moving average of the daily number of unlinked local cases is more than five for either Singapore or Hong Kong, the ATB arrangement will be suspended after two days (including the day on which the exceedance of the threshold is announced) for a two-week period. If the seven-day moving average of the daily number of unlinked local cases reported on the last day of the suspension period does not exceed five for both Singapore and Hong Kong, the ATB arrangement can resume on the next day.

For details of the ATB, please refer to the designated website: www.tourism.gov.hk/travelbubble.

Issued at HKT 18:07

Public hospitals daily update on COVID-19 cases

****

The following is issued on behalf of the Hospital Authority:

As at 9am today (November 21), nine COVID-19 confirmed patients were discharged from hospital in the last 24 hours. So far, a total of 5 248 patients with confirmed or probable infection have been discharged.

At present, there are 577 negative pressure rooms in public hospitals with 1 060 negative pressure beds activated. A total of 132 confirmed patients are currently hospitalised in 19 public hospitals, among which eight patients are in critical condition, two are in serious condition and the remaining 122 patients are in stable condition.

The Hospital Authority will maintain close contact with the Centre for Health Protection to monitor the latest developments and to inform the public and healthcare workers on the latest information in a timely manner.

Details of the above-mentioned patients are as follows:

Patient condition	Case numbers
Discharged	5302, 5340, 5384, 5392, 5399, 5432, 5447, 5460, 5491
Critical	1989, 3496, 4706, 4833, 5110, 5185, 5409, 5433
Serious	5273, 5439

Issued at HKT 18:52

FEHD steps up inspections and reminds catering business operators and public to continue complying with anti-epidemic regulations

****

The Food and Environmental Hygiene Department (FEHD) and the Police conducted joint operations last night (November 20) and at small hours today (November 21) to step up inspections at catering premises including bars in Lan Kwai Fong in Central and reminded the catering business operators to strictly comply with the requirements and directions under the Prevention and Control of Disease (Requirements and Directions) (Business and Premises) Regulation (Cap. 599F) (the Regulation), and the public to comply with the various restrictions in relation to group gatherings and mask-wearing under the anti-epidemic regulations and directions when patronising catering premises.

During the operations, the FEHD and the Police inspected 52 catering premises (including bars). A total of 12 verbal warnings were given, while procedures on prosecution were initiated against two catering business operators for breaching the requirement on the number of persons allowed at one table in the premises under the Regulation.

A spokesman for the FEHD said, "According to the latest directions issued by the Secretary for Food and Health yesterday in relation to catering business under the Regulation that are applicable to the five-day period from November 22 to November 26, live performance/dancing must not be allowed in any catering premises (including bars or pubs) as well as clubs or nightclubs. The following requirements and restrictions will continue to apply: dining-in must cease from 0.00am to 4.59am every day; no more than two persons may be at one table for a bar/pub or night establishment/nightclub while no more than four persons may be at one table for other catering premises; the total number of customers allowed in catering premises must not exceed 50 per cent of the normal seating capacity; a mask must be worn within the premises except when the person is consuming food or drink at a table therein; tables must be arranged in a way to ensure there is a distance of at least 1.5m or some form of partition which could serve as effective buffer between one table and another table; body temperature screening must be conducted before the person is allowed to enter the catering premises; and hand sanitisers must be provided, etc."

In addition, to actively promote the participation of bar/pub staff in the voluntary free COVID-19 testing, the FEHD will arrange its testing agency, Prenetics Limited, to deliver specimen bottles at bar area in Lan Kwai Fong and a mobile van will be parked near the bar area tomorrow afternoon to encourage practitioners in bars/pubs and their patrons to undergo the voluntary testing.

The testing agency will be responsible for the provision of one-stop service covering specimen collection and testing. The testing agency will deliver specimen bottles to operators of bars/pubs for collecting deep throat saliva samples of their staff, and then collect the samples in the subsequent one to two days for testing. Moreover, the testing agency will also deliver the specimen bottles to patrons of bars/pubs who are interested in taking the test and they can return their specimen bottles by themselves to the mobile collection van of the testing agency parked at Hoi Chak Street in Quarry Bay from 9am to 5pm between November 23 and November 28. Specimens with preliminary positive results will be relayed to the Public Health Laboratory Services Branch of the Department of Health to re-test and confirm the result. Confirmed cases will be followed up and announced by the Centre for Health Protection.

Since October 1, the testing agency has delivered over 15 000 specimen bottles at over 1 000 bars and pubs, and collected about 8 000 specimens for testing.

The spokesman stressed that the FEHD will continue to step up inspections at catering premises across the territory and conduct joint operations with the Police if necessary, to ensure that catering business operators and the public strictly comply with relevant regulations. Enforcement actions will be taken against offenders so as to minimise the risk of transmission of COVID-19 in food premises.

If catering business operators contravene the Regulation, they are liable to a maximum fine of $50,000 and imprisonment for six months. Persons who violate the group gathering restriction of the Prevention and Control of Disease (Prohibition in Group Gathering) Regulation (Cap. 599G) are subject to a fixed penalty of $2,000.

The spokesman appealed to catering business operators to comply with relevant regulations on prevention and control of disease in a concerted and persistent manner, with a view to keeping their staff, customers and the public safe. Members of the public also have to comply with the related regulations and directions on group gatherings and mask-wearing at catering premises.

Issued at HKT 19:54

CHP investigates 43 additional confirmed cases of COVID-19

****

The Centre for Health Protection (CHP) of the Department of Health has announced that as of 0.00am, November 21, the CHP was investigating 43 additional confirmed cases of coronavirus disease 2019 (COVID-19), taking the number of cases to 5 561 in Hong Kong so far (comprising 5 560 confirmed cases and one probable case).

Among the newly reported cases announced, seven had a travel history during the incubation period.

A total of 156 cases have been recorded in the past 14 days (November 7 – 20), including 55 local cases of which 29 are from unknown sources.

The CHP's epidemiological investigations and relevant contact tracing on the confirmed cases are ongoing. For case details and contact tracing information, please see the Annex One or the list of buildings with confirmed cases of COVID-19 in the past 14 days and the latest local situation of COVID-19 available on the website "COVID-19 Thematic Website" (www.coronavirus.gov.hk).

As a number of cases confirmed recently claimed that they had visited dancing venues, the CHP strongly appealed to those who had visited the dancing venues as listed in Annex Two on or after November 1 to visit the Hospital Authority's designated general out-patient clinics (www.ha.org.hk/haho/ho/covid-19/GOPC_extend_EN.pdf) and collect deep throat saliva specimen collection packs for free COVID-19 testing as soon as possible. The public are also urged to seek medical attention early if symptoms develop.

In view of the severe epidemic situation, the CHP called on members of the public to avoid going out, having social contact and dining out. They should put on a surgical mask and maintain stringent hand hygiene when they need to go out. The CHP strongly urged the elderly to stay home as far as possible and avoid going out. They should consider asking their family and friends to help with everyday tasks such as shopping for basic necessities.

The spokesman said, "Given that the situation of COVID-19 infection remains severe and that there is a continuous increase in the number of cases reported around the world, members of the public are strongly urged to avoid all non-essential travel outside Hong Kong.

"The CHP also strongly urges the public to maintain at all times strict personal and environmental hygiene, which is key to personal protection against infection and prevention of the spread of the disease in the community. On a personal level, members of the public should wear a surgical mask when having respiratory symptoms, taking public transport or staying in crowded places. They should also perform hand hygiene frequently, especially before touching the mouth, nose or eyes.

"As for household environmental hygiene, members of the public are advised to maintain drainage pipes properly, regularly pour water into drain outlets (U-traps) and cover all floor drain outlets when they are not in use. After using the toilet, they should put the toilet lid down before flushing to avoid spreading germs."

Moreover, the Government has launched the website "COVID-19 Thematic Website" (www.coronavirus.gov.hk) for announcing the latest updates on various news on COVID-19 infection and health advice to help the public understand the latest updates. Members of the public may also gain access to information via the COVID-19 WhatsApp Helpline launched by the Office of the Government Chief Information Officer. Simply by saving 9617 1823 in their phone contacts or clicking the link wa.me/85296171823?text=hi, they will be able to obtain information on COVID-19 as well as the "StayHomeSafe" mobile app and wristband via WhatsApp.

Issued at HKT 20:05

Government responds to media enquiries about virus testing

****

On reports that three taxi drivers and a rehab bus driver that were confirmed cases of COVID-19 earlier were subsequently tested negative after being followed up by the Hospital Authority and have been discharged from the hospital, a government spokesman today (November 21) responded as follows:

The four cases were preliminarily confirmed by the private laboratory responsible for the Targeted Group Testing Scheme (TGTS) arranged by the Transport Department as one positive and three "indeterminate". They were sent to the Public Health Laboratory Services Branch of the Department of Health (DH) for confirmatory test according to established procedures and subsequently confirmed as four positive cases. The test results at that time showed that the viral load of the specimens was very low. These cases were later tested negative for the virus and met the discharge criteria hence were arranged to be discharged. This does not affect the confirmation as positive cases earlier.

The private laboratory responsible for the related TGTS is KingMed Diagnostics (Hong Kong) Limited. This laboratory has participated with satisfactory performance in the external quality assurance programme of the DH, and has the medical testing accreditation of the Hong Kong Laboratory Accreditation Scheme (HOKLAS). The Public Health Laboratory Services Branch of the Centre for Health Protection of the DH has been designated by the World Health Organization (WHO) this year as the WHO COVID-19 Reference Lab and WHO COVID-19 external quality assessment programme provider. The Public Health Laboratory Services Branch also provides a quality assessment programme for local laboratories.

Taking into account that multiple cases were tested positive at the same time, the Public Health Laboratory Services Branch has earlier conducted follow-up investigations, including obtaining relevant information, visiting the laboratory and reviewing their sample handling and testing procedures. The Public Health Laboratory Services Branch has so far found no definite evidence that cross-contamination of specimens occurred during the process. The Public Health Laboratory Services Branch has also provided some suggestions to the private laboratory in accordance with good laboratory practice. The Government will continue to follow up and closely monitor the quality of service provided by the laboratory to the Government so as to ensure its service quality.

Issued at HKT 20:10

SCED speaks on Hong Kong-Singapore Air Travel Bubble

****

Following is the transcript of remarks by the Secretary for Commerce and Economic Development, Mr Edward Yau, on the Hong Kong-Singapore Air Travel Bubble at a media session today (November 21):

Secretary for Commerce and Economic Development: We have planned to launch the Hong Kong-Singapore Air Travel Bubble tomorrow, but in the light of the recent upsurge of local cases, we have decided together with the Singapore Government to defer the launching of the Air Travel Bubble by two weeks. Under the agreed arrangement, we have got certain mechanisms and dialogues on this. In the interest of making a good start and avoiding confusion for passengers, we have decided to put this back for two weeks. So doing is necessary to avoid any inconvenience caused by the abrupt changes of the scheme to passengers, particularly those who need to return to Hong Kong in short time. We will review the situation and keep each other well informed of the epidemic situation, so as to decide the way forward. We will make a further announcement by early December on the formal launching of the scheme.

Reporter: Do you have an estimate of how many passengers will be affected by the delay of the travel bubble scheme? Are you worried that there will be further delay given the worsening situation of COVID-19 pandemic in Hong Kong? You earlier said that Hong Kong is in talks with over 11 countries over possible travel bubble scheme, how's the progress of these talks and do they have to be suspended as well?

Secretary for Commerce and Economic Development: First and foremost, we are talking about deferring and putting back the inaugural flights of the scheme by two weeks. We still aim at putting the scheme in place, provided that we are satisfied with the public health considerations being fulfilled. We will continue to review the situation with the Singapore Government.

As for talks with other places, they are also watching the progress of the Hong Kong-Singapore one. I believe the most important thing is that for any scheme to be successful, it must fulfill the condition of securing public health and making sure that both sides would be comfortable and feel safe about the scheme. In the light of the situation in Hong Kong, I think it is a responsible way to put this back for a while and then relaunch it at a suitable juncture.

Reporter: How many passengers will be affected?

Secretary for Commerce and Economic Development: Under the scheme, our original plan is that in the initial two weeks, there will one flight per day with a capacity of up to 200 (passengers). That's roughly the situation, depending on when we can relaunch it. That's the calculation.

Reporter: Who initiated the deferral of the travel bubble, is it by Hong Kong or Singapore as Singapore asked to have the PCR test upon landing this morning? Are you sure that the Air Travel Bubble can take flights after two weeks? Do you think that the two authorities are doing enough to safeguard the public health and safety of passengers? For the people who bought tickets right now, what will happen to them? Are they still allowed to travel and if they still proceed with their journey, what are the measures they need to take upon landing in Singapore?

Secretary for Commerce and Economic Development: We have been talking about the launching of Air Travel Bubble with Singapore for some months. We agreed in principle, worked out the details and made suitable announcements recently. At the same time, both governments are also looking at the situation on a daily basis. Particularly in the light of Hong Kong's situation, I think it is a responsible way for us to touch base again. At this particular moment, we have mutually agreed to put this scheme back by two weeks. This would allow us to review the situation and to have Hong Kong's new wave (of COVID-19 outbreak) settled a bit. This is also in line with the spirit of the entire arrangement that if circumstances do not permit, we will have to make suitable adjustments. I think we have made in the outset. That is exactly to fulfill the very important purpose of taking public health as the pre-requisite and making sure that this arrangement will be safe and comfortable by both sides.

As to the passengers affected, there are usual arrangements for refund or ticket adjustments to be made by the travel agents or the airlines. This will be taken care of in the usual manner.

Issued at HKT 20:13

Response on trial run of COVID-19 testing technique at airport
****

In response to media reports on discordant results between different tests conducted under the trial run of a COVID-19 nucleic acid testing technique at the Hong Kong International Airport (HKIA), a spokesman for the Food and Health Bureau (FHB) made the following response today (November 21):

The Government has been monitoring the latest developments of COVID-19 testing techniques, and would assess such testing techniques with reference to scientific studies around the world and in Hong Kong, practical experience, and expert advice.

The Government started on October 28 at HKIA a trial run of a nucleic acid test using reverse transcription loop-mediated isothermal amplification (RT-LAMP) technique using gargle as the specimen collection method, while also testing that technique using deep throat saliva (DTS) specimen. The RT-LAMP trial run was conducted in parallel with the reverse transcription polymerase chain reaction (RT-PCR) nucleic acid test used by the Department of Health (DH) with DTS as the specimen collection method for comparison, so as to examine the sensitivity and reliability of the RT-LAMP technique. During the trial, DH and the organisation participating in the trial also conducted RT-PCR tests on the gargle and DTS samples respectively for reference purpose. The three-week trial ended on November 17.

The Government is carefully examining the data collected from the trial, and will assess the efficacy of the testing technique including specimen collection method and the feasibility of applying it to different uses, including testing for arriving passengers.

Regarding the discordant results in the airport trial, FHB confirms that there were 25 cases in the trial that produced varying discordant results from tests conducted by different organisations, using different testing techniques, and with specimen collected using different methods, of which six cases' DTS specimens collected at the DH's Temporary Specimen Collection Centre at the airport were tested negative, while the gargle specimens separately collected by the organisation participating in the trial run returned positive, negative or indeterminate results using RT-PCR and RT-LAMP tests, among which four of the DTS specimens were tested positive when re-screened by DH using RT-PCR test. Among the other cases in the trial, there were also situations where the gargle specimens were tested negative using RT-PCR or RT-LAMP tests by the organisation participating in the trial, while the DTS specimens were tested positive by DH. The detailed results will need to be further assessed after the analysis of the trial data, and the Government has yet to come to a conclusion on the trial at this stage.

We stress that all relevant travellers who were re-screened as positive cases had been admitted to hospital for isolation in accordance with existing procedures. There are advantages and limitations to different testing techniques and specimen collection methods for COVID-19 tests, and it is not uncommon that different testing techniques or specimen collection methods would generate discordant results, which might be due to the sensitivity and specificity of the testing technique, the viral load in the specimens provided by a sampling method or laboratory technical issues, etc. Specifically, the RT-PCR nucleic acid test is still the "gold standard" in COVID-19 tests, and is also the reference test employed by DH's Public Health Laboratory Services Branch (PHLSB) in confirming positive cases.

As for sampling methods, DTS, nasopharyngeal swab (NPS) and combined nasal and throat swab (CNTS) are more commonly used in Hong Kong for specimen collection, and the three methods are generally similar in accuracy and sensitivity, and could all effectively identify COVID-19 cases. DH's PHLSB has also been monitoring whether other specimen collection methods (such as gargle specimens) would be suitable. Scientifically, there is no single testing technique or specimen collection method that can ensure complete accuracy. The airport trial aimed to compare different testing techniques or specimen collection methods with the current arrangements. The Government will continue to analyse the trial data and review the suitability of different testing techniques and specimen collection methods.

Issued at HKT 22:43

Government further tightens testing and isolation arrangement for crew members of aircraft and other exempted persons

****

The Government today (November 21) announced that testing and isolation arrangement for air crew members and other exempted persons who are exempted from quarantine requirement upon arriving Hong Kong will be tightened with effect from tomorrow (November 22).

A Government spokesman pointed out that in view of the development and severity of the global epidemic situation, the Government announced its plan on November 14 to tighten the epidemic control measures on all inbound travellers comprehensively based on the prevention and risk assessment. In addition to the tightening of the testing and isolation arrangement for consular and diplomatic officers as announced on November 17, the Government will, starting from tomorrow (November 22), further tighten the testing and isolation arrangement for air crew members and other exempted persons. With effect from tomorrow, air crew and other exempted persons who are exempted from compulsory quarantine arrangement under the Compulsory Quarantine of Certain Persons Arriving at Hong Kong Regulation (Cap. 599C) and the Compulsory Quarantine of Persons Arriving at Hong Kong from Foreign Places Regulation (Cap. 599E) arriving at Hong Kong at the Hong Kong International Airport (HKIA) must subject to compliance with certain conditions, with details as follows:

All air crew members who have visited very high risk places (i.e. the specified very high-risk places gazetted under the Prevention and Control of Disease (Regulation of Cross-boundary Conveyances and Travellers) Regulation (Cap.599H)) during the 14 days prior to arrival in Hong Kong:

- All air crew members must possess a negative result of SARS-CoV-2 nucleic acid test done at an ISO15189-accredited laboratory or a laboratory recognised by the Government where the laboratory is located with the specimen collected within 48 hours prior to the scheduled departure time of the flight to Hong Kong for duty (except local based air crew members and freight crew members);
- All air crew members must take a post-arrival SARS-CoV-2 nucleic acid test at the Department of Health's (DH) Temporary Specimen Collection Centre (TSCC) and wait for the results there or any other location as designated by DH upon arrival at HKIA;
- All non-local based air crew members, including freight crew members, must self-isolate at the hotel room arranged by the airline until departure from Hong Kong on their next duty flight upon availability of their test results;
- All local based air crew members must take point-to-point transfer and self-isolate until their next duty flight at the hotel room arranged by the airline for the duration of their stay when laying over at the very high risk place;
- Respective airlines must arrange point-to-point transportation for their air crew members between the airport (or holding location) and their accommodation. The use of public transport is prohibited; and
- All air crew members must collect and return their deep throat saliva sample at Day-12 upon their arrival in accordance with the instructions for SARS-CoV-2 nucleic acid test again if their duration of stay is more than 12 days.

Air crew members who have not visited very high risk places during the 14 days prior to arrival in Hong Kong:

- Non-local based air crew members who possess a negative result of SARS-CoV-2 nucleic acid test done at an ISO15189-accredited laboratory or a laboratory recognised by the Government where the laboratory is located with the specimen collected within 48 hours prior to the scheduled departure time of the flight to Hong Kong are required to take a post-arrival SARS-CoV-2 nucleic acid test at the DH's TSCC before leaving HKIA for self-isolation at the hotel room arranged by the airline until departure from Hong Kong on their next duty flight upon availability of the test results. Otherwise, they have to wait for the results at the TSCC or any other location as designated by DH;

- Local based air crew members must take a post-arrival SARS-CoV-2 nucleic acid test at the DH's TSCC upon arrival at HKIA and subject to self-isolation at their accommodation until their test results are available;
- Respective airlines must arrange point-to-point transportation for their air crew members between the airport (or holding location) and their accommodation whilst in Hong Kong. The use of public transport is prohibited; and
- All air crew members must collect and return their deep throat saliva sample at Day-12 upon their arrival in accordance with the instructions for SARS-CoV-2 nucleic acid test again if their duration of stay is more than 12 days.

Other exempted persons (all exempted persons other than air crew and sea crew) who have visited very high risk places during the 14 days prior to arrival in Hong Kong:

- They must possess a negative result of SARS-CoV-2 nucleic acid test done at an ISO15189-accredited laboratory or a laboratory recognised by the Government where the laboratory is located with the specimen collected within 48 hours prior to the scheduled departure time of the flight to Hong Kong;
- They must take a post-arrival SARS-CoV-2 nucleic acid test at the DH's TSCC and wait for the results there or any other location as designated by DH upon arrival at HKIA;
- Specimen bottles will be distributed to the exempted persons upon arrival. They must collect and return their deep throat saliva sample at Day-12 upon their arrival in accordance with the instructions for SARS-CoV-2 nucleic acid test again;
- Except Consul Generals or representatives in Hong Kong and government officials at equivalent/higher level, all other officers must be subject to self-isolation for 14 days at an accommodation arranged by respective organisations; and
- Respective organisations must arrange point-to-point transportation for the exempted persons. The use of public transport is prohibited.

Other exempted persons (all exempted persons other than air crew and sea crew) who have not visited very high risk places during the 14 days prior to arrival in Hong Kong:

- If they possess a negative result of SARS-CoV-2 nucleic acid test done at an ISO15189-accredited laboratory or a laboratory recognised by the Government where the laboratory is located with the specimen collected within 48 hours prior to the scheduled departure time of the flight to Hong Kong, they are required to take a post-arrival SARS-CoV-2 nucleic acid test at the DH's TSCC before leaving HKIA;

- If they do not possess a negative result of SARS-CoV-2 nucleic acid test done at an ISO15189-accredited laboratory or a laboratory recognised by the Government where the laboratory is located with the specimen collected within 48 hours prior to the scheduled departure time of the flight to Hong Kong, they must take a post-arrival SARS-CoV-2 nucleic acid test at the DH's TSCC and wait for the results there or any other location as designated by DH upon arrival at HKIA;
- Specimen bottles will be distributed to the exempted persons upon arrival. They must collect and return their deep throat saliva sample at Day-12 upon their arrival in accordance with the instructions for SARS-CoV-2 nucleic acid test again; and
- Respective organisations must arrange point-to-point transportation for the exempted persons. The use of public transport is prohibited.

Currently, crew change arrangement for passenger vessels and goods vessels without cargo operation in Hong Kong has been suspended. As for those with cargo operation, the Government has requested shipping companies to arrange all crew members of goods vessels to undergo nucleic acid tests at the point of departure within 48 hours and possess a negative result before embarking to travel to Hong Kong. They will also be required to conduct another test at the TSCC again upon arrival in Hong Kong and may only leave for their vessels upon availability of results. If the above conditions are not met, the crew member will not be granted exemption and will be denied entry into Hong Kong. The shipping agents must ensure that the crew members would go on-board the vessel immediately and directly upon arrival in Hong Kong and should not stay in public places. Point-to-point transfers to and from the vessel for the sea crew members must be arranged. For details, please refer to the press release issued on July 26 by the Government.

The spokesman added that the above measures aim to further tighten the exemption conditions following the previous round of tightening measures targeting at exempted persons as announced by the Government in mid-July, taking into risk assessment of the epidemic situation. The spokesman emphasised that the exemption arrangement was essential for maintaining the necessary operation of society and the economy, and for ensuring an uninterrupted supply of all daily necessities to the public. According to the latest daily average number of exempted persons arriving at Hong Kong at HKIA, air crew members accounts for 93 per cent which represents the largest group amongst all. Sea crew members arriving in Hong Kong for crew change currently make up around 5 per cent of exempted persons arriving from HKIA. The rest of the 2 per cent represents other exempted persons, such as officers of Consulates General and other government officials.

The spokesman said, "Upon the introduction of the tightened measures, all exempted persons having visited very high risk places must be subject to 'test-and-hold' arrangement. In addition, the scope of activity of the exempted person in Hong Kong is limited to the purpose as designated in the exemption, and they may only take point-to-point transportation. The use of public transport is prohibited. Exempted persons must also avoid unnecessary social contact during the period they are exempted from quarantine. These measures are introduced with a view to minimising the chance of transmission of virus from imported cases into the community."

The spokesman added, "Based on risk-level assessment by the Centre for Health Protection, the Government has been adjusting its anti-epidemic measures under the 'suppress and lift' strategy. The Government will stay vigilant and adopt necessary mechanism in guarding against the importation of cases and curbing the transmission of diseases on the one hand, whilst ensuring as far as possible the essential operation of our city on the other."

Issued at HKT 23:22

November 22[53]

Compulsory testing notice gazetted

****

The Government today (November 22) exercised the power under the Prevention and Control of Disease (Compulsory Testing for Certain Persons) Regulation (Cap. 599J) for the first time and published in the gazette a compulsory testing notice, which requires any person who had been present at 14 specified dance premises (see Annex) during the period from November 1 to 21 to undergo a COVID-19 nucleic acid test by November 24.

A spokesman for the Food and Health Bureau said, "The local epidemic situation is worsening rapidly. The number of confirmed cases of a cluster related to dancing activities and dancing venues continued to increase significantly in the past few days, with cases distributed all over the territory and some confirmed cases are asymptomatic. It indicates the existence of many silent transmission chains in the community. The Government must act swiftly. To cut the transmission chains as quickly as possible, the Centre for Health Protection has been tracing possibly infected persons who had been to the relevant dancing venues. Meanwhile, it is necessary for the Government to issue a compulsory testing notice targeting specified dance premises under Cap. 599J immediately, in order to require the relevant persons to get tested promptly to avoid delay in treatment."

According to the notice, all persons who had been to any of the 14 specified dance premises during the period from November 1 to 21, must undergo a COVID-19 nucleic acid test by November 24 through designated means. Persons who are subject to compulsory testing may choose to undergo testing as below:

---

[53] https://www.info.gov.hk/gia/general/202011/22.htm

(1) To attend any of the four Community Testing Centres (see the list at https://www.communitytest.gov.hk/en/) by November 24. The relevant testing charges can be waived;

(2) To collect a deep throat saliva specimen collection pack from any of the 47 designated general outpatient clinics of the Hospital Authority (see the list at https://www.ha.org.hk/haho/ho/covid-19/GOPC_extend_EN.pdf) and return the specimen to designated specimen collection points by November 24;

(3) To undergo testing at any healthcare facilities of the Hospital Authority (including general outpatient clinics and accident and emergency departments) as instructed by a medical professional of the Hospital Authority by November 24; or

(4) To self-arrange testing provided by private laboratories recognised by the Department of Health (see the list at https://www.coronavirus.gov.hk/pdf/List_of_recognised_laboratories.pdf).

Persons who are subject to compulsory testing must also report the result of the test or submit the test report to the Government by phone (6275 6901), fax (2530 5872) or email (ct@csb.gov.hk) by November 27.

The spokesman said, "To reduce transmission risk, persons who underwent testing are advised to stay at home and avoid going out when waiting for test results."

Any enquiries on compulsory testing arrangements may be addressed to the hotline at 6275 6901 (to commence operation today, operating daily from 9am to 6pm). The Government will continue to trace possibly infected persons who had been to the relevant dancing venues, and seriously verify whether they had complied with the testing notice. Any person who fails to comply with the testing notice commits an offence and may be fined a fixed penalty of $2,000. The person would also be issued with a compulsory testing order requiring him/her to undergo testing within a specified timeframe. Failure to comply with the order is an offence and the offender would be liable to a fine at level 4 ($25,000) and imprisonment for six months.

The spokesman said, "The 14 specified dance premises adopted the mode of operation of party rooms. In accordance with the directions and specifications by the Secretary for Food and Health under the Prevention and Control of Disease (Requirements and Directions) (Business and Premises) Regulation (Cap. 599F) on November 20, these premises must be closed from November 22 for a period of five days till November 26. Furthermore, within this period, live performance and dancing must not be allowed in any catering premises (including bars or pubs) as well as clubs or nightclubs."

"Strengthening COVID-19 testing is an integral part of the epidemic control strategy, which can help to slow down the transmission of the virus by early identification, early isolation and early treatment. The Government will later require other high risk groups or high exposure groups to undergo compulsory testing, including symptomatic persons, staff of residential care homes for the elderly and taxi drivers, etc. The relevant policy bureaux are actively working on the implementation of the relevant compulsory testing and will announce the details later."

"Understanding that some members of the public are concerned about their livelihood if they are tested positive, the Government will provide a one-off grant of $5,000 to local citizens who have been confirmed COVID-19 positive. Details will be announced by the Labour and Welfare Bureau later."

"The Government urges all individuals who are in doubt about their own health conditions, or individuals with infection risks (such as individuals who visited places with epidemic outbreaks or contacted confirmed cases) to undergo testing promptly for early identification of infected persons. The Food and Health Bureau will publish compulsory testing notices regarding particular groups when necessary taking into account the epidemic development and the testing participation rate."

Issued at HKT 6:00

Latest arrangements for services of HAD

****

In view of the latest developments of the COVID-19 epidemic, the Home Affairs Department (HAD) announced today (November 22) its service arrangements from tomorrow (November 23). The details are set out below.

The Home Affairs Enquiry Centres (HAECs) in 18 districts will open from 10am to 5pm, Monday to Friday (from 10am to 5pm on Monday, Wednesday and Friday only for the HAEC in Mui Wo) to provide services for the public.

Counter services of the Estate Beneficiaries Support Unit (EBSU) will be provided Monday to Friday, from 10am to 1pm and from 2pm to 5pm. The EBSU hotline (2835 1535) will continue to operate from 8.45am to 1pm and from 2pm to 6pm, Monday to Friday.

The services provided by the Office of the Licensing Authority will remain normal. The opening hours will be from 9am to 6pm from Monday to Friday (except public holidays). All licensing applications in connection with hotels, guesthouses and other premises as well as entertainment are encouraged to be submitted by post or using e-submission. Application forms and submission details can be found on the webpage of the Office of the Licensing Authority: www.hadla.gov.hk.

The multi-purpose halls, conference rooms, classrooms, meeting rooms, activity rooms, study rooms and covered play areas of community halls and community centres (except from those used as community testing centres) will remain open to organisations with approved bookings. However, there will be limits on the number of participants for activities to be held and precautionary measures in order to ensure that appropriate social distancing and avoidance of infection.

The HAD's hotlines for persons under home quarantine will operate between 9am and 6pm from Monday to Friday. For phone numbers of the hotlines, please visit the website of the HAD at www.had.gov.hk/file_manager/docs/district_hotline_en.pdf. For other enquiries, please call the HAD's enquiry hotline at 2835 2500 between 9am and 7pm from Monday to Friday.

Issued at HKT 12:00

Transcript of remarks by SFH at media session

****

Following is the transcript of remarks made by the Secretary for Food and Health, Professor Sophia Chan, after attending a radio programme today (November 22):

Reporter: Could you also tell us more about the five new testing centres that the Government is proposing?

Secretary for Food and Health: Virus testing is a very important strategy, especially when we are now facing a very severe situation in Hong Kong. The number of unlinked cases has been increasing in the past few days and we are now testing more people. In terms of the compulsory testing order that we issued just this morning, we envisaged that there will be more people coming out, especially the compulsory testing order is for the 14 places whereby the dancing gatherings have taken place. So we urge people who have been there since November 1 to come out to test before next Tuesday, so that we can identify more people if they require hospitalisation or quarantine.

Reporter: Where will the five new testing centres be and when will they be in use?

Secretary for Food and Health: We will be increasing the number of testing centres in the coming week. Obviously it will be in different districts in Hong Kong. On top of the five testing centres, we will also be assessing the situation of different districts. If there are a lot of cases in a particular district, not only are we putting on or setting up more centres, but we can, like what we have done in Tai Po District, we can set up mobile swabbing stations, or send mobile vans to distribute specimen bottles.

Issued at HKT 13:14

FEHD continues to step up inspections and reminds catering business operators and public to continue complying with anti-epidemic regulations

****

The Food and Environmental Hygiene Department (FEHD) continues to step up inspections at catering premises (including bars) across the territory and reminds the catering business operators to strictly comply with the requirements and directions under the Prevention and Control of Disease (Requirements and Directions) (Business and Premises) Regulation (Cap. 599F) (the Regulation), and the public to comply with the various restrictions in relation to group gatherings and mask-wearing under the anti-epidemic regulations and directions when patronising catering premises.

The FEHD and the Police conducted a joint operation last night (November 21) again and inspected 48 catering premises (including bars) in Soho area in Central. Procedure on prosecution was initiated against one catering business operator for beaching the requirement on the distance between tables under the Regulation.

Inclusive of the cases in the above paragraph, the FEHD conducted a total of 3 066 inspections at catering premises (including bars) across the territory on Friday (November 20) and yesterday (November 21), while procedures on prosecution were initiated against nine catering business operators for breaching the Regulation, mainly about violating the requirements on the number of persons at one table and the distance between tables, as well as not wearing a mask at all times within the premises except when consuming food or drink at a table therein.

A spokesman for the FEHD said, "According to the current directions issued by the Secretary for Food and Health in relation to catering business under the Regulation, food business operators must strictly comply with a series of requirements and restrictions, including live performance/dancing must not be allowed in any catering premises (including bars / pubs) as well as clubs / nightclubs; dining-in must cease from 0.00am to 4.59am every day; no more than two persons may be at one table for a bar/pub or night establishment/nightclub while no more than four persons may be at one table for other catering premises; the total number of customers allowed in catering premises must not exceed 50 per cent of the normal seating capacity; a mask must be worn within the premises except when the person is consuming food or drink at a table therein; tables must be arranged in a way to ensure there is a distance of at least 1.5m or some form of partition which could serve as effective buffer between one table and another table; body temperature screening must be conducted before the person is allowed to enter the catering premises; and hand sanitisers must be provided, etc."

The spokesman stressed that the FEHD will continue to proactively take stringent enforcement actions in the coming week, stepping up inspections at catering premises across the territory and conducting joint operations with the Police if necessary, to ensure that catering business operators and the public strictly comply with relevant regulations. Enforcement actions will be taken against offenders so as to minimise the risk of transmission of COVID-19 in food premises.

If catering business operators contravene the Regulation, they are liable to a maximum fine of $50,000 and imprisonment for six months. Persons who violate the group gathering restriction of the Prevention and Control of Disease (Prohibition in Group Gathering) Regulation (Cap. 599G) are subject to a fixed penalty of $2,000.

The spokesman appealed to catering business operators to comply with relevant regulations on prevention and control of disease in a concerted and persistent manner, with a view to keeping their staff, customers and the public safe. Members of the public also have to comply with the related regulations and directions on group gatherings and mask-wearing at catering premises.

Issued at HKT 18:30

Public hospitals daily update on COVID-19 cases

****

The following is issued on behalf of the Hospital Authority:

As at 9am today (November 22), 11 COVID-19 confirmed patients were discharged from hospital in the last 24 hours. So far, a total of 5 259 patients with confirmed or probable infection have been discharged.

At present, there are 577 negative pressure rooms in public hospitals with 1 060 negative pressure beds activated. A total of 164 confirmed patients are currently hospitalised in 19 public hospitals, among which eight patients are in critical condition, two are in serious condition and the remaining 154 patients are in stable condition.

The Hospital Authority will maintain close contact with the Centre for Health Protection to monitor the latest developments and to inform the public and healthcare workers on the latest information in a timely manner.

Details of the above-mentioned patients are as follows:

Patient condition	Case numbers
Discharged	5321, 5327, 5351, 5360, 5366, 5379, 5382, 5443, 5495, 5519, 5540
Critical	1989, 3496, 4706, 4833, 5110, 5185, 5409, 5433
Serious	5273, 5439

Issued at HKT 18:47

CHP investigates 68 additional confirmed cases of COVID-19

****

The Centre for Health Protection (CHP) of the Department of Health has announced that as of 0.00am, November 22, the CHP was investigating 68 additional confirmed cases of coronavirus disease 2019 (COVID-19), taking the number of cases to 5 629 in Hong Kong so far (comprising 5 628 confirmed cases and one probable case).

Among the newly reported cases announced, seven had a travel history during the incubation period.

A total of 196 cases have been recorded in the past 14 days (November 8 – 21), including 90 local cases of which 40 are from unknown sources.

The CHP's epidemiological investigations and relevant contact tracing on the confirmed cases are ongoing. For case details and contact tracing information, please see the Annex One or the list of buildings with confirmed cases of COVID-19 in the past 14 days and the latest local situation of COVID-19 available on the website "COVID-19 Thematic Website" (www.coronavirus.gov.hk).

As a number of cases confirmed recently claimed that they had visited dancing venues, the CHP strongly appealed to those who had visited the dancing venues as listed in Annex Two on or after November 1 to visit the Hospital Authority's designated general out-patient clinics (www.ha.org.hk/haho/ho/covid-19/GOPC_extend_EN.pdf) and collect deep throat saliva specimen collection packs for free COVID-19 testing as soon as possible. The public are also urged to seek medical attention early if symptoms develop.

In view of the severe epidemic situation, the CHP called on members of the public to avoid going out, having social contact and dining out. They should put on a surgical mask and maintain

stringent hand hygiene when they need to go out. The CHP strongly urged the elderly to stay home as far as possible and avoid going out. They should consider asking their family and friends to help with everyday tasks such as shopping for basic necessities.

The spokesman said, "Given that the situation of COVID-19 infection remains severe and that there is a continuous increase in the number of cases reported around the world, members of the public are strongly urged to avoid all non-essential travel outside Hong Kong.

"The CHP also strongly urges the public to maintain at all times strict personal and environmental hygiene, which is key to personal protection against infection and prevention of the spread of the disease in the community. On a personal level, members of the public should wear a surgical mask when having respiratory symptoms, taking public transport or staying in crowded places. They should also perform hand hygiene frequently, especially before touching the mouth, nose or eyes.

"As for household environmental hygiene, members of the public are advised to maintain drainage pipes properly, regularly pour water into drain outlets (U-traps) and cover all floor drain outlets when they are not in use. After using the toilet, they should put the toilet lid down before flushing to avoid spreading germs."

Moreover, the Government has launched the website "COVID-19 Thematic Website" (www.coronavirus.gov.hk) for announcing the latest updates on various news on COVID-19 infection and health advice to help the public understand the latest updates. Members of the public may also gain access to information via the COVID-19 WhatsApp Helpline launched by the Office of the Government Chief Information Officer. Simply by saving 9617 1823 in their phone contacts or clicking the link wa.me/85296171823?text=hi, they will be able to obtain information on COVID-19 as well as the "StayHomeSafe" mobile app and wristband via WhatsApp.

Issued at HKT 21:36

Various means for public to undergo virus testing

****

The Government reminds the public that all persons who had been to any of the 14 specified dance premises during the period from November 1 to 21 can undergo a COVID-19 nucleic acid test through various means. Designated general outpatient clinics of the Hospital Authority will continue to open from 9am tomorrow for public to collect deep throat saliva specimen collection packs.

Various means for conducting COVID-19 nucleic acid test include the followings:

* To collect a deep throat saliva specimen collection pack from any of the 47 designated

general outpatient clinics of the Hospital Authority (time slots for distribution of specimen collection packs and specimen collection, see www.ha.org.hk/haho/ho/covid-19/GOPC_extend_EN.pdf);

* To self-arrange testing provided by private laboratories recognised by the Department of Health (see the list at www.coronavirus.gov.hk/pdf/List_of_recognised_laboratories.pdf);

* To attend any of the four Community Testing Centres (see the list at www.communitytest.gov.hk/en);

* To undergo testing at any healthcare facilities of the Hospital Authority (including general outpatient clinics and accident and emergency departments) as instructed by a medical professional of the Hospital Authority.

A Government spokesman said, "We notice that quite a number of people who had been to the dance premises take the initiative to undergo virus testing in order to comply with the requirements of the Compulsory Testing Notice under the Prevention and Control of Disease (Compulsory Testing for Certain Persons) Regulation. We would like to thank them for their co-operation."

"The testing centres will increase the test quota and extend operation hours when necessary, and reserve certain test quota for persons who are subject to compulsory testing. If members of the public plan to conduct testing at any of the testing centres, they can check the centre's appointment status in advance."

"If persons who are subject to compulsory testing have symptoms, they should seek medical attention immediately instead of going to the community testing centres. To reduce transmission risk, persons who underwent testing are advised to stay at home and avoid going out when waiting for test results."

If persons who are subject to compulsory testing have previously undergone the above mentioned test between November 18 and 21, they would be taken to have complied with the requirements set out in the Compulsory Testing Notice.

Any enquiries on compulsory testing arrangements may be addressed to the hotline at 6275 6901 which operates daily from 9am to 6pm. The hotlines of the community testing centres are as follows:

Quarry Bay Community Hall, Eastern District (Prenetics)	3008 8325
Henry G Leong Yaumatei Community Centre (Kingmed Diagnostics (Hong Kong) Limited)	9869 3603

Lek Yuen Community Hall, Sha Tin (Hong Kong Molecular Pathology Diagnostic Centre Limited)	2986 1272 2986 1270
Yuen Long Town East Community Hall (BGI)	2818 9690

Persons who are subject to compulsory testing must report the result of the test or submit the test report to the Government by phone (6275 6901), fax (2530 5872) or email (ct@csb.gov.hk) on or before November 27.

Issued at HKT 23:49

November 23[54]

Mobile specimen collection stations and specimen bottle distribution point to be set up in Tsuen Wan, Sai Kung and Tai Po from today

****

The local epidemic situation is worsening rapidly. The confirmed cases distributed all over the territory. Some of the confirmed cases are asymptomatic and this has indicated the existence of many silent transmission chains in the community. In view of a number of confirmed COVID-19 cases relating to residents in Tsuen Wan, Sai Kung and Tai Po recently, in order to identify cases in the community as early as possible to help cut the transmission chains, the Government arranges testing agencies to provide free testing services through mobile specimen collection stations and specimen bottle distribution point in Tsuen Wan, Sai Kung and Tai Po starting today (November 23), with a view to facilitating and encouraging residents of the districts or individuals who perceive themselves as having a higher risk of exposure to undergo COVID-19 testing.

The testing agencies (BGI and Hong Kong Molecular Pathology Diagnostic Centre Limited) will set up a total of seven mobile specimen collection stations / specimen bottle distribution point in Tsuen Wan, Sai Kung and Tai Po (see Annex). The mobile stations / distribution point operate starting from November 23. Members of the public may visit the mobile specimen collection stations direct for on-site registration and specimen collections, or the specimen bottle distribution point to obtain specimen bottle and submit deep throat saliva specimens for free COVID-19 testing.

[54] https://www.info.gov.hk/gia/general/202011/23.htm

A government spokesman said, "The testing agencies will provide specimen collection services by combined nasal and throat swab at the mobile specimen collection stations; or distribute specimen bottles to members of the public and collect deep throat saliva specimens at the specimen bottle distribution point for testing free of charge. Persons who are subject to compulsory testing and undergo testing at the mobile specimen collection stations or through the services provided at specimen bottle distribution point will be deemed to have undergone a test at a community testing centre. People whose test results are negative will be informed by SMS through their mobile phones. If any specimen tested shows a positive COVID-19 result, the specimen will be referred to the Public Health Laboratory Services Branch of the Department of Health (DH) for a confirmatory test. Confirmed cases will be followed up and announced by the Centre for Health Protection of the DH."

The spokesman urges all individuals who are in doubt about their own health conditions, or individuals with infection risks (such as individuals who visited places with epidemic outbreaks or contacted confirmed cases) to undergo testing promptly for early identification of infected persons.

Issued at HKT 9:14

Horticulture staff officer of Housing Department tests positive for COVID-19

****

The Housing Department today (November 23) learnt that a staff officer of its Horticulture Unit has tested positive for coronavirus disease 2019 (COVID-19). She is staying at a hospital for treatment.

The officer concerned works on the sixth floor of Block 1 at the Hong Kong Housing Authority Headquarters in Ho Man Tin. The floor concerned is not a public floor and is not open to the public. She last performed duties on November 20.

She has no recent travel history, and has been wearing facial masks when performing duties. She followed relevant disease prevention measures at work. The department will continue to closely co-operate with the Centre for Health Protection (CHP) on disease prevention measures. The workplace of the officer concerned, including the common areas, will be fully cleaned and sterilised in accordance with the guidelines of the CHP.

During the pandemic, the department has been strictly implementing various disease prevention measures, including measuring the body temperature of people entering the buildings, providing facial masks and other personal protective equipment for staff, and requesting staff to wear facial masks when in contact with others and at public places. Cleaning and sterilising measures for the working environment of the department have also been stepped up.

The department will continue to maintain close liaison with the CHP and co-operate with its quarantine work.

Issued at HKT 15:00

Engineering laboratory technician of Water Supplies Department tested positive for COVID-19

****

The Water Supplies Department (WSD) today (November 23) said an engineering laboratory technician of its Pak Kong Water Treatment Works Laboratory had tested positive for COVID-19 last night (November 22).

The staff member last came to work on November 17. Her job duties did not involve water treatment. There is no effect on drinking water safety.

She has been admitted to hospital for medical treatment. Staff who had close contact with her at work have undergone COVID-19 testing and the results were all negative. The WSD has thoroughly cleaned and sterilised the Pak Kong Water Treatment Works Laboratory. The department will maintain close liaison with the Centre for Health Protection. Staff have been reminded to pay attention to personal hygiene and to stay vigilant. They should seek medical advice immediately if feeling unwell.

Issued at HKT 16:00

Hong Kong Customs-outsourced security guard tests positive for COVID-19

****

Hong Kong Customs today (November 23) learned that an outsourced male security guard has tested positive for the coronavirus disease 2019 (COVID-19).

The outsourced security guard concerned worked at the Customs Headquarters Building and mainly performed supporting duties. He last performed his duties last Saturday (November 21) and is now under medical treatment.

The officer has no recent travel history. He has been wearing surgical masks when performing duties and has properly maintained social distancing with people he has had contact with. His body temperature was normal when undergoing temperature screening before work every day.

The department has been closely co-operating with the Centre for Health Protection (CHP) on the CHP's epidemiological investigations to follow up on the situations of the colleagues working with him. The concerned working places have also undergone a thorough cleaning and sterilisation.

Customs is highly concerned about the epidemic of COVID-19. Apart from continuing to step up the cleaning and sterilising measures for all working locations, the department also reminds all officers to strictly comply with the hygienic measures of infectious diseases provided by the CHP. The officers will also be reminded to consult a doctor promptly if they have any discomforting symptoms.

Issued at HKT 18:00

Public hospitals daily update on COVID-19 cases

****

The following is issued on behalf of the Hospital Authority:

As at 9am today (November 23), eight COVID-19 confirmed patients were discharged from hospital in the last 24 hours. So far, a total of 5 267 patients with confirmed or probable infection have been discharged.

At present, there are 584 negative pressure rooms in public hospitals with 1 085 negative pressure beds activated. A total of 224 confirmed patients are currently hospitalised in 19 public hospitals, among which eight patients are in critical condition, two are in serious condition and the remaining 214 patients are in stable condition.

The Hospital Authority will maintain close contact with the Centre for Health Protection to monitor the latest developments and to inform the public and healthcare workers on the latest information in a timely manner.

Details of the above-mentioned patients are as follows:

Patient condition	Case numbers
Discharged	5300, 5421, 5431, 5445, 5470, 5477, 5508, 5522
Critical	1989, 3496, 4706, 4833, 5110, 5185, 5409, 5433
Serious	5273, 5439

Issued at HKT 18:20

Transcript of remarks by SLW on one-off grant to local citizens confirmed COVID-19 positive
****

Following is the transcript of remarks by the Secretary for Labour and Welfare, Dr Law Chi-kwong, this afternoon (November 23) on the one-off grant to local citizens who have been confirmed COVID-19 positive:

Reporter: Mr Law, Secretary. First of all, from what you said earlier, you are hoping to help people from low-income families who may have their income cut because of their infection, but can you clarify whether there will be any means test? If there is no means test, how can you ensure these people are actually from low-income families that they actually have their income slashed because of COVID-19 infection? Looking at that, aside from the impact after they were infected, there is also the issue of close contacts. If they are from low-income families, they are required to take a two-week mandatory quarantine. They also have their income affected. Why are these people not benefitting from the subsidy? My third question is how you would ensure that there will not be abuse. Can you also clarify whether there will be any age limits? Thank you.

Secretary for Labour and Welfare: Let us go back to the question about means test. There will be no means test. That is what I have just described the conditions (of eligibility of the one-off grant), namely those who have substantial reduction in income and will be suffering from financial difficulties. They will be eligible to apply for this ex-gratia payment (one-off grant). I do not expect that some high-income groups will be entitled to such circumstances. The strictest way is to do a means test, but then you understand that doing a means test will prolong the application process. It can be hard for the applicants, too, because they may have to provide such a lot of information before the application is approved, and they are already suffering from COVID-19. To balance all these considerations, we consider that these broad considerations or conditions eligible for the grant will be sufficient to cover primarily those who are grassroots.

As for the issue about close contacts, we have actually considered whether we should provide some benefits for those who are classified as close contacts. In fact, to look at the discussion in the past couple of days, not just in the past few days – because the idea was actually raised to us by some of the experts during the meeting of the expert advisory group more than a week ago on a Saturday, so we have been thinking about this particular measure for slightly more than a week's time. One of the major considerations of any government action to provide any benefits is to consider the possibility of abuse. For this one-off grant for those who are COVID-19 positive and hospitalised, we do consider that the risk (of abuse) is quite minimal. In fact, we are just targeting at those who belong to the grassroots, who are employed or self-employed, and who suffer from the loss of income. So, we do not expect that will create any substantial abuse.

But for the case of close contacts, it can be more volatile I would say. The way to deal with abuse can be even far more complicated and expensive than a process of providing such a benefit to such an individual. So, we have decided not to include those who are classified as close contacts into the circumstances.

Issued at HKT 20:56

CHP investigates 73 additional confirmed cases of COVID-19

****

The Centre for Health Protection (CHP) of the Department of Health has announced that as of 0.00am, November 23, the CHP was investigating 73 additional confirmed cases of coronavirus disease 2019 (COVID-19), taking the number of cases to 5 702 in Hong Kong so far (comprising 5 701 confirmed cases and one probable case).

A total of 254 cases have been recorded in the past 14 days (November 9 – 22), including 149 local cases of which 45 are from unknown sources.

The CHP's epidemiological investigations and relevant contact tracing on the confirmed cases are ongoing. For case details and contact tracing information, please see the Annex One or the list of buildings with confirmed cases of COVID-19 in the past 14 days and the latest local situation of COVID-19 available on the website "COVID-19 Thematic Website" (www.coronavirus.gov.hk).

As a number of cases confirmed recently claimed that they had visited venues for dancing or singing, the CHP strongly appealed to those who had visited the venues as listed in Annex Two on or after November 1 to visit the Hospital Authority's designated general out-patient clinics (www.ha.org.hk/haho/ho/covid-19/GOPC_extend_EN.pdf) and collect deep throat saliva specimen collection packs for free COVID-19 testing as soon as possible. The public are also urged to seek medical attention early if symptoms develop.

In view of the severe epidemic situation, the CHP called on members of the public to avoid going out, having social contact and dining out. They should put on a surgical mask and maintain stringent hand hygiene when they need to go out. The CHP strongly urged the elderly to stay home as far as possible and avoid going out. They should consider asking their family and friends to help with everyday tasks such as shopping for basic necessities.

The spokesman said, "Given that the situation of COVID-19 infection remains severe and that there is a continuous increase in the number of cases reported around the world, members of the public are strongly urged to avoid all non-essential travel outside Hong Kong.

"The CHP also strongly urges the public to maintain at all times strict personal and environmental hygiene, which is key to personal protection against infection and prevention of the spread of the disease in the community. On a personal level, members of the public should wear a surgical mask when having respiratory symptoms, taking public transport or staying in crowded places. They should also perform hand hygiene frequently, especially before touching the mouth, nose or eyes.

"As for household environmental hygiene, members of the public are advised to maintain drainage pipes properly, regularly pour water into drain outlets (U-traps) and cover all floor drain outlets when they are not in use. After using the toilet, they should put the toilet lid down before flushing to avoid spreading germs."

Moreover, the Government has launched the website "COVID-19 Thematic Website" (www.coronavirus.gov.hk) for announcing the latest updates on various news on COVID-19 infection and health advice to help the public understand the latest updates. Members of the public may also gain access to information via the COVID-19 WhatsApp Helpline launched by the Office of the Government Chief Information Officer. Simply by saving 9617 1823 in their phone contacts or clicking the link wa.me/85296171823?text=hi, they will be able to obtain information on COVID-19 as well as the "StayHomeSafe" mobile app and wristband via WhatsApp.

Issued at HKT 23:30

Over 2 140 people returned to Hong Kong on first day of implementation of Return2hk Scheme
****

"Return2hk - Travel Scheme for Hong Kong Residents returning from Guangdong Province or Macao without being subject to quarantine under the Compulsory Quarantine of Certain Persons Arriving at Hong Kong Regulation (Cap. 599C)" (Return2hk Scheme) commenced today (November 23). Up to 6pm, a total of about 2 140 people returned to Hong Kong under the Scheme, of which around 1 810 people returned through the Shenzhen Bay Port while around 330 people made use of the Hong Kong-Zhuhai-Macao Bridge (HZMB) Hong Kong Port to return.

A Government spokesman said, "Many Hong Kong residents with a quota have, before their entry into Hong Kong, obtained a 'Green' QR code by transmitting the negative nucleic test result to the electronic health declaration system of the Department of Health through 'Yuekang code' (粵康碼) or 'Macao health code' (澳康碼). They could use the dedicated channel at the boundary control point and the clearance process was smooth."

"To expedite the clearance process, reduce waiting time and avoid network connection problems at the boundary control points, Hong Kong residents who intend to return to Hong Kong under the Return2hk Scheme are strongly advised to, apart from returning on the date and at the boundary control point as specified in their booking, complete the code conversion process through 'Yuekang code' (粵康碼) or 'Macao health code' (澳康碼) within 24 hours before setting off to obtain a 'Green' QR code. They would then be exempted from the compulsory quarantine requirement upon their entry into Hong Kong."

"If the code conversion process generates QR code of a different colour (e.g. a 'Pink' QR code), it means the traveller has yet to fulfil all the specified conditions, and he/she may still be subject to the 14-day compulsory quarantine requirement upon entry into Hong Kong."

The Government has produced user guides on "code conversion" for the easy reference of returning Hong Kong residents. They are available at the links below:

Transmission of the valid negative COVID-19 nucleic acid test result to the electronic health declaration system of the Department of Health through "Yuekang code" (粵康碼):

Video (in Chinese only): youtu.be/ccq9-3FzDr8

PDF version (English version):
www.coronavirus.gov.hk/pdf/Return2hk_Code_Conversion_Use_Guide_en.pdf

Transmission of the valid negative COVID-19 nucleic acid test result to the electronic health declaration system of the Department of Health through "Macao health code" (澳康碼)

PDF version (English version):
www.coronavirus.gov.hk/pdf/Return2hk_Code_Conversion_Use_Guide_en.pdf

Hong Kong residents who have successfully reserved a quota should return to Hong Kong on the date and at the boundary control point as specified in the booking, and bring along their Hong Kong Identity Card or other identification documents, the confirmation of a successful booking (i.e. a printout of the booking confirmation page) as well as the proof of a valid negative nucleic acid test result (paper or electronic copy are both acceptable).

Re-entry into Guangdong Province or Macao

The Government spokesman specifically reminded that, if returning Hong Kong residents would subsequently enter the Guangdong Province or Macao again, they would still be subject to the prevailing quarantine arrangement of the two places (e.g. 14-day compulsory quarantine), unless exemption has been granted for them separately. They should therefore take note of the latest quarantine arrangements of Guangdong Province and Macao, and make necessary preparations.

Self-monitoring of health conditions after returning Hong Kong

The spokesman stressed that Hong Kong residents who can fulfil all the specified conditions and are returning to Hong Kong under the Return2hk Scheme should still exercise self-monitoring of their health conditions for at least 14 days after their entry into Hong Kong. They should observe the points listed in the "Health-monitoring Checklist for Inbound Travellers". If they feel unwell, they should seek medical advice promptly and reveal their travel history to medical practitioners. They may proactively make a request to their doctor for testing when there is any suspicion.

Details about the Return2hk Scheme are available at the "COVID-19 Thematic Website" (return2hk.gov.hk or 回港易.政府.香港). Members of the public may also call the Return2hk Scheme hotline at 3142 2330 for enquiries.

Issued at HKT 23:42

November 24[55]

Compulsory testing notice gazetted
****

The Government has exercised the power under the Prevention and Control of Disease (Compulsory Testing for Certain Persons) Regulation (Cap. 599J) and published in the Gazette a compulsory testing notice, which requires any person who had been present at seven specified premises (see Annex 1) during the period from November 1 to 23 to undergo a COVID-19 nucleic acid test by November 26.

A spokesman for the Food and Health Bureau said today (November 24), "The local epidemic situation is worsening rapidly. The number of confirmed cases related to group gathering activities in indoor premises continues to rise significantly. As such, the Government published in the Gazette a compulsory testing notice under the Regulation for the first time on November 21, requiring persons who had been to 14 specified dance premises to undergo compulsory testing.

"Upon further contact tracing by the Centre for Health Protection, we found that large group gathering activities in other premises were involved for some recent confirmed cases. Therefore, the Government published another compulsory testing notice, which requires persons who had been to seven other premises to undergo testing."

[55] https://www.info.gov.hk/gia/general/202011/24.htm

According to the latest notice, all persons who had been to any of the seven specified premises during the period from November 1 to 23 must undergo a COVID-19 nucleic acid test by November 26 through designated means.

Persons subject to compulsory testing may choose to undergo testing as below:

1. To obtain a deep throat saliva specimen collection pack from any of the 47 designated general outpatient clinics (GOPCs) of the Hospital Authority and return the specimen to designated specimen collection points (see the specimen collection packs distribution time and specimen collection time at www.ha.org.hk/haho/ho/covid-19/GOPC_extend_TC.pdf);

2. To self-arrange testing provided by private laboratories recognised by the Department of Health (see the list at www.coronavirus.gov.hk/pdf/List_of_recognised_laboratories.pdf);

3. To attend any of the four Community Testing Centres (see the list at www.communitytest.gov.hk/en/);

4. To visit any of the seven mobile specimen collection stations/specimen bottle distribution points (see the list at Annex 2) for testing, or obtain and submit specimen bottles; or

5. To undergo testing at any healthcare facilities of the Hospital Authority (including GOPCs and accident and emergency departments) as instructed by a medical professional of the Hospital Authority.

The spokesman said, "We encourage persons who are subject to compulsory testing to obtain deep throat saliva specimen collection packs from designated GOPCs. No reservation is needed. As long as their specimens are submitted on or before November 26, they would be taken to have complied with the requirements set out in the compulsory testing notice."

"If persons who are subject to compulsory testing have symptoms, they should seek medical attention immediately and undergo testing as instructed by a medical professional. They should not attend the Community Testing Centres."

Persons who are subject to compulsory testing must report the result of the test or submit the test report to the Government by phone (6275 6901), fax (2530 5872) or email (ct@csb.gov.hk) by November 29. If persons who are subject to compulsory testing have previously undergone the above mentioned test between November 20 and 23, they would be taken to have complied with the requirements set out in the compulsory testing notice.

The spokesman said, "To reduce transmission risk, persons who underwent testing are advised to stay at home and avoid going out when waiting for test results."

Any enquiries on compulsory testing arrangements may be addressed to the hotline at 6275

6901 which operates daily from 9am to 6pm. If persons who are subject to compulsory testing plan to conduct testing at any of the Community Testing Centres, they can check the centre's appointment status in advance. The hotlines of the Community Testing Centres are as follows:

Quarry Bay Community Hall, Eastern District (Prenetics)	3008 8325
Henry G Leong Yaumatei Community Centre (Kingmed Diagnostics (Hong Kong) Limited)	9869 3603
Lek Yuen Community Hall, Sha Tin (Hong Kong Molecular Pathology Diagnostic Centre Limited)	2986 1272 2986 1270
Yuen Long Town East Community Hall (BGI)	2818 9690

The Government will continue to trace possibly infected persons who had been to the relevant venues, and seriously verify whether they had complied with the testing notice. Any person who fails to comply with the testing notice commits an offence and may be fined a fixed penalty of $2,000. The person would also be issued with a compulsory testing order requiring him/her to undergo testing within a specified timeframe. Failure to comply with the order is an offence and the offender would be liable to a fine at level 4 ($25,000) and imprisonment for six months.

The spokesman said, "The Government urges all individuals who are in doubt about their own health conditions, or individuals with infection risks (such as individuals who visited places with epidemic outbreaks or contacted confirmed cases) to undergo testing promptly for early identification of infected persons. The Food and Health Bureau will publish compulsory testing notices regarding particular groups when necessary taking into account the epidemic development and the testing participation rate."

Issued at HKT 6:00

CAD-outsourced workman tests positive for COVID-19

****

The Civil Aviation Department (CAD) learned that an outsourced workman had tested positive for the coronavirus disease 2019 (COVID-19) last night (November 23). He is being treated in a hospital.

The outsourced workman worked at the CAD Headquarters and performed support duties without contact with members of the public at work. He last performed his duties on November 21 and has no recent travel history. He has been wearing surgical masks while performing his duties and has properly maintained social distancing with people he has had contact with. His body temperature was normal when undergoing temperature screening during work.

The CAD has been closely liaising and cooperating with the Centre for Health Protection (CHP) in the epidemiological investigation. The outsourced staff working with the workman are asymptomatic and have been arranged to undergo COVID-19 testing. The concerned work places have also been fully cleaned and sterilised.

The CAD is concerned about the COVID-19 epidemic. All staff have been highly vigilant since the epidemic broke out. Relevant hygienic measures for infectious diseases provided by the CHP have been strictly adopted. All staff have their body temperatures checked before performing their duties, and wear proper personal protective equipment.

The department will continue to step up the cleaning and sterilising measures for all work locations and remind all staff to strictly comply with the hygienic measures for infectious diseases provided by the CHP. The staff will also be reminded to consult a doctor promptly if they have any discomforting symptoms.

Issued at HKT 12:15

Transcript of remarks by CE at media session before ExCo meeting
****

Following is the transcript of remarks by the Chief Executive, Mrs Carrie Lam and the Secretary for Food and Health, Professor Sophia Chan, at a media session before the Executive Council meeting today (November 24):

Reporter: Research has shown that vaccines developed in the US and the UK have a 90 per cent success rate and may be rolled out next month, while Brazil is expecting regulatory approval for the vaccine developed by Sinovac. What is your administration's plan to secure vaccines for Hong Kong and when will you have the details of when a vaccine will be made available? Second question, Hong Kong has not been able to stamp out COVID-19 cases. Experts point to loopholes in the current system of contact tracing, quarantine and testing of incoming travellers that allowed infected individuals to enter the territory. How would mandatory testing be implemented effectively if the Government cannot identify all close contacts and would the Government consider tightening existing measures such as extending the quarantine period to 21 days as Professor Yuen Kwok-yung recommended? And, third question, you have spoken about consulting Beijing on the Policy Address, and as of this month, there are no opposition forces left in the legislature, opposition candidates have been banned, parties banned, annual town hall public forums and regular legislative Q&As were axed. In light of this, how will you prevent yourself from being isolated from hearing any opposition or voices of the general public? Thank you.

Chief Executive: There are three questions. First is on a vaccine, we are very delighted to learn about the positive news coming out from the World Health Organization and also from individual research institutions about the development in the COVID-19 vaccine. As the Secretary for Food and Health has mentioned many times and we have got the money from the Finance Committee some time ago, we have enough money to procure vaccines to safeguard the health of the Hong Kong people. It's on a dual track. One is we have joined the international arrangement, the COVAX. The other is we have been discussing, negotiating and signing advance purchase agreements with some of these research companies and drug production companies, but I'm not supposed to give you the details, that is to be preserved, to be kept on a confidential basis. As you know some of the vaccines are being developed in the Mainland and I have also asked the Central People's Government that, we will be on our own to procure, but if needed, then the Central Government will also lend us a helping hand in supply of vaccine.

The second question is made up of many parts. I could only respond by sharing with you that this COVID-19 pandemic is of a magnitude that one has not seen, is a major challenge for humanity all over the world, perhaps except our own country, which has through very vigorous measures managed to control the pandemic and hence, the economy has rebounded and other things have been happening. As far as Hong Kong is concerned, we continue in a very vigilant manner to fight the epidemic and also to introduce various measures that are necessary. This morning, I have described to you how we will step up testing on a mandatory basis and also on a target-group basis. I've also given you a preview that later today we will announce measures to tighten the social distancing measures in order to control the spread of the disease, especially in light of this big cluster arising from the dancing halls. If our experts and our evidence, whether it is local or international, clearly show that there are more effective means to do it, or we need to adjust our measures, then of course we will do it.

But I just want to give Hong Kong people a general sit-rep of where we stand. Globally-we have to look at it globally because this is a global pandemic-Hong Kong is not doing bad at all. There are several indicators of how a territory or country is handling this COVID-19 pandemic. One is the confirmed cases per one million population, the other is deaths per one million population and the third is the tests per one million population. If one looks at all those international statistical compilations, you will realise that Hong Kong is not doing bad at all. Let's have confidence in ourselves that by putting in our best efforts, by government taking the lead and by individual citizens playing their part. This is still the time for avoiding close contact. This is still the time for not going into high-risk places. If people are not complying, then I will find it very difficult to manage the situation. But we will try. We'll never give up because this is concerning the health and the safety and the well-being of people of Hong Kong.

On the third question, if I may correct you, I am not consulting Beijing on the Policy Address. I am compiling my own Policy Address as the Chief Executive of the Hong Kong Special

Administrative Region (HKSAR). But it is clear to everyone that if we want our economy to bounce back, there is no better place than the Mainland of China for us to tap into because other parts of the world are still struggling with the pandemic and with high unemployment rate, with economic slowdown and so on. A couple of months ago, I have put to the Central Government a list of issues that I feel are important to help Hong Kong's economy to revive. They may not be immediate measures, but they are the measures which will help Hong Kong's economy to grow and hence give Hong Kong people more confidence at this difficult time, so consulting Beijing was on those individual measures that the HKSAR Chief Executive have put forth. It's not on the Policy Address. I don't think they have any interest in other things which concern maybe livelihood and others.

To answer your final thing about whether I will continue to hear from the people, I would say that with a more rational Legislative Council, it actually provides a much better platform for myself and my senior officials and my departmental colleagues to be engaged with the Legislative Councillors on issues of mutual concern. And where that project or that piece of legislation is doing good for Hong Kong, then it should be approved as soon as possible. Similarly, I would very much like to go into the community to organise more sessions, to meet with the people. But you would remember what has happened since June last year. Whenever there was any news about the Chief Executive going to a place, there will be on the social media this mobilisation of the rioters to meet me. Now that with the national security law, law and order has been restored. Chaos has been replaced by peacefulness. I am very willing, very ready to go to meet the people of Hong Kong.

Issued at HKT 15:20

Further anti-epidemic measure for performing venues implemented by Government to protect audiences

****

A Government spokesman said today (November 24) that the Leisure and Cultural Services Department (LCSD) will implement a further anti-epidemic measure at its performance venues from November 30. If performers are not able to wear masks during a performance with a live audience, they must take a Government-recognised coronavirus disease 2019 (COVID-19) test 72 hours prior to their performance. They can only participate in the performance after they have obtained a negative test result in order to protect audiences.

Since October 1, all performance venues of the LCSD have resumed performances or programmes with live audiences with the following anti-epidemic measures:

(a) The number of audience members in performance venues such as concert halls, theatres, auditoria, cultural activities halls and arenas is limited to 75 per cent of their original capacity. Consecutive seats are limited to four with seats evenly distributed;

(b) In activities to be held in minor facilities of the performance venues such as rehearsal rooms, music/dance studios and lecture/conference/function rooms, no more than four participants, including the instructor in a cluster, can be conducted, with appropriate distance maintained between groups. The number of users in minor facilities is limited to 75 per cent of their original capacity;

(c) Audiences must wear their own masks in the venues; and

(d) Backstage staff must wear masks in the venues at all times.

To strike a balance between anti-epidemic efforts and conducting live performances in light of the fluctuating epidemic situation of COVID-19, the Centre for Health Protection issued the Health Advice for Performing Arts on November 5. In response to the advice, the LCSD will implement a further anti-epidemic measure at its performance venues starting from November 30. In addition to the abovementioned requirement that performers who cannot wear masks during a performance with a live audience must take a test 72 hours prior to their performance and obtain a negative result before participating in the performance, depending on the number of days of the performance, a performer has to provide an updated negative test result every 10 days. In case of violation, the LCSD will reserve the right to ban the performers concerned from performing. Relevant details are set out in the Notes to Hirers to be distributed to venue hirers.

Meanwhile, the Government will issue letters to operators of other major non-government performance venues including the West Kowloon Cultural District Authority, the Hong Kong Academy for Performing Arts and the Hong Kong Arts Centre to inform them of the latest arrangements at LCSD performance venues. The Government appeals to all relevant venue operators to require performers who cannot wear masks during a performance to take a test before the performance.

Performers can undergo the COVID-19 test by various means:

• Collect a deep throat saliva specimen collection pack from any of the designated general outpatient clinics of the Hospital Authority (for time slots for distribution of specimen collection packs and specimen collection, see www.ha.org.hk/haho/ho/covid-19/GOPC_extend_EN.pdf);

• Self-arranged testing provided by private laboratories recognised by the Department of Health (see the list at www.coronavirus.gov.hk/pdf/List_of_recognised_laboratories.pdf); or

• Attend any of the Community Testing Centres (see the list at www.communitytest.gov.hk/en).

Issued at HKT 17:30

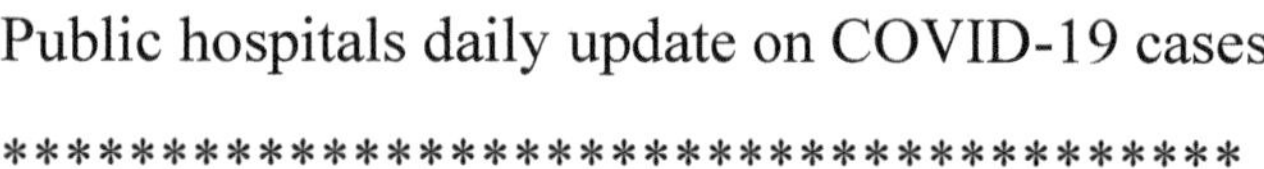

Public hospitals daily update on COVID-19 cases

****

The following is issued on behalf of the Hospital Authority:

As at 9am today (November 24), seven COVID-19 confirmed patients were discharged from hospital in the last 24 hours. So far, a total of 5 274 patients with confirmed or probable infection have been discharged.

At present, there are 607 negative pressure rooms in public hospitals with 1 126 negative pressure beds activated. A total of 290 confirmed patients are currently hospitalised in 19 public hospitals, among which seven patients are in critical condition, two are in serious condition and the remaining 281 patients are in stable condition.

The Hospital Authority will maintain close contact with the Centre for Health Protection to monitor the latest developments and to inform the public and healthcare workers on the latest information in a timely manner.

Details of the above-mentioned patients are as follows:

Patient condition	Case numbers
Discharged	5371, 5437, 5446, 5450, 5463, 5526, 5635
Critical	1989, 3496, 4833, 5110, 5185, 5409, 5433
Serious	5273, 5439

Issued at HKT 18:16

Man sentenced for breaching compulsory quarantine order

****

A 23-year-old man was sentenced to immediate imprisonment for six days by the Kwun Tong Magistrates' Courts today (November 24) for violating the Compulsory Quarantine of Certain Persons Arriving at Hong Kong Regulation (Cap 599C) (the Regulation).

The man was earlier issued a compulsory quarantine order stating that he must conduct quarantine at home for 14 days. Before the expiry of the quarantine order, he was found to have taken off his wristband during a surprise check on May 20 without reasonable excuse nor permission given by an authorised officer. He was charged with contravening Sections 8(4) and 8(5) of the Regulation and was sentenced by the Kwun Tong Magistrates' Courts today to immediate imprisonment for six days.

Pursuant to the Regulation, starting from February 8, save for exempted persons, all persons who have stayed in the Mainland, Macao or Taiwan in the 14 days preceding arrival in Hong Kong, regardless of their nationality or travel documents, will be subject to compulsory quarantine for 14 days. Moreover, pursuant to the Compulsory Quarantine of Persons Arriving at Hong Kong from Foreign Places Regulation (Cap 599E), starting from March 19, all persons arriving from countries or territories outside China would also be subject to compulsory quarantine for 14 days. Breaching a quarantine order is a criminal offence and offenders are subject to a maximum fine of $25,000 and imprisonment for six months.

A spokesman for the Department of Health said the sentence sends a clear message to the community that breaching a compulsory quarantine order is a criminal offence that the Government will not tolerate, and solemnly reminded the public to comply with the Regulation. As of today, a total of 71 persons have been convicted by the courts for breaching compulsory quarantine orders and have received sentences including immediate imprisonment for up to three months or a fine of $15,000. The spokesman reiterated that resolute actions will be taken against anyone who has breached the relevant regulations.

Issued at HKT 20:10

CHP investigates 80 additional confirmed cases of COVID-19

****

The Centre for Health Protection (CHP) of the Department of Health has announced that as of 0.00am, November 24, the CHP was investigating 80 additional confirmed cases of coronavirus disease 2019 (COVID-19), taking the number of cases to 5 782 in Hong Kong so far (comprising 5 781 confirmed cases and one probable case).

Among the newly reported cases announced, 11 had a travel history during the incubation period.

A total of 321 cases have been recorded in the past 14 days (November 10 – 23), including 212 local cases of which 52 are from unknown sources.

The CHP's epidemiological investigations and relevant contact tracing on the confirmed cases are ongoing. For case details and contact tracing information, please see the Annex One or the list of buildings with confirmed cases of COVID-19 in the past 14 days and the latest local situation of COVID-19 available on the website "COVID-19 Thematic Website" (www.coronavirus.gov.hk).

In view of the latest epidemic developments in the Mainland, starting tomorrow (November 25), inbound travellers who have been to Inner Mongolia in the past 14 days arriving via land boundary control points will be provided with specimen collection containers. They are required to collect their deep throat saliva samples by themselves in accordance with the instructions and return the samples for conducting COVID-19 testing. The arrangement of distributing specimen collection containers to inbound travellers who have been to Shandong Province, Xinjiang, Shanghai and Tianjin in the past 14 days arriving via land boundary control points, which has come into effect earlier, remains unchanged.

As a number of cases confirmed recently claimed that they had visited venues for dancing or singing, the CHP strongly appealed to those who had visited the venues as listed in Annex Two on or after November 1 to visit the Hospital Authority's designated general out-patient clinics (www.ha.org.hk/haho/ho/covid-19/GOPC_extend_EN.pdf) and collect deep throat saliva specimen collection packs for free COVID-19 testing as soon as possible. The public are also urged to seek medical attention early if symptoms develop.

In view of the severe epidemic situation, the CHP called on members of the public to avoid going out, having social contact and dining out. They should put on a surgical mask and maintain stringent hand hygiene when they need to go out. The CHP strongly urged the elderly to stay home as far as possible and avoid going out. They should consider asking their family and friends to help with everyday tasks such as shopping for basic necessities.

The spokesman said, "Given that the situation of COVID-19 infection remains severe and that there is a continuous increase in the number of cases reported around the world, members of the public are strongly urged to avoid all non-essential travel outside Hong Kong.

"The CHP also strongly urges the public to maintain at all times strict personal and environmental hygiene, which is key to personal protection against infection and prevention of the spread of the disease in the community. On a personal level, members of the public should wear a surgical mask when having respiratory symptoms, taking public transport or staying in crowded places. They should also perform hand hygiene frequently, especially before touching the mouth, nose or eyes.

"As for household environmental hygiene, members of the public are advised to maintain drainage pipes properly, regularly pour water into drain outlets (U-traps) and cover all floor drain outlets when they are not in use. After using the toilet, they should put the toilet lid down before flushing to avoid spreading germs."

Moreover, the Government has launched the website "COVID-19 Thematic Website" (www.coronavirus.gov.hk) for announcing the latest updates on various news on COVID-19 infection and health advice to help the public understand the latest updates. Members of the public may also gain access to information via the COVID-19 WhatsApp Helpline launched by the Office of the Government Chief Information Officer. Simply by saving 9617 1823 in their phone contacts or clicking the link wa.me/85296171823?text=hi, they will be able to obtain information on COVID-19 as well as the "StayHomeSafe" mobile app and wristband via WhatsApp.

Issued at HKT 21:52

November 25[56]

Government further tightens social distancing measures

****

In view of the development of COVID-19 in Hong Kong, the Government announced on November 24 to further tighten social distancing measures under the Prevention and Control of Disease (Requirements and Directions) (Business and Premises) Regulation (Cap. 599F).

A spokesman for the Food and Health Bureau said, "The COVID-19 epidemic situation has been worsening drastically. There have been over a hundred confirmed cases reported from the large outbreak cluster caused by group gathering activities in indoor premises. At the same time, there have been a number of local cases with unknown source reported in the last few days, indicating the existence of many silent transmission chains in the community. The Secretary for Food and Health has been tightening various social distancing measures since November 14. However, given the serious epidemic situation, we need to further tighten the social distancing measures under Cap. 599F, targeting those closed, crowded, closely-contacted, and mask-off leisure and entertainment group activities."

The latest details of requirements and restrictions are as follows:

(I) Catering premises and scheduled premises (details at Annex 1)

1. All bars or pubs, bath-houses, clubs or nightclubs must be closed. Party rooms will continue to be closed;

2. The number of people participating in any one banquet in catering premises will be limited to 40;

3. Apart from catering premises, live performance and dancing must not be allowed in meeting rooms or function rooms of clubhouses;

[56] https://www.info.gov.hk/gia/general/202011/25.htm

4. For hotels and guesthouses, restrictions will be imposed on gathering activities and infection control measures will be strengthened, including no more than four persons in a guest room, no more than eight persons in a suite with more than one bedroom, and no more than 20 persons during any religious or cultural ritual in relation to a wedding. Operators of hotels must arrange for persons under quarantine to be segregated from other persons not under quarantine, and must take reasonable steps to ensure that persons under quarantine cannot leave their guest rooms and cannot receive any visitors into their guest rooms during the quarantine period;

5. Persons responsible for carrying on catering businesses providing dine-in services and scheduled premises must apply for a "LeaveHomeSafe" venue QR code from the Government on or before December 2, and display the QR code obtained at the entrance of the premises or at a conspicuous position within two working days upon receipt of the QR code; and

6. Other requirements and restrictions on catering business and scheduled premises will be maintained, including no dine-in service from 0.00am to 4.59am and no more than four persons per table in catering premises with the number of customers not exceeding 50% of the seating capacity. Persons must not consume food or drink and must wear a mask when they are away from the table in catering premises. Facilities involving higher health risks such as steam and sauna facilities and ball pits will continue to be closed.

"In view of the recent development of the epidemic, the Government considers it necessary to prohibit high-risk dancing activities, particularly dancing parties in entertainment catering venues. Specifically, under the latest direction of Cap. 599F, live performance and dancing must not be allowed in all catering premises (including catering premises in hotels), meeting rooms and function rooms in hotels/guesthouses, as well as clubhouses. Party rooms, clubs or nightclubs must be closed. Meanwhile, dancing schools which fulfil the definition of fitness centres under Cap. 599F have to follow the relevant infection control measures to continue their operation. Such measures include coaches/staff to wear masks all the time, other persons to wear masks when doing exercise unless there are 1.5 meters or effective partitions between each of them, no more than four persons in each training group or class, and training groups or classes of more than four persons must be arranged in sub-groups of no more than four persons and keeping 1.5 meters between each sub-group etc.. As for the other public places not regulated under Cap. 599F, they are subject to the restrictions under the Prevention and Control of Disease (Prohibition on Group Gathering) Regulation (Cap. 599G) and the Prevention and Control of Disease (Wearing of Mask) Regulation (Cap. 599I) where, unless exempted, group gatherings of more than four persons are prohibited and a person must wear a mask at any time in specified public places.

The Government gazetted the directions and specification under Cap. 599F to implement the above measures. The above measures will take effect from November 26 for a period of seven days till December 2, 2020.

Persons responsible for carrying on catering businesses and managers of scheduled premises that contravene the statutory requirements under Cap. 599F would have committed a criminal offence. Offenders are subject to a maximum fine of $50,000 and imprisonment for six months.

(II) Group gatherings

7. Unless exempted, the prohibition on group gatherings of more than four persons in public places will continue during the seven-day period from November 26 to December 2, 2020.

Any person who participates in a prohibited group gathering; organises a prohibited group gathering; owns, controls or operates the place of such a gathering; and knowingly allows the taking place of such gathering commits an offence under Cap. 599G. Offenders are liable to a maximum fine of $25,000 and imprisonment for six months. Persons who participate in a prohibited group gathering may discharge liability for the offence by paying a fixed penalty of $2,000.

(III) Mask-wearing requirement

8. The mandatory mask-wearing requirement under Cap. 599I will be extended for a period of seven days from November 26 to December 2, 2020. During the aforementioned period, a person must wear a mask all the time when the person is boarding or on board a public transport carrier, is entering or present in an MTR paid area, or is entering or present in a specified public place (i.e. all public places, save for outdoor public places in country parks and special areas as defined in section 2 of the Country Parks Ordinance (Cap. 208)).

Under Cap. 599I, if a person does not wear a mask in accordance with the requirement, an authorised person may deny that person from boarding a public transport carrier or entering the area concerned, as well as require that person to wear a mask and disembark from the carrier or leave the said area. A person in contravention of the relevant provision commits an offence and the maximum penalty is a fine at level 2 ($5,000). In addition, authorised public officers may issue fixed penalty notices to persons who do not wear a mask in accordance with the requirement and such persons may discharge liability for the offence by paying a fixed penalty of $2,000.

The spokesman said, "The Government urges all members of the public to stay at home as much as possible, go out or dine out less often, and reduce the frequency of social activities with friends outside co-living family members to prevent getting themselves infected and subsequent transmission to their family members, in order to safeguard themselves and their family at this key moment. Maintaining good personal and environmental hygiene at all times is key to prevention of infection and the spread of the virus in the community."

"The Government will review the various measures in place from time to time in accordance with the development of the epidemic situation, and make suitable adjustments taking into account all relevant factors."

Issued at HKT 2:52

Security guard employed by Housing Department contractor at Fu Shan Estate tests positive for COVID-19

****

The Housing Department today (November 25) learned that a security guard employed by its contractor tested positive for COVID-19. The security guard concerned worked at Fu Fai House, Fu Shan Estate. He is now in hospital for treatment.

The security guard normally works on the night shift and is responsible for patrolling the public areas of Fu Fai House. He last performed duties on November 20. The Centre for Health Protection (CHP) notified him yesterday (November 24) that he had tested positive for COVID-19.

The security guard has no recent travel history. He has been wearing a face mask and has been observing relevant disease prevention measures at work. When performing duties, he has been undergoing temperature checks and his body temperature was normal.

The security guard is also a tenant residing at Fu Shun House of the estate.

The common areas of Fu Fai House and Fu Shun House as well as the estate management office of Fu Shan Estate have been thoroughly cleaned and disinfected in accordance with the guidelines of the CHP.

The Housing Department will continue to keep close liaison with the CHP and co-operate with its quarantine work.

Issued at HKT 15:26

Pet dog tests positive for COVID-19 virus

****

A spokesman for the Agriculture, Fisheries and Conservation Department (AFCD) said today (November 25) that samples from a pet dog sent to the AFCD have tested positive for the COVID-19 virus.

The case involves a poodle that lived in Tsuen Wan. When the owner was found to be a close contact of a confirmed COVID-19 case, the dog was sent to the AFCD for quarantine on

November 20. Samples collected from the dog by the department tested positive for the COVID-19 virus. However, the dog currently has not shown any symptoms. The AFCD will continue to closely monitor the dog and conduct repeat testing.

The spokesman reminded pet owners to adopt good hygiene practices (including hand washing before and after being around or handling animals, their food or supplies, as well as avoiding kissing them) and to maintain a clean and hygienic household environment. People who have taken ill should restrict contact with animals. If any changes in the health condition of pets are spotted, advice from a veterinarian should be sought as soon as possible.

The spokesman emphasised that currently there is no evidence to show that pets are playing a role in the spread of infection with the COVID-19 virus among humans. Pet owners should always maintain good hygiene practices and under no circumstances should they abandon their pets.

Issued at HKT 18:00

Public hospitals daily update on COVID-19 cases

****

The following is issued on behalf of the Hospital Authority:

As at 9am today (November 25), 20 COVID-19 confirmed patients were discharged from hospital in the last 24 hours. Including a patient (case number: 5705) discharged on November 23, a total of 5 295 patients with confirmed or probable infection have been discharged.

At present, there are 607 negative pressure rooms in public hospitals with 1 126 negative pressure beds activated. A total of 349 confirmed patients are currently hospitalised in 21 public hospitals, among which seven patients are in critical condition, three are in serious condition and the remaining 339 patients are in stable condition.

The Hospital Authority will maintain close contact with the Centre for Health Protection to monitor the latest developments and to inform the public and healthcare workers on the latest information in a timely manner.

Details of the above-mentioned patients are as follows:

Patient condition	Case numbers
Discharged	5374, 5381, 5388, 5390, 5404, 5422, 5427, 5435, 5449, 5452, 5478, 5506,

	5509, 5538, 5562, 5566, 5580, 5650, 5654, 5705, 5712
Critical	1989, 3496, 4833, 5110, 5185, 5409, 5433
Serious	5273, 5439, 5713

Issued at HKT 18:10

Probationary Customs Officer preliminarily tests positive for COVID-19

****

Hong Kong Customs today (November 25) learned that a female probationary Customs Officer has preliminarily tested positive for the coronavirus disease 2019 (COVID-19). The officer's specimen for COVID-19 testing has been sent to the Department of Health (DH) for a confirmatory test.

The officer had started to receive induction training at the Hong Kong Customs College (HKCC) since November 16 and was notified today through the Targeted Group Testing Scheme that she had preliminarily tested positive for the virus. She is now under medical treatment. Her specimen for COVID-19 testing has also been sent to the DH for a confirmatory test according to the established procedures.

The officer has no recent travel history. She has been wearing surgical masks during training and has properly maintained social distancing with people she has had contact with. Her body temperature was normal when undergoing temperature screening before training every day.

The department has been closely co-operating with the Centre for Health Protection (CHP) on the CHP's epidemiological investigations to follow up on the situations of other trainees and trainers. They have also been arranged to conduct virus tests. In view of the situation, the HKCC has arranged a thorough cleaning and sterilisation at relevant training venues and facilities.

Customs has all along been highly concerned about the epidemic of COVID-19. Apart from continuing to step up the cleaning and sterilising measures, the department also reminds all officers to strictly comply with the hygienic measures of infectious diseases provided by the CHP at all times. The officers will also be reminded to consult a doctor promptly if they have any discomforting symptoms.

Issued at HKT 19:15

LCSD imposes further restriction on dancing activities

****

The Leisure and Cultural Services Department (LCSD) announced today (November 25) that the following anti-epidemic measures will be introduced in view of the latest situation of COVID-19.

Starting from tomorrow (November 26), processing of application for dancing activities in indoor facilities managed by the LCSD , except rehearsals before performances, will be suspended. From November 28 (Saturday), dancing activities, except rehearsals before performances, will be temporarily prohibited in these indoor facilities until further notice. Besides, all users of dance rooms, activity rooms, multi-purpose rooms and fitness rooms managed by the LCSD have to wear face masks at all times from this Friday (November 27) except when the person is playing designated sports as specified in Cap 599F gazette notice.

For recreation and sports programmes, with effect from November 28, LCSD will suspend the enrolment for dancing activities as well as cancelling all dance training courses and fun days. Full or partial refund will be arranged for affected participants of paid activities.

Regarding cultural venues, all museums, including the Hong Kong Science Museum and the Hong Kong Space Museum, will temporarily suspend some of their interactive exhibits and all children facilities. All museums will continue to apply visitor quotas.

For refund arrangements in relation to these measures, the hirer may submit a completed refund application form together with the original booking permit to the LCSD booking office at a District Leisure Services Office or to relevant leisure venues in person or by post. The application form can be downloaded from www.lcsd.gov.hk/en/aboutlcsd/forms/refund.html. For performance venues, staff of facility booking section at related venues will contact affected hirers for rescheduling or refund.

The LCSD will continue to monitor the situation closely and review the arrangements in a timely manner.

Issued at HKT 21:30

CHP investigates 85 additional confirmed cases of COVID-19

****

The Centre for Health Protection (CHP) of the Department of Health has announced that as of 0.00am, November 25, the CHP was investigating 85 additional confirmed cases of coronavirus disease 2019 (COVID-19), taking the number of cases to 5 867 in Hong Kong so far (comprising 5 866 confirmed cases and one probable case).

Among the newly reported cases announced, one is an imported case.

A total of 392 cases have been recorded in the past 14 days (November 11 – 24), including 279 local cases of which 63 are from unknown sources.

The CHP's epidemiological investigations and relevant contact tracing on the confirmed cases are ongoing. For case details and contact tracing information, please see the Annex One or the list of buildings with confirmed cases of COVID-19 in the past 14 days and the latest local situation of COVID-19 available on the website "COVID-19 Thematic Website" (www.coronavirus.gov.hk).

As a number of cases confirmed recently claimed that they had visited venues for dancing or singing, the CHP strongly appealed to those who had visited the venues as listed in Annex Two on or after November 1 to visit the Hospital Authority's designated general out-patient clinics (www.ha.org.hk/haho/ho/covid-19/GOPC_extend_EN.pdf) and collect deep throat saliva specimen collection packs for free COVID-19 testing as soon as possible. The public are also urged to seek medical attention early if symptoms develop.

In view of the severe epidemic situation, the CHP called on members of the public to avoid going out, having social contact and dining out. They should put on a surgical mask and maintain stringent hand hygiene when they need to go out. The CHP strongly urged the elderly to stay home as far as possible and avoid going out. They should consider asking their family and friends to help with everyday tasks such as shopping for basic necessities.

The spokesman said, "Given that the situation of COVID-19 infection remains severe and that there is a continuous increase in the number of cases reported around the world, members of the public are strongly urged to avoid all non-essential travel outside Hong Kong.

"The CHP also strongly urges the public to maintain at all times strict personal and environmental hygiene, which is key to personal protection against infection and prevention of the spread of the disease in the community. On a personal level, members of the public should wear a surgical mask when having respiratory symptoms, taking public transport or staying in crowded places. They should also perform hand hygiene frequently, especially before touching the mouth, nose or eyes.

"As for household environmental hygiene, members of the public are advised to maintain drainage pipes properly, regularly pour water into drain outlets (U-traps) and cover all floor drain outlets when they are not in use. After using the toilet, they should put the toilet lid down before flushing to avoid spreading germs."

Moreover, the Government has launched the website "COVID-19 Thematic Website" (www.coronavirus.gov.hk) for announcing the latest updates on various news on COVID-19 infection and health advice to help the public understand the latest updates. Members of the public may also gain access to information via the COVID-19 WhatsApp Helpline launched by the Office of the Government Chief Information Officer. Simply by saving 9617 1823 in their phone contacts or clicking the link wa.me/85296171823?text=hi, they will be able to obtain information on COVID-19 as well as the "StayHomeSafe" mobile app and wristband via WhatsApp.

Issued at HKT 21:40

Transcript of CE's press conference on "The Chief Executive's 2020 Policy Address"
****

Following is the transcript of remarks by the Chief Executive, Mrs Carrie Lam, at the press conference on "The Chief Executive's 2020 Policy Address" at Central Government Offices, Tamar, today (November 25):

Reporter: Two questions. Firstly about the teachers. So you said the Government will enhance the quality of teachers through measures in respect of entry to the profession. What sort of measures are you talking about and does that mean there will be political screening for people who want to become a teacher? And secondly about the possible city-wide COVID testing, under what circumstances will the Government roll out a new round and when will the testing be made compulsory? Will a lockdown be imposed during the process, and how can Hong Kong manage on its own when you said the Government would not ask for help from the Mainland?

Chief Executive: Of the two questions, first let me just repeat that I attach utmost importance to education and education in Hong Kong. In the past three years or so we have devoted huge resources, and they are permanent resources because I don’t want the teachers to be under a lot of anxiety and worries about the positions in schools and the teaching ratios and so on. But it is time for us to take a very serious look at the various aspects of our education system, and the point you mentioned about the quality of teachers is one of the very important components because how students learn from their school much depends on the quality, the commitment, the dedication and the professionalism of our teaching staff. When we said that we will enhance the quality of teachers, first we would expect the education institutes to do their part because teachers are trained in universities, and so we expect the teaching institutions to do their part in preparing graduates to come in to the teaching profession. And then we expect the school sponsoring bodies and the school management committees of the schools in recruiting and appointing teachers. They have to look not only for academic excellence; they have to look at the character of these teachers. And the third is in-service training. Whether the teacher is a fresh teacher, a teacher upon promotion or a teacher undergoing some specialty training, the Education Bureau will take on a role to arrange and to support all these training programmes for teachers. We also have a role in the discipline of teachers because the education authority is the registration authority of all teachers in Hong Kong. There is no involvement whatsoever of political screening, but of course as a teacher, which more or less comes into what we call a public service, we expect the teachers to uphold the Basic Law and Support the Hong Kong Special Administrative Region of the People's Republic of China.

As far as COVID-19 testing, I have explained yesterday about the regime that we are going to adopt in rolling out more COVID-19 testing. One is when we have a cluster then we need to do very vigorous testing in order to find out and identify all those confirmed cases because they may be asymptomatic, so they will not be seeing a doctor yet. In the first instance we should try to find them out and isolate them and then treat them and prevent them from spreading the virus in the community. In future and including at the moment this dancing hall cluster, they will be subject to mandatory testing. In other words, if they don't come forward with a test result within a period of time, then they will be offending the regulation. In future we will adopt the same approach in mandatory testing for these high-risk clusters. The second type of testing is for target groups. For people in professions who are high-risk in contacting the virus, because they are working in airport or working in air cargo, for example; people in positions which will make other people very vulnerable if they are infected, for example, the elderly homes, the container terminals and the slaughterhouse and so on; and other frontline staff in the Government and as well as in the retail industry, we will advise them and arrange for them to undertake voluntary testing, but under a very targeted manner. The third approach is perhaps what you are asking. That is people have no symptom whatsoever and they have not come into contact with a confirmed case but they are worried about their own situation. We are also happy to provide a free-of-charge test for them, which is now available in 47 general outpatient clinics of the Hospital Authority and we will make the distribution network much wider after arranging the bottles to be distributed at over 100 post offices and perhaps in time to come in the MTR stations. That's the testing regime that the Hong Kong SAR Government is adopting right now. What the Policy Address said is we did not rule out that, because the pandemic situation is changing very rapidly in future we may have to do a wider sort of universal testing like what we have done previously. But at the moment we don't have that plan yet because that would not be very effective, especially under the present circumstances when we have other priority groups that we need to tackle.

You also questioned about lockdown. In recent days I notice there are a lot of people advocating – it's just like a slogan, advocating – that we should have mandatory universal testing of everyone in Hong Kong. Now, we have to ask ourselves, one, is it based on science? Is it based on evidence that it is a good arrangement? And then we have to look at the practicality of doing so. And then we have to look at, in order for it to have the effect of finding out everyone that is infected in Hong Kong, we need to lock down. So if I go through a test today, there's no point if I'm allowed to go out, to go to work, to go to a restaurant. Arrangements have to be put in place to lock me down at home for a long period when everybody, the 7 million people, have gone through the tests. You can imagine that would require locking down the whole city, no in, no out. Airport will have to be closed. The land borders will have to suspended and then a stay home mandatory order for everyone, until everybody has been cleared and the infected being found out and that would at least take four to eight weeks. Last time we did it in two weeks, hundreds of laboratory technicians in over a hundred centres, testing 1.7 million people. We're going to test 7 million, assuming that we are doubly effective, that will still be four weeks instead of two weeks. Can Hong Kong survive with a city lockdown of four weeks? Can you as an individual tolerate a stay-home mandatory order for four weeks? Can we as a government find ways to feed you, being locked down at home for four weeks? Do we have that system? Do we have that capacity? Do we have that law-abiding compliant population to follow that requirement? I think these are very pertinent questions that everyone who advocate universal mandatory testing should try to answer. Thank you.

Reporter: Hello Mrs Lam. Following is a question for the external voting, is it the case that Beijing is reluctant to have the polling station being set up in major Mainland cities so that you didn't mention anything about it in the Policy Address? You just now said that you won't proceed with it. Was it you won't proceed with it if there are obstacles that the Government cannot overcome at the end? So, do you mean there are legality issues or logistics ones? The second question is, could you please give more details on the Mainland vaccines you have mentioned in the Policy Address? When will they be ready? And, how do you ensure the public confidence over the safety of Mainland doses? Thank you.

Chief Executive: Thank you for the two questions. First of all, in the Policy Address I mentioned that although the LegCo elections have been deferred for one year, we have received quite a lot of views about improvements to the electoral arrangements, like special queue for elderly people, like using electronic means to dish out the ballot papers, and so on, including a desire especially by Hong Kong people now living, working and studying in the Mainland to be able to cast their vote on the voting day. All these are now being considered by the Constitutional and Mainland Affairs Bureau. Of course, in the course of considering these proposals to come up with a piece of legislation, we have to address the issues that you have highlighted, that is the legal, the logistics and so on. For every government initiative, we want to proceed with consensus. But unfortunately, in every place, particularly in Hong Kong, it's quite a luxury to ask for a complete consensus. There will be differences in opinion given Hong Kong's diversity, for example, if you ask me, I would say the Lantau Tomorrow Vision is wonderful for Hong Kong. I have outlined the six advantages and the economic benefits of Lantau Tomorrow Vision, still there is a lot of objection, but we still proceed. I wouldn't agree that whenever there are obstacles, I would not proceed, because that would mean a very lame duck SAR Government, if whenever there are obstacles, one would not proceed. Similarly, for the voting in Mainland, we are considering the various factors. There is no CPG (Central People's Government) angle, let me make it very clear, this is a Hong Kong issue. But when we have decided to implement, then we need some support and advice from the Central Government, on whether it is possible in a Mainland city to set up polling stations and so on. Allowing Hong Kong permanent residents who are registered voters to cast their vote is an idea of the HKSAR Government based on the aspirations of Hong Kong people living, working in the Mainland, conveyed to us over the years.

As far as the Mainland vaccine, I have no detailed information to provide. What I have got from the Central Government is, if there comes a day that despite the efforts made by the HK

SAR Government in vaccine procurement, that you still face problem - if you read very carefully the actual articulation- then the Central Government has promised to help us by earmarking a certain proportion of vaccine either developed or produced- it's not entirely developed, it could be developed elsewhere but produced- in the Mainland for us to use. The ultimate objective is to ensure and safeguard the health of the Hong Kong people. At the moment, I have no more to disclose about the vaccines now being produced and developed in the Mainland of China.

Issued at HKT 23:07

Discrepancy in COVID- 19 Test Result SMS Message

****

The following is issued on behalf of the Hospital Authority:

To tie in with the "Enhanced Laboratory Surveillance Programme" of the Centre for Health Protection (CHP) of the Department of Health, the Hospital Authority (HA) contracted a test service vendor since July to arrange COVID-19 test and to enhance service recently by notifying negative test results via SMS message to the members of the public concerned. The HA was informed by the vendor today (November 25) that discrepancy of personal identification information was found during the SMS message handling process, resulting in the receipt of other people's negative test result.

Among the 2972 participants involved in the incident, six of them were tested positive, but negative SMS test result messages were sent to them wrongly by the system. Upon notification of the error, the HA has immediately contacted the CHP to follow up with the six patients concerned.

The HA spokesperson said, "All cases tested positive are reported to the CHP separately through an established mechanism. The CHP will inform the patients and arrange their admission for treatment. The HA has confirmed with the CHP that the six patients concerned have already been admitted under isolation treatment. Patient management is not affected and no patient has unduly stayed in the community."

The vendor has sent clarification SMS messages to the remaining recipients to amend the personal identification information and to reconfirm the test results. The vendor has verified that no other positive test results were notified as negative cases wrongly.

The HA is very concerned about the incident, which has been reported to the Office of the Privacy Commissioner for Personal Data. The HA has requested the vendor to review the system and to fix the error so as to avoid the occurrence of similar incident. The HA expresses apology to the members of the public affected.

Issued at HKT 23:58

November 26[57]

HAD imposes further restriction on dancing and singing activities

****

The Home Affairs Department (HAD) today (November 26) announced that in view of the latest situation of COVID-19, dancing and singing classes in community halls/community centres have been suspended starting from today. Starting from tomorrow (November 27), all dancing and singing activities, except performances, will also be suspended until further notice.

All users of community halls/community centres have to wear face masks at all times except when a person is playing designated sports as specified in the Prevention and Control of Disease (Requirements and Directions) (Business and Premises) Regulation (Cap. 599F) Gazette notice.

Issued at HKT 17:38

Public hospitals daily update on COVID-19 cases

****

The following is issued on behalf of the Hospital Authority:

As of 9am today (November 26), five COVID-19 confirmed patients were discharged from hospital in the last 24 hours. So far, a total of 5 300 patients with confirmed or probable infection have been discharged.

At present, there are 607 negative pressure rooms in public hospitals with 1 126 negative pressure beds activated. A total of 429 confirmed patients are currently hospitalised in 20 public hospitals and a community treatment facility, among whom seven patients are in critical condition, four are in serious condition and the remaining 418 patients are in stable condition.

The Hospital Authority will maintain close contact with the Centre for Health Protection to monitor the latest developments and will inform the public and healthcare workers of the latest developments in a timely manner.

[57] https://www.info.gov.hk/gia/general/202011/26.htm

Details of the above-mentioned patients are as follows:

Patient condition	Case numbers
Discharged	3764, 5386, 5479, 5686, 5784
Critical	1989, 3496, 4833, 5110, 5185, 5409, 5735
Serious	5273, 5433, 5439, 5713

Issued at HKT 17:50

LCSD-outsourced cleaning worker tests positive for COVID-19 as Kowloon Park Sports Centre temporarily closed

****

The Leisure and Cultural Services Department (LCSD) today (November 26) said that an outsourced cleaning service contractor worker has tested positive for coronavirus disease 2019 (COVID-19).

The outsourced cleaning worker concerned worked at Kowloon Park Sports Centre in Yau Tsim Mong District. He last performed his duties on November 23. He had contact with a person with a confirmed case earlier. He sought medical treatment in a hospital on November 24 and has been treated under isolation since that day. He was notified today that he had tested positive for COVID-19. The worker has no recent travel history. He wore a surgical mask when performing duties and his body temperature was normal when he underwent temperature screening during work.

The LCSD has arranged a thorough cleaning and sterilisation at Kowloon Park Sports Centre according to guidelines provided by the Centre for Health Protection (CHP). The Sports Centre has been temporarily closed from 5pm today and will reopen at 7am on November 28.

The LCSD is highly concerned about the COVID-19 epidemic and will continue to maintain close liaison with the CHP. Staff are reminded to pay attention to personal hygiene and to stay vigilant. They should seek medical advice immediately if feeling unwell.

Issued at HKT 18:47

Four persons sentenced for breaching compulsory quarantine order

****

Four persons were sentenced by Kowloon City magistrates' courts today (November 26) for violating the Compulsory Quarantine of Certain Persons Arriving at Hong Kong Regulation (Cap. 599C) or the Compulsory Quarantine of Persons Arriving at Hong Kong from Foreign Places Regulation (Cap. 599E) respectively.

The first case involved a woman aged 26, who was earlier issued a compulsory quarantine order stating that she must conduct quarantine at home for 14 days. Before the expiry of the quarantine order, she was found to have taken off her wristband during a surprise check on May 7 without reasonable excuse nor permission given by an authorised officer. She was charged with contravening Sections 8(4) and 8(5) of the Compulsory Quarantine of Certain Persons Arriving at Hong Kong Regulation (Cap. 599C) and was fined $10,000.

The second case involved a man aged 61. Before the expiry of the quarantine order, he left the place of quarantine on March 30 without reasonable excuse nor permission given by an authorised officer. He was charged with contravening Sections 8(1) and 8(5) of the Compulsory Quarantine of Persons Arriving at Hong Kong from Foreign Places Regulation (Cap. 599E) and was fined $10,000.

The remaining two cases involved two men aged 80 and 46. Before the expiry of the quarantine order, they left the place of quarantine on March 27 and July 3 respectively without reasonable excuse nor permission given by an authorised officer. They were charged with contravening Sections 8(1) and 8(5) of the Compulsory Quarantine of Certain Persons Arriving at Hong Kong Regulation (Cap. 599C) and were fined $12,000 and sentenced to immediate imprisonment for seven days.

Pursuant to the Compulsory Quarantine of Certain Persons Arriving at Hong Kong Regulation (Cap. 599C) starting from February 8, save for exempted persons, all persons who have stayed in the Mainland, Macao or Taiwan in the 14 days preceding arrival in Hong Kong, regardless of their nationality or travel documents, will be subject to compulsory quarantine for 14 days. Moreover, pursuant to the Compulsory Quarantine of Persons Arriving at Hong Kong from Foreign Places Regulation (Cap. 599E), starting from March 19, all persons arriving from countries or territories outside China would also be subject to compulsory quarantine for 14 days. Breaching a quarantine order is a criminal offence and offenders are subject to a maximum fine of $25,000 and imprisonment for six months.

A spokesman for the Department of Health said the sentence sends a clear message to the community that breaching a compulsory quarantine order is a criminal offence that the Government will not tolerate, and solemnly reminded the public to comply with the Regulation. As of today, a total of 75 persons have been convicted by the courts for breaching compulsory quarantine orders and have received sentences including immediate imprisonment for up to three months or a fine of $15,000. The spokesman reiterated that resolute actions will be taken against anyone who has breached the relevant regulations.

Issued at HKT 19:39

Security guard employed by Housing Department contractor at Sun Chui Estate tests positive for COVID-19

****

The Housing Department today (November 26) learned that a security guard employed by its contractor tested positive for COVID-19. The security guard concerned worked at Sun Wai House, Sun Chui Estate. She is now in hospital for treatment.

The security guard normally works on morning shift and stays at the guard counter of Sun Wai House. She last performed duties on November 24. The Centre for Health Protection (CHP) notified her today that she had tested positive for COVID-19.

The security guard has no recent travel history. She has been wearing a face mask and has been observing relevant disease prevention measures at work. When performing duties, she has been undergoing temperature checks and her body temperature was normal.

The common areas of Sun Wai House and the estate management office of Sun Chui Estate have been thoroughly cleaned and disinfected in accordance with the guidelines of the CHP.

The Housing Department will continue to keep close liaison with the CHP and co-operate with its quarantine work.

Issued at HKT 21:05

CHP investigates 81 additional confirmed cases of COVID-19

****

The Centre for Health Protection (CHP) of the Department of Health has announced that as of 0.00am, November 26, the CHP was investigating 81 additional confirmed cases of coronavirus disease 2019 (COVID-19), taking the number of cases to 5 948 in Hong Kong so far (comprising 5 947 confirmed cases and one probable case).

Among the newly reported cases announced, six had a travel history during the incubation period.

A total of 459 cases have been recorded in the past 14 days (November 12 – 25), including 359 local cases of which 74 are from unknown sources.

The CHP's epidemiological investigations and relevant contact tracing on the confirmed cases are ongoing. For case details and contact tracing information, please see the Annex One or the list of buildings with confirmed cases of COVID-19 in the past 14 days and the latest local situation of COVID-19 available on the website "COVID-19 Thematic Website" (www.coronavirus.gov.hk).

As a number of cases confirmed recently claimed that they had visited venues for dancing or singing, bars or gyms, the CHP reminded those who had visited the specified venues (Annex Two) under the Prevention and Control of Disease (Compulsory Testing for Certain Persons) Regulation (Cap. 599J) to receive COVID-19 nucleic acid test according to the compulsory testing notice. The public are also urged to seek medical attention early if symptoms develop.

In view of the severe epidemic situation, the CHP called on members of the public to avoid going out, having social contact and dining out. They should put on a surgical mask and maintain stringent hand hygiene when they need to go out. The CHP strongly urged the elderly to stay home as far as possible and avoid going out. They should consider asking their family and friends to help with everyday tasks such as shopping for basic necessities.

The spokesman said, "Given that the situation of COVID-19 infection remains severe and that there is a continuous increase in the number of cases reported around the world, members of the public are strongly urged to avoid all non-essential travel outside Hong Kong.

"The CHP also strongly urges the public to maintain at all times strict personal and environmental hygiene, which is key to personal protection against infection and prevention of the spread of the disease in the community. On a personal level, members of the public should wear a surgical mask when having respiratory symptoms, taking public transport or staying in crowded places. They should also perform hand hygiene frequently, especially before touching the mouth, nose or eyes.

"As for household environmental hygiene, members of the public are advised to maintain drainage pipes properly, regularly pour water into drain outlets (U-traps) and cover all floor drain outlets when they are not in use. After using the toilet, they should put the toilet lid down before flushing to avoid spreading germs."

Moreover, the Government has launched the website "COVID-19 Thematic Website" (www.coronavirus.gov.hk) for announcing the latest updates on various news on COVID-19 infection and health advice to help the public understand the latest updates. Members of the public may also gain access to information via the COVID-19 WhatsApp Helpline launched by the Office of the Government Chief Information Officer. Simply by saving 9617 1823 in their phone contacts or clicking the link wa.me/85296171823?text=hi, they will be able to obtain information on COVID-19 as well as the "StayHomeSafe" mobile app and wristband via WhatsApp.

Issued at HKT 23:33

Government to gazette compulsory testing notice
****

The Government will exercise the power under the Prevention and Control of Disease (Compulsory Testing for Certain Persons) Regulation (Cap. 599J) and will publish in the Gazette a compulsory testing notice, which requires any person who had been present at seven specified premises (see Annex 1) during the period from November 1 to 26 to undergo a COVID-19 nucleic acid test by November 29.

A spokesman for the Food and Health Bureau (FHB) said today (November 26), "The local epidemic situation is continuously worsening. The number of confirmed cases related to group gathering activities in indoor premises continues to rise significantly. Upon further contact tracing by the Centre for Health Protection, we found that some recently confirmed cases were involved in large group gathering activities in certain premises. Therefore, the Government will publish a compulsory testing notice, which requires persons who had been to seven specified premises to undergo testing."

Persons subject to compulsory testing may choose to undergo testing as below:

1. To obtain a deep throat saliva specimen collection pack from any of the 47 designated general outpatient clinics (GOPCs) of the Hospital Authority and return the specimen to designated specimen collection points (see the specimen collection packs distribution time and specimen collection time at www.ha.org.hk/haho/ho/covid-19/GOPC_extend_en.pdf)

2. To self-arrange testing provided by private laboratories recognised by the Department of Health (see the list at www.coronavirus.gov.hk/pdf/List_of_recognised_laboratories_RTPCR.pdf);

3. To attend any Community Testing Centres (see the list at www.communitytest.gov.hk/en/);

4. To visit any of the seven mobile specimen collection stations/specimen bottle distribution points (see the list at Annex 2) for testing, or obtain and submit specimen bottles; or

5. To undergo testing at any healthcare facilities of the Hospital Authority (including GOPCs and accident and emergency departments) as instructed by a medical professional of the Hospital Authority.

"If persons who are subject to compulsory testing have symptoms, they should seek medical attention immediately and undergo testing as instructed by a medical professional. They should not attend the Community Testing Centres."

Persons who are subject to compulsory testing must report the result of the test or submit the test report to the Government by phone (6275 6901), fax (2530 5872) or email (ct@csb.gov.hk) by December 2. If persons who are subject to compulsory testing have previously undergone the above mentioned test between November 21 and 26, they would be taken to have complied with the requirements set out in the compulsory testing notice.

The spokesman said, "To reduce transmission risk, persons who underwent testing are advised to stay at home and avoid going out when waiting for test results."

Any enquiries on compulsory testing arrangements may be addressed to the hotline at 6275 6901 which operates daily from 9am to 6pm. If persons who are subject to compulsory testing plan to conduct testing at any of the Community Testing Centres, they can check the centre's appointment status in advance. The hotlines of the Community Testing Centres are at www.communitytest.gov.hk/en/info/ .

The Government will continue to trace possibly infected persons who had been to the relevant venues, and seriously verify whether they had complied with the testing notice. Any person who fails to comply with the testing notice commits an offence and may be fined a fixed penalty of $2,000. The person would also be issued with a compulsory testing order requiring him/her to undergo testing within a specified timeframe. Failure to comply with the order is an offence and the offender would be liable to a fine at level 4 ($25,000) and imprisonment for six months.

The spokesman said, "The Government urges all individuals who are in doubt about their own health conditions, or individuals with infection risks (such as individuals who visited places with epidemic outbreaks or contacted confirmed cases) to undergo testing promptly for early identification of infected persons. The FHB will publish compulsory testing notices regarding particular groups when necessary taking into account the epidemic development and the testing participation rate."

Issued at HKT 23:44

November 27[58]

CAD officer tests positive for COVID-19

****

The Civil Aviation Department (CAD) learned that an officer had tested positive for the coronavirus disease 2019 (COVID-19) last night (November 26).

The officer worked at the CAD Headquarters office building and performed support duties without contact with members of the public while at work. He last performed his duties on November 26 and has no recent travel history. He has been wearing surgical masks while

[58] https://www.info.gov.hk/gia/general/202011/27.htm

performing his duties and has properly maintained social distancing with people he has had contact with. His body temperature was normal when undergoing temperature screening during work.

The CAD will cooperate with the Centre for Health Protection (CHP) in the epidemiological investigation and will arrange the staff working with the officer to undergo COVID-19 testing. The concerned work places will also be fully cleaned and sterilised.

The CAD is concerned about the COVID-19 epidemic. Relevant hygienic measures for infectious diseases provided by the CHP have been strictly adopted. All staff have their body temperatures checked before performing their duties, and wear proper personal protective equipment.

The department will continue to step up the cleaning and sterilising measures for all work locations and remind all staff to strictly comply with the hygienic measures for infectious diseases provided by the CHP. The staff will also be reminded to consult a doctor promptly if they have any discomforting symptoms.

Issued at HKT 12:15

One-off ex-gratia cash allowance for locally confirmed COVID-19 patients opens for application from today

****

The Social Welfare Department (SWD) today (November 27) announced that the one-off ex-gratia cash allowance for locally confirmed COVID-19 patients is open for eligible Hong Kong residents to apply from today. The one-off ex-gratia allowance of $5,000 aims to remove the concern of potentially infected persons from coming forward to take COVID-19 tests that they would suffer from financial hardship whilst being hospitalised in public hospitals for COVID-19 treatment.

Applicants have to meet the following eligibility criteria:

they are Hong Kong residents who are confirmed by the Department of Health to have contracted COVID-19 locally on or after November 22, 2020; and

they are currently employed but not entitled to paid sick leave or are self-employed and face financial hardship whilst being hospitalised in public hospitals for COVID-19 treatment.

Applicants are not required to undergo any specific means test, but they have to declare that they meet the aforementioned eligibility criteria and provide basic information about their current employment. The SWD will assess the applications and may seek to verify relevant information with concerned government departments, the Hospital Authority and/or the applicants' employers as appropriate.

Eligible applicants may apply for the ex-gratia allowance starting from today through medical social workers of the hospitals where they are receiving or have received treatment for COVID-19. Applicants may submit the applications themselves or, if need be, appoint a family member/relative or agent to submit applications on their behalf. For applicants who cannot complete their applications whilst receiving treatment, they may do so as soon as possible after they have been discharged from hospital.

For enquiries, applicants, or their appointed family member/relative or agent, may contact the medical social services units of respective hospitals during office hours. For contact information of the related medical social services units, please refer to the Annex.

Issued at HKT 16:59

Public hospitals daily update on COVID-19 cases

****

The following is issued on behalf of the Hospital Authority:

As of 9am today (November 27), 13 COVID-19 confirmed patients were discharged from hospital in the previous 24 hours. So far, a total of 5 313 patients with confirmed or probable infection have been discharged.

At present, there are 618 negative pressure rooms in public hospitals with 1 138 negative pressure beds activated. A total of 495 confirmed patients are currently hospitalised in 20 public hospitals and a community treatment facility, among whom six patients are in critical condition, six are in serious condition and the remaining 483 patients are in stable condition.

The Hospital Authority will maintain close contact with the Centre for Health Protection to monitor the latest developments and will inform the public and healthcare workers of the latest developments in a timely manner.

Details of the above-mentioned patients are as follows:

Patient condition	Case numbers
Discharged	1779, 5400, 5444, 5468, 5485, 5489, 5496, 5628, 5687,

	5732, 5785, 5860, 5871
Critical	1989, 3496, 4833, 5110, 5185, 5735
Serious	5273, 5409, 5433, 5439, 5713, 5745

Issued at HKT 18:05

All post offices to distribute COVID-19 specimen collection packs from tomorrow

****

Under the Government's Enhanced Laboratory Surveillance Programme, to assist individuals who perceive themselves as having a higher risk of exposure and who experience mild discomfort to undergo a COVID-19 test, the Hospital Authority (HA) provides specimen collection packs and collects specimens through its 47 general out-patient clinics (GOPCs). In order to facilitate individuals to obtain specimen collection packs, the Government will extend the distribution points for specimen collection packs to 121 post offices (except mobile post offices) starting from tomorrow (November 28).

Members of the public can visit the post offices during the respective office hours to collect specimen collection packs for free. The specimen collection pack contains a deep throat saliva specimen collection bottle, plastic packaging bags and specimen collection guidelines. Only one pack will be distributed to each person while stocks last. Depending on the number allocated by the Government and the size of each post office, the number of specimen collection packs distributed by each post office each day will vary. Please browse the following webpage for details: www.hongkongpost.hk/en/about_us/network/SpecimenCollection/index.html.

The public should note that all post offices will not collect specimens. Participants can return the deep throat saliva specimen to the 47 GOPCs of the HA or 13 clinics of the Department of Health (DH) within the designated time. Details of the clinics and submission times are provided in the following website: www.coronavirus.gov.hk/eng/early-testing.html. Those who have a negative test result for COVID-19 will receive an SMS notification within three days after submitting the specimen. If the test result is positive, the DH will follow up immediately.

Issued at HKT 18:52

Princess Margaret Hospital announces a nurse tested preliminarily positive for COVID-19

****

The following is issued on behalf of the Hospital Authority:

Princess Margaret Hospital (PMH) made an announcement today (November 27) regarding a nurse tested preliminarily positive for COVID-19:

A female nurse of the Paediatrics and Adolescent Medicine Department yesterday (November 26) learnt that a person she had been in contact in the community was confirmed COVID-19. She was classified as a close contact and required to quarantine. She informed the hospital immediately. COVID-19 deep throat saliva test was immediately arranged for her and the test result was preliminarily positive. The nurse is asymptomatic and currently in stable condition.

The nurse concerned performed general clinical nursing care duties in the Paediatrics and Adolescent Medicine ward and was equipped with appropriate personal protective equipment during her work. She did not come into contact with any COVID-19 patients over the past 28 days in the hospital and was not required to perform high-risk medical procedures for patients. As a precautionary measure, admission, discharge of patients as well as visiting arrangement based on compassionate ground of the concerned ward has been suspended.

The hospital's infection control team initiated contact tracing. So far, four infant patients in the ward have been classified as close contacts and have been transferred to the isolation ward for treatment. Their COVID-19 tests are preliminarily negative. In addition, a colleague who had meals together with the nurse is classified as a close contact and is required to quarantine for 14 days. The hospital is conducting COVID-19 tests for another 20 patients of the concerned ward. The hospital will follow up with the Centre for Health Protection (CHP) and will arrange 28-day medical surveillance for patients and staff in the ward.

The hospital has arranged thorough cleansing and disinfection for the ward concerned, staff pantry and changing room. PMH will continue to closely monitor the health of our staff and patients and communicate with the CHP about the latest situation.

Issued at HKT 20:50

New Territories South Animal Management Centre of AFCD launched to be another quarantine facility for animals related to COVID-19 cases

****

In light of the latest developments of COVID-19, there has been a sharp increase in both the numbers of confirmed and close contact human cases that required pet owners to send their pet animals to the Agriculture, Fisheries and Conservation Department (AFCD) for quarantine and veterinary monitoring. Hence, the Department needs to have more room to cater for such needs. The AFCD today (November 27) announced that the New Territories South Animal Management Centre (NTSAMC) would be launched next Monday (November 30) as another quarantine facility for pet animals related to COVID-19 cases. All animals originally kept in the NTSAMC will be transferred to other Animal Management Centres for follow-up, and the NTSAMC will not open to public until further notice.

The animal keeping facility at the Hong Kong Port of the Hong Kong-Zhuhai-Macao Bridge will only be used for quarantine and veterinary monitoring for animals tested positive for the COVID-19 virus.

An AFCD spokesman reminded pet owners to adopt good hygiene practices (including hand washing before and after being around or handling animals, their food or supplies, as well as avoiding kissing them) and to maintain a clean and hygienic household environment. People who are sick should restrict contact with animals. If any changes in the health condition of the pets are spotted, advice from a veterinarian should be sought as soon as possible.

The spokesman emphasised that currently there is no evidence that pets are playing a role in the spread of human infection with the COVID-19. Pet owners should always maintain good hygiene practices and under no circumstances should they abandon their pets.

Issued at HKT 21:06

Tuen Mun Hospital announces a patient tested preliminarily positive for COVID-19

****

The following is issued on behalf of the Hospital Authority:

The spokesperson for Tuen Mun Hospital (TMH) made the following announcement today (November 27) regarding a case tested preliminarily positive for COVID-19:

A 21-year-old male patient was admitted to an Orthopaedics and Traumatology (O&T) ward of TMH yesterday (November 26) afternoon. He was arranged to take the viral test for COVID-19 and the preliminary result available in the late evening was positive. The patient has been transferred to an isolation ward. He remains asymptomatic and in stable condition.

The patient underwent a surgery in October and required regular follow-up consultation. He attended the O&T specialist-out-patient clinic on November 24. In yesterday afternoon, the patient attended the Accident and Emergency Department (A&E) of TMH because of wound bleeding. He was arranged to be admitted to an O&T ward after initial assessment.

Upon learning the patient's test result, the Infection Control Unit conducted investigation to trace the healthcare workers and patients who had been in contact with him. The contact tracing identified that five patients who stayed in the same cubicle with the patient concerned as close contacts and required quarantine for 14 days. They were arranged to take the viral test for COVID-19 and all results were negative. All staff members who have been in contact with the patient concerned were equipped with appropriate personal protective equipment, therefore no staff member is required to be put under quarantine nor medical surveillance.

TMH had arranged thorough cleansing and disinfection in the ward concerned, A&E and the specialist out-patient clinic. The hospital will fully cooperate with the Centre for Health Protection on follow up actions.

Issued at HKT 21:08

CHP investigates 92 additional confirmed cases of COVID-19

****

The Centre for Health Protection (CHP) of the Department of Health has announced that as of 0.00am, November 27, the CHP was investigating 92 additional confirmed cases of coronavirus disease 2019 (COVID-19), taking the number of cases to 6 040 in Hong Kong so far (comprising 6 039 confirmed cases and one probable case).

Among the newly reported cases announced, three had a travel history during the incubation period.

A total of 517 cases have been recorded in the past 14 days (November 13 – 26), including 427 local cases of which 81 are from unknown sources.

The CHP's epidemiological investigations and relevant contact tracing on the confirmed cases are ongoing. For case details and contact tracing information, please see the Annex One or the list of buildings with confirmed cases of COVID-19 in the past 14 days and the latest local situation of COVID-19 available on the website "COVID-19 Thematic Website" (www.coronavirus.gov.hk).

As a number of cases confirmed recently claimed that they had visited venues for dancing or singing, bars or gyms, the CHP reminded those who had visited the specified venues (Annex Two) under the Prevention and Control of Disease (Compulsory Testing for Certain Persons) Regulation (Cap. 599J) to receive COVID-19 nucleic acid test according to the compulsory testing notice. The public are also urged to seek medical attention early if symptoms develop.

In view of the severe epidemic situation, the CHP called on members of the public to avoid going out, having social contact and dining out. They should put on a surgical mask and maintain stringent hand hygiene when they need to go out. The CHP strongly urged the elderly to stay home as far as possible and avoid going out. They should consider asking their family and friends to help with everyday tasks such as shopping for basic necessities.

The spokesman said, "Given that the situation of COVID-19 infection remains severe and that there is a continuous increase in the number of cases reported around the world, members of the public are strongly urged to avoid all non-essential travel outside Hong Kong.

"The CHP also strongly urges the public to maintain at all times strict personal and environmental hygiene, which is key to personal protection against infection and prevention of the spread of the disease in the community. On a personal level, members of the public should wear a surgical mask when having respiratory symptoms, taking public transport or staying in crowded places. They should also perform hand hygiene frequently, especially before touching the mouth, nose or eyes.

"As for household environmental hygiene, members of the public are advised to maintain drainage pipes properly, regularly pour water into drain outlets (U-traps) and cover all floor drain outlets when they are not in use. After using the toilet, they should put the toilet lid down before flushing to avoid spreading germs."

Moreover, the Government has launched the website "COVID-19 Thematic Website" (www.coronavirus.gov.hk) for announcing the latest updates on various news on COVID-19 infection and health advice to help the public understand the latest updates. Members of the public may also gain access to information via the COVID-19 WhatsApp Helpline launched by the Office of the Government Chief Information Officer. Simply by saving 9617 1823 in their phone contacts or clicking the link wa.me/85296171823?text=hi, they will be able to obtain information on COVID-19 as well as the "StayHomeSafe" mobile app and wristband via WhatsApp.

Issued at HKT 22:00

Government gazetted specifications under Prevention and Control of Disease (Compulsory Testing for Certain Persons) Regulation

****

The Government has today (November 27) gazetted the specifications under the Prevention and Control of Disease (Compulsory Testing for Certain Persons) Regulation (Cap. 599J), which during a period of 14 days from November 28 to December 11, 2020 empower a registered medical practitioner to require any person whom he clinically suspects has contracted COVID-19 to undergo a test.

A spokesman for the Food and Health Bureau said, "According to expert advice, compulsory testing for symptomatic patients can effectively slow down the transmission of the virus by early identification, early isolation and early treatment. As the recent epidemic situation is deteriorating rapidly, the Government considers it necessary to solicit help from medical practitioners in identifying possibly infected persons as soon as possible."

During the period of 14 days from November 28 to December 11, 2020, registered medical practitioners may, by a written direction, require a person whom the medical practitioner attends to in the course of professional practice and clinically suspects to have contracted COVID-19 to undergo a COVID-19 nucleic acid test. Persons who receive the written direction should undergo a test within two days after the issue date of the written direction (the testing deadline).

Persons who are subject to such testing may choose to undergo a test as below:

(1) To use the specimen bottle provided by the registered medical practitioner who issued the written direction to collect a deep throat saliva specimen and submit the specimen bottle to one of the Government designated collection points set up at 13 clinics of the Department of Health (DH) and 47 General Out-patient Clinics of the Hospital Authority by the testing deadline (see the specimen collection points and time at www.chp.gov.hk/files/pdf/list_of_collection_points_en.pdf and gia.info.gov.hk/general/202011/19/P2020111900497_354653_1_1605778457666.pdf). Having reported the case to the DH, the registered medical practitioner who issued the written direction will be notified of the test result; or

(2) To self-arrange testing provided by private laboratories recognised by the DH (see the list at www.coronavirus.gov.hk/pdf/List_of_recognised_laboratories_RTPCR.pdf) by the testing deadline and submit the test result to the medical practitioner who issued the written direction or his clinic staff by electronic mail, fax, or by hardcopy within four days after the testing deadline.

For example, if the written direction is issued on Monday, the person subject to testing should undergo a test via one of the above options on or before Wednesday, the testing deadline. If the test result of the specimen is preliminary positive, the specimen will be referred to the Public Health Laboratory Services Branch of the DH for a confirmatory test. Confirmed cases will be followed up and announced by the Centre for Health Protection of the DH.

The spokesman said, "Persons who are subject to testing are suspected to be infected and should not attend the Community Testing Centres for testing. To reduce transmission risk, persons who underwent testing are advised to stay at home and avoid going out when waiting for test results. The Government urges all individuals who are in doubt about their own health conditions, or individuals with infection risks (such as individuals who visited places with epidemic outbreaks or contacted confirmed cases) to seek medical consultation and undergo testing promptly for early and effective identification of possible infections."

Failure to comply with the direction is an offence and the offender would be liable to a fine of $2,000 and would be served with a compulsory testing order. Failure to comply with a compulsory testing order is also an offence and the offender would be liable to a fine at level 4 ($25,000) and imprisonment for six months.

Issued at HKT 23:19

Mobile specimen collection stations continue to provide virus testing service to residents of Tsuen Wan, Sai Kung and Tai Po

****

As of yesterday (November 26), the Government had provided free COVID-19 nucleic acid testing service to more than 12 300 persons through seven mobile specimen collection stations and specimen bottle distribution point in Tsuen Wan, Sai Kung and Tai Po.

A Government spokesman said today (November 27) that after reviewing the usage and public demand for the testing service, the Government has decided to extend the services at the following mobile specimen collection stations to continue to provide urgent cluster testing service for citizens until further notice:

• Sha Tsui Road Playground, Tsuen Wan

• Carpark of the Sai Kung Jockey Club Town Hall, 8 Chan Man Street, Sai Kung

• Basketball Court, Tai Po Community Centre, No. 2 Heung Sze Wui Street, Tai Po

• Open area outside Tai Wo Neighbourhood Community Centre, Tai Wo Estate, Tai Po

All the above mobile specimen collection stations will operate daily from 10am to 8pm. The specimen bottle distribution point set up at the Platform outside Tsuen King Circuit Sports Centre, Tsuen Wan will cease operation after November 27, while the mobile specimen collection stations set up at the Amphitheatre, Hong Kong Velodrome Park, 105-107 Po Hong Road, Tseung Kwan O and the Hard-surfaced Soccer Pitch, Po Hong Park, 10 Wan Lung Road, Tseung Kwan O will maintain operations until November 29.

Persons who are subject to compulsory testing and undergo testing at the mobile specimen collection stations will be deemed to have undergone a test at a community testing centre. People whose test results are negative will be informed by SMS through their mobile phones. If any specimen tested shows a positive COVID-19 result, the specimen will be referred to the Public Health Laboratory Services Branch of the Department of Health (DH) for a confirmatory test.

Confirmed cases will be followed up and announced by the Centre for Health Protection of the DH.

The spokesman urges all individuals who are in doubt about their own health conditions, or individuals with infection risks (such as individuals who visited places with epidemic outbreaks or contacted confirmed cases) to undergo testing promptly for early identification of infected persons.

Issued at HKT 23:46

November 28[59]

Government's response to registration of COVID-19 vaccines
****

The Food and Health Bureau (FHB) made a statement in response to an online media report about the FHB claiming that COVID-19 vaccines developed and approved for use in the Mainland cannot be used in the healthcare system of Hong Kong. The media report did not give an accurate account of the overall situation. The Government regrets that the report created a biased image that the Hong Kong Special Administrative Region's regulatory system for pharmaceutical products was prejudiced against Mainland vaccines.

Hong Kong's regulatory framework and registration system for pharmaceutical products are long-established and have been effective. They were further strengthened and enhanced in 2015, so as to ensure that Hong Kong citizens are provided with effective and safe products that are of good quality. The relevant regulatory regime is generic in nature and is applicable to all pharmaceutical products provided and used in Hong Kong, including vaccines.

The COVID-19 epidemic is a public health emergency. The Government is adopting a "two-pronged" strategy to procure vaccines that meet the criteria of safety, efficacy and quality for Hong Kong citizens. Depending on need, the Government will consider implementing necessary measures to enable the emergency use of vaccines with proven safety and efficacy. The Government would not rule out the possibility of introducing legislation on emergency basis if necessary.

Issued at HKT 1:07

[59] https://www.info.gov.hk/gia/general/202011/28.htm

Public hospitals daily update on COVID-19 cases

****

The following is issued on behalf of the Hospital Authority:

As at 9am today (November 28), 15 COVID-19 confirmed patients were discharged from hospital in the last 24 hours. So far, a total of 5 328 patients with confirmed or probable infection have been discharged.

At present, there are 619 negative pressure rooms in public hospitals with 1 137 negative pressure beds activated. A total of 567 confirmed patients are currently hospitalised in 20 public hospitals and community treatment facility, among which seven patients are in critical condition, four are in serious condition and the remaining 556 patients are in stable condition.

The Hospital Authority will maintain close contact with the Centre for Health Protection to monitor the latest developments and to inform the public and healthcare workers on the latest information in a timely manner.

Details of the above-mentioned patients are as follows:

Patient condition	Case numbers
Discharged	5383, 5389, 5397, 5406, 5407, 5412, 5448, 5455, 5456, 5465, 5488, 5559, 5651, 5674, 5683
Critical	1989, 3496, 4833, 5110, 5185, 5409, 5735
Serious	5273, 5439, 5713, 5745

Issued at HKT 17:20

DoJ staff member preliminarily tests positive for COVID-19

****

The Department of Justice (DoJ) today (November 28) said a staff member has preliminarily tested positive for COVID-19.

The staff member concerned worked at the West Kowloon Law Courts Building. She last came to work on November 26 and has no recent travel history. She has been wearing surgical masks while performing her duties and has properly maintained social distancing with people she has had contact with. Her body temperature was normal when undergoing temperature screening during work.

Thorough cleaning and disinfection for relevant places at the West Kowloon Law Courts Building has been arranged.

The DoJ is concerned about the COVID-19 epidemic. The department will continue to remind all staff to strictly comply with the hygienic measures for infectious diseases provided by the Centre for Health Protection. The staff will also be reminded to consult a doctor promptly if they have any discomforting symptoms.

Issued at HKT 18:26

CHP investigates 84 additional confirmed cases of COVID-19

****

The Centre for Health Protection (CHP) of the Department of Health has announced that as of 0.00am, November 28, the CHP was investigating 84 additional confirmed cases of coronavirus disease 2019 (COVID-19), taking the number of cases to 6 124 in Hong Kong so far (comprising 6 123 confirmed cases and one probable case).

Among the newly reported cases announced, three had a travel history during the incubation period.

A total of 603 cases have been recorded in the past 14 days (November 14 – 27), including 512 local cases of which 96 are from unknown sources.

The CHP's epidemiological investigations and relevant contact tracing on the confirmed cases are ongoing. For case details and contact tracing information, please see the Annex One or the list of buildings with confirmed cases of COVID-19 in the past 14 days and the latest local situation of COVID-19 available on the website "COVID-19 Thematic Website" (www.coronavirus.gov.hk).

As a number of cases confirmed recently claimed that they had visited venues for dancing or singing, bars or gyms, the CHP reminded those who had visited the specified venues (Annex Two) under the Prevention and Control of Disease (Compulsory Testing for Certain Persons) Regulation (Cap. 599J) to receive COVID-19 nucleic acid test according to the compulsory testing notice. The public are also urged to seek medical attention early if symptoms develop.

In view of the severe epidemic situation, the CHP called on members of the public to avoid going out, having social contact and dining out. They should put on a surgical mask and maintain

stringent hand hygiene when they need to go out. The CHP strongly urged the elderly to stay home as far as possible and avoid going out. They should consider asking their family and friends to help with everyday tasks such as shopping for basic necessities.

The spokesman said, "Given that the situation of COVID-19 infection remains severe and that there is a continuous increase in the number of cases reported around the world, members of the public are strongly urged to avoid all non-essential travel outside Hong Kong.

"The CHP also strongly urges the public to maintain at all times strict personal and environmental hygiene, which is key to personal protection against infection and prevention of the spread of the disease in the community. On a personal level, members of the public should wear a surgical mask when having respiratory symptoms, taking public transport or staying in crowded places. They should also perform hand hygiene frequently, especially before touching the mouth, nose or eyes.

"As for household environmental hygiene, members of the public are advised to maintain drainage pipes properly, regularly pour water into drain outlets (U-traps) and cover all floor drain outlets when they are not in use. After using the toilet, they should put the toilet lid down before flushing to avoid spreading germs."

Moreover, the Government has launched the website "COVID-19 Thematic Website" (www.coronavirus.gov.hk) for announcing the latest updates on various news on COVID-19 infection and health advice to help the public understand the latest updates. Members of the public may also gain access to information via the COVID-19 WhatsApp Helpline launched by the Office of the Government Chief Information Officer. Simply by saving 9617 1823 in their phone contacts or clicking the link wa.me/85296171823?text=hi, they will be able to obtain information on COVID-19 as well as the "StayHomeSafe" mobile app and wristband via WhatsApp.

Issued at HKT 22:03

November 29[60]

FEHD continues to step up inspections and reminds catering business operators and public to comply with anti-epidemic regulations

****

The Food and Environmental Hygiene Department (FEHD) and the Police conducted joint operations last night (November 28) to step up inspections at catering premises at Yuk Wah Crescent in Wong Tai Sin District and Kau Wah Keng in Kwai Tsing District, as well as

[60] https://www.info.gov.hk/gia/general/202011/29.htm

stepping up inspections at catering premises in Yuen Long town centre on the night of November 27 till small hours of November 28, and reminded the catering business operators to strictly comply with the requirements and directions under the Prevention and Control of Disease (Requirements and Directions) (Business and Premises) Regulation (Cap. 599F) (the Regulation), and the public to comply with the various restrictions in relation to group gatherings and mask-wearing under the anti-epidemic regulations and directions when patronising catering premises.

During the operations, the FEHD and the Police inspected 51 catering premises. A total of 28 verbal warnings were given. The FEHD initiated procedures on prosecution against five catering business operators for breaching the requirements on the number of persons allowed at one table in the premises, distance or partition between tables and mask-wearing under the Regulation. The FEHD also initiated procedures on prosecution against two catering business operators at Yuk Wa Crescent in Wong Tai Sin District for violating the Food Business Regulation (Cap. 132X) (FBR) by extending business area illegally and on-street storage of food preparation utensils. The FEHD also issued fixed penalty notices to 15 persons in Yuen Long town centre for violating the requirement on group gatherings.

In addition, the FEHD also initiated procedures on prosecution against two barbeque site operators at Kau Wah Keng in Kwai Tsing District for violating the FBR by operating food business without a licence. Apart from arresting the concerned operators, a total of about 97 kilogrammes of barbeque food were also seized.

An FEHD spokesman said, "According to the current directions issued by the Secretary for Food and Health in relation to catering business under the Regulation, food business operators must strictly comply with a series of requirements and restrictions, including all bars or pubs, clubs or nightclubs must be closed; live performance and dancing must not be allowed in catering premises; dining-in must cease from 0.00am to 4.59am every day; no more than four persons may be at one table in catering premises; the total number of customers allowed in catering premises must not exceed 50 per cent of the normal seating capacity; a mask must be worn within the premises except when the person is consuming food or drink at a table therein; tables must be arranged in a way to ensure there is a distance of at least 1.5m or some form of partition which could serve as effective buffer between one table and another table; body temperature screening must be conducted before the person is allowed to enter the catering premises; and hand sanitisers must be provided, etc."

The spokesman stressed that the FEHD will continue to proactively take stringent enforcement actions, step up inspections at catering premises across the territory and conduct joint operations with the Police if necessary, to ensure that catering business operators and the public strictly comply with relevant regulations. Enforcement actions will be taken against offenders so as to minimise the risk of transmission of COVID-19 in food premises.

If catering business operators contravene the Regulation, they are liable to a maximum fine of $50,000 and imprisonment for six months. Persons who violate the group gathering restriction of the Prevention and Control of Disease (Prohibition in Group Gathering) Regulation (Cap. 599G) or the mask-wearing requirement under the Prevention and Control of Disease (Wearing of Mask) Regulation (Cap. 599I) are subject to a fixed penalty of $2,000.

In addition, the spokesman made the following appeals:

(1) the frontline staff of catering businesses should actively participate in the voluntary free Targeted Group Testing Scheme. The deadline for online registration has been extended to December 21. Restaurant operators may register through the FEHD's website before the deadline for the testing service. High-exposure groups who had already registered and undergone voluntary testing may register again. For details, please visit the FEHD's website (www.fehd.gov.hk/english/events/covid19_test/info_20200926.html); and

(2) with respect to the FEHD's announcement on November 16 to provide voluntary free testing services for cold stores staff, operators of licensed cold stores who have not yet accepted invitations from the testing agency (Prenetics Limited) should proactively participate in the scheme as early as possible for prudency sake.

The spokesman appealed to catering business operators to comply with relevant regulations on prevention and control of disease in a concerted and persistent manner, with a view to keeping their staff, customers and the public safe. Members of the public also have to comply with the related regulations and directions on group gatherings and mask-wearing at catering premises.

Issued at HKT 12:42

Correctional Officer of Rehabilitation Unit of Lai King Correctional Institution preliminarily tests positive for COVID-19

****

The Lai King Correctional Institution last night (November 28) learned that a correctional officer of Rehabilitation Unit has preliminarily tested positive for the coronavirus disease 2019 (COVID-19).

The staff member last performed her duties this Tuesday (November 24) and was notified by Centre for Health Protection (CHP) on the same day that she had visited an outside hospital ward where a confirmed case was hospitalised thereat when she was off duty last week, she was therefore regarded as close contact of the case. She was arranged to undergo quarantine at Penny's Bay Quarantine Centre the next day (November 25) and was notified last night to have preliminarily tested positive for COVID-19. The staff member is now admitted to Pamela Youde Nethersole Eastern Hospital for treatment. The staff member has no recent travel history. She has been wearing surgical masks when performing duties and has properly maintained social distancing with people she has had contact with. Her body temperature was normal when undergoing temperature screening at work.

Having noticed that the staff member was arranged to undergo quarantine this midweek, the Correctional Services Department (CSD) instantly arranged all persons in custody in the institution and relevant correctional officers having close contact with her to take COVID-19 testing and all specimens were tested negative.

The CSD has liaised with the CHP and follow up the advice given. Thorough cleaning and disinfection has also been arranged immediately by the institution for the locations concerned, testing will again be arranged for all persons in custody and staff of the institution.

CSD is highly concerned about the epidemic of COVID-19 and has remained highly vigilant since the epidemic broke out. Relevant hygienic measures for prevention of infectious diseases have been strictly implemented in accordance with the established mechanism. In addition, a series of disease prevention and disinfection measures have been put in place, including requiring staff members to check body temperatures and wear masks before and when performing duties. All working locations in the institution also undergo cleaning and disinfection regularly. The persons in custody and staff members are also reminded by the management to have medical consultation promptly if they have any discomforting symptoms.

Issued at HKT 14:02

Transcript of remarks by SLW on requiring staff of residential care homes to undergo compulsory testing

****

Following is the transcript of remarks by the Secretary for Labour and Welfare, Dr Law Chi-kwong, on requiring staff of residential care homes to undergo compulsory testing after attending a radio programme this morning (November 29):

Reporter: Secretary, eventually how would you make sure that these staff (members) maybe can get tested once a week and also what is the consequences this time if they don't have enough time to go to get tested? Would they be prevented from going to work?

Secretary for Labour and Welfare: Under the current regulations, if they are required to do the COVID-19 test but they don't, they are violating the regulations and will have a penalty of $2,000 fine. They will also be given an order to do it within a given number of days and if they don't, the penalty will be even more severe. It will be like (a maximum penalty of) $25,000 and also imprisonment. So I really hope that the people will comply and do so. The idea is if it is needed and when the system works smoothly, definitely we will contemplate that for those who don't comply they should not be working. That is the instruction we will be giving to the residential service operators. We will see how it goes. Anyway, this is the first time. The aim is in the long run it will be once every week and also only those having a valid negative test result will be able to go back to work.

Issued at HKT 15:27

Public hospitals daily update on COVID-19 cases

****

The following is issued on behalf of the Hospital Authority:

As at 9am today (November 29), 12 COVID-19 confirmed patients were discharged from hospital in the last 24 hours. So far, a total of 5 340 patients with confirmed or probable infection have been discharged.

At present, there are 619 negative pressure rooms in public hospitals with 1 137 negative pressure beds activated. A total of 642 confirmed patients are currently hospitalised in 20 public hospitals and community treatment facility, among which 11 patients are in critical condition, three are in serious condition and the remaining 628 patients are in stable condition.

The Hospital Authority will maintain close contact with the Centre for Health Protection to monitor the latest developments and to inform the public and healthcare workers on the latest information in a timely manner.

Details of the above-mentioned patients are as follows:

Patient condition	Case numbers
Discharged	5398, 5426, 5459, 5492, 5501, 5546, 5558, 5565, 5567, 5576, 5706, 5764
Critical	1989, 3496, 4833, 5110, 5185, 5409, 5511, 5723, 5735, 5739, 5745
Serious	5273, 5439, 5713

Issued at HKT 17:41

Government announces suspension of face-to-face classes
****

Further to the Government's earlier separate announcements on suspension of face-to-face classes and school activities for all kindergartens and Primary 1 to Primary 3 levels of primary schools until December 6, the Government announced today (November 29) that in light of the worsening situation of the COVID-19 epidemic, all kindergartens as well as primary and secondary schools (including special schools and schools offering non-local curriculum) will suspend face-to-face classes and school activities starting from this Wednesday (December 2) until the beginning of school Christmas holidays. Private schools offering non-formal curriculum (commonly known as "tutorial schools") will suspend face-to-face classes for two weeks.

A spokesman for the Education Bureau (EDB) said, "The EDB has earlier discussed with the sector about the related arrangements, and understands that schools would need time to make preparations for face-to-face class suspension, including students' home learning arrangements, Primary 6 internal assessment for the purpose of Secondary School Places Allocation and the learning arrangements for graduate classes. We will issue a letter to inform schools of the details tomorrow so that schools can make advance preparations."

He added, "The EDB understands that the sector and parents are deeply concerned about the arrangements of the primary school internal assessment for the purpose of Secondary School Places Allocation and that Secondary 6 students have to face public examinations soon. With suspension of face-to-face classes and school activities, the EDB will discuss with the sector possible options to allow schools to consider arranging students of Primary 6 to take internal assessment for the purpose of Secondary School Places Allocation and graduate classes to attend on-campus lessons to prepare for the public examinations or take internal examinations."

The EDB reminds schools of the related arrangements and measures that schools should implement during the period of suspension of face-to-face classes to sustain students' learning at home through flexible use of various learning modes. During such period, schools should remain open to take care of those students who have to go back to schools because of the lack of carers at home. They should arrange staff to be on duty to handle school affairs, answer parents' enquiries and take care of those students who have returned to schools. Schools should also ensure that the campus environment is clean and hygienic.

Parents should take precautionary measures for COVID-19 and pay close attention to the health conditions of their children. They should avoid bringing their children to crowded places with poor ventilation. Students should maintain a balanced diet, exercise regularly and take adequate rest in order to strengthen their immunity. If students are feeling unwell (even if the symptoms are very mild), they must not return to schools and should seek medical advice promptly to receive appropriate diagnoses and treatments.

Issued at HKT 18:57

Engineer of Transport Department tests positive for COVID-19

****

The Transport Department (TD) today (November 29) learnt that an engineer has tested positive for COVID-19.

The officer concerned works on 16/F, South Tower, West Kowloon Government Offices, 11 Hoi Ting Road, Yau Ma Tei, Kowloon. The floor concerned is not open to the public. She last performed duties on November 26.

She has no recent travel history, and has been wearing facial masks when performing duties. She followed relevant disease prevention measures at work. The TD will continue to closely co-operate with the Centre for Health Protection (CHP) on disease prevention measures. The workplace of the officer concerned, including the common areas, will be fully cleaned and sterilised in accordance with the guidelines of the CHP.

During the pandemic, the TD has been strictly implementing various disease prevention measures, including measuring the body temperature of people entering the buildings, providing facial masks and other personal protective equipment for staff, and requesting staff to wear facial masks when in contact with others and at public places. Cleaning and sterilising measures for the working environment of the department have also been stepped up. Staff have been reminded to pay attention to personal hygiene and to stay vigilant. They should seek medical advice immediately if feeling unwell.

The TD will continue to maintain close liaison with the CHP and co-operate with its quarantine work.

Issued at HKT 19:05

Government to gazette compulsory testing notice

****

The Government will exercise the power under the Prevention and Control of Disease (Compulsory Testing for Certain Persons) Regulation (Cap. 599J) and will publish in the Gazette a compulsory testing notice, which requires any person who had been present at three specified premises during the period from November 15 to 29 to undergo a COVID-19 nucleic acid test by December 3.

A spokesman for the Food and Health Bureau (FHB) said today (November 29), "The local epidemic situation is continuously worsening. The number of confirmed cases related to group gathering activities in indoor premises continues to rise significantly. Upon further contact tracing by the Centre for Health Protection, we found that some recently confirmed cases involved certain premises. Therefore, the Government will publish a compulsory testing notice, which requires persons who had been to three specified premises to undergo testing."

Details of the three specified premises are as follows:

1. Stellar House (Address: 3/F, Chuang's Enterprises Building, No. 382 Lockhart Road, Wan Chai)

2. Otto e Mezzo 8½ BOMBANA (Address: Shop No. 202, 2/F, Alexandra House, 18 Chater Road, Central)

3. Chuen Cheung Kui Restaurant (Sheung Wan) (Address: Shop C, G/F. & 1/F, Alliance Building, 130-136 Connaught Road Central, Sheung Wan)

Persons subject to compulsory testing may choose to undergo testing as below:

1. To obtain a deep throat saliva specimen collection pack from any of the 121 post offices or 47 designated general outpatient clinics (GOPCs) of the Hospital Authority (see the distribution points and time at www.hongkongpost.hk/en/about_us/network/SpecimenCollection/index.html#list and www.coronavirus.gov.hk/pdf/HA_clinics_submission_time_bilingual.pdf) and return the specimen to designated specimen collection points (see the specimen collection points and time at www.chp.gov.hk/files/pdf/list_of_collection_points_en.pdf and www.coronavirus.gov.hk/pdf/HA_clinics_submission_time_bilingual.pdf);

2. To self-arrange testing provided by private laboratories recognised by the Department of Health (see the list at www.coronavirus.gov.hk/pdf/List_of_recognised_laboratories_RTPCR.pdf);

3. To attend any Community Testing Centres (see the list at www.communitytest.gov.hk/en/);

4. To visit any mobile specimen collection stations (see the list at www.info.gov.hk/gia/general/202011/27/P2020112700934.htm) for testing; or

5. To undergo testing at any healthcare facilities of the Hospital Authority (including GOPCs and accident and emergency departments) as instructed by a medical professional of the Hospital Authority.

"If persons who are subject to compulsory testing have symptoms, they should seek medical attention immediately and undergo testing as instructed by a medical professional. They should not attend the Community Testing Centres."

Persons who are subject to compulsory testing must report the result of the test or submit the test report to the Government by phone (6275 6901), fax (2530 5872) or email (ct@csb.gov.hk) by December 6. If persons who are subject to compulsory testing have previously undergone the above mentioned test between November 24 and 29, they would be taken to have complied with the requirements set out in the compulsory testing notice.

The spokesman said, "To reduce transmission risk, persons who underwent testing are advised to stay at home and avoid going out when waiting for test results."

Any enquiries on compulsory testing arrangements may be addressed to the hotline at 6275 6901 which operates daily from 9am to 6pm. If persons who are subject to compulsory testing plan to conduct testing at any of the Community Testing Centres, they can check the centre's appointment status in advance. The hotlines of the Community Testing Centres are at www.communitytest.gov.hk/en/info/ .

The Government will continue to trace possibly infected persons who had been to the relevant venues, and seriously verify whether they had complied with the testing notice. Any person who fails to comply with the testing notice commits an offence and may be fined a fixed penalty of $2,000. The person would also be issued with a compulsory testing order requiring him/her to undergo testing within a specified timeframe. Failure to comply with the order is an offence and the offender would be liable to a fine at level 4 ($25,000) and imprisonment for six months.

The spokesman said, "The Government urges all individuals who are in doubt about their own health conditions, or individuals with infection risks (such as individuals who visited places with epidemic outbreaks or contacted confirmed cases) to undergo testing promptly for early identification of infected persons. The FHB will publish compulsory testing notices regarding particular groups when necessary taking into account the epidemic development and the testing participation rate."

Issued at HKT 22:30

AFCD staff tests positive for COVID-19

****

The Agriculture, Fisheries and Conservation Department (AFCD) said that a staff member had tested positive for the coronavirus disease 2019 (COVID-19) on November 28.

A spokesman for the AFCD said, "The staff worked at the Tung Chung Au Country Park Management Centre on Lantau Island and mainly performed general cleansing duties inside the Centre without contact with members of the public while at work. She last performed her duties on November 24 and has no recent travel history. She wore surgical masks while performing her duties and properly maintained social distancing with people she had contacted. Her body temperature was normal when undergoing temperature screening during work."

The spokesman noted that the AFCD would cooperate with the Centre for Health Protection (CHP) in the epidemiological investigation and arrange other staff working with the affected to take COVID-19 tests. The concerned work place will also be thoroughly cleaned and sterilised. The management centre in question will be closed until further notice. Visitors to the country park will not be affected.

The AFCD has all along been concerned about the COVID-19 epidemic. Relevant hygienic measures for infectious diseases provided by the CHP have been strictly observed. All staff have their body temperatures checked before performing their duties, and wear proper personal protective equipment.

The department will continue to step up cleaning and sterilising all work locations and remind all staff to strictly comply with the hygienic measures for infectious diseases provided by the CHP. Should they feel unwell, medical advice should be sought.

Issued at HKT 23:15

CHP investigates 115 additional confirmed cases of COVID-19

****

The Centre for Health Protection (CHP) of the Department of Health has announced that as of 0.00am, November 29, the CHP was investigating 115 additional confirmed cases of coronavirus disease 2019 (COVID-19), taking the number of cases to 6 239 in Hong Kong so far (comprising 6 238 confirmed cases and one probable case).

Among the newly reported cases announced, six had a travel history during the incubation period.

A total of 679 cases have been recorded in the past 14 days (November 15 – 28), including 590 local cases of which 120 are from unknown sources.

The CHP's epidemiological investigations and relevant contact tracing on the confirmed cases are ongoing. For case details and contact tracing information, please see the Annex One or the list of buildings with confirmed cases of COVID-19 in the past 14 days and the latest local situation of COVID-19 available on the website "COVID-19 Thematic Website" (www.coronavirus.gov.hk).

As a number of cases confirmed recently claimed that they had visited venues for dancing or singing, bars or gyms, and food premises, the CHP reminded those who had visited the specified venues (Annex Two) under the Prevention and Control of Disease (Compulsory Testing for Certain Persons) Regulation (Cap. 599J) to receive COVID-19 nucleic acid test according to the compulsory testing notice. The public are also urged to seek medical attention early if symptoms develop.

In view of the severe epidemic situation, the CHP called on members of the public to avoid going out, having social contact and dining out. They should put on a surgical mask and maintain stringent hand hygiene when they need to go out. The CHP strongly urged the elderly to stay home as far as possible and avoid going out. They should consider asking their family and friends to help with everyday tasks such as shopping for basic necessities.

The spokesman said, "Given that the situation of COVID-19 infection remains severe and that there is a continuous increase in the number of cases reported around the world, members of the public are strongly urged to avoid all non-essential travel outside Hong Kong.

"The CHP also strongly urges the public to maintain at all times strict personal and environmental hygiene, which is key to personal protection against infection and prevention of the spread of the disease in the community. On a personal level, members of the public should wear a surgical mask when having respiratory symptoms, taking public transport or staying in crowded places. They should also perform hand hygiene frequently, especially before touching the mouth, nose or eyes.

"As for household environmental hygiene, members of the public are advised to maintain drainage pipes properly, regularly pour water into drain outlets (U-traps) and cover all floor drain outlets when they are not in use. After using the toilet, they should put the toilet lid down before flushing to avoid spreading germs."

Moreover, the Government has launched the website "COVID-19 Thematic Website" (www.coronavirus.gov.hk) for announcing the latest updates on various news on COVID-19 infection and health advice to help the public understand the latest updates. Members of the public may also gain access to information via the COVID-19 WhatsApp Helpline launched by the Office of the Government Chief Information Officer. Simply by saving 9617 1823 in their phone contacts or clicking the link wa.me/85296171823?text=hi, they will be able to obtain information on COVID-19 as well as the "StayHomeSafe" mobile app and wristband via WhatsApp.

Issued at HKT 23:58

November 30[61]

[61] https://www.info.gov.hk/gia/general/202011/30.htm

Public hospitals daily update on COVID-19 cases

****

The following is issued on behalf of the Hospital Authority:

As at 9am today (November 30), four COVID-19 confirmed patients were discharged from hospital in the last 24 hours. So far, a total of 5 344 patients with confirmed or probable infection have been discharged.

At present, there are 625 negative pressure rooms in public hospitals with 1 161 negative pressure beds activated. A total of 752 confirmed patients are currently hospitalised in 21 public hospitals and community treatment facility, among which 11 patients are in critical condition, five are in serious condition and the remaining 736 patients are in stable condition.

The Hospital Authority will maintain close contact with the Centre for Health Protection to monitor the latest developments and to inform the public and healthcare workers on the latest information in a timely manner.

Details of the above-mentioned patients are as follows:

Patient condition	Case numbers
Discharged	5554, 5878, 6096, 6101
Critical	1989, 3496, 4833, 5110, 5185, 5409, 5511, 5723, 5735, 5739, 5745
Serious	5273, 5439, 5607, 5713, 5987

Issued at HKT 18:56

Latest arrangements for Hongkong Post services

****

In view of the Government's announcement made today (November 30) on the special work arrangements for government employees, Hongkong Post announced the arrangements for Hongkong Post services starting from tomorrow (December 1).

To strike a balance between the public demand for counter services of post offices and the need to reduce the epidemic from further spreading in the community as far as possible, all post offices will maintain their normal opening hours from Monday to Friday while their closing hours will be advanced to 4pm; business hours on Saturdays will remain the same (General Post Office and Tsim Sha Tsui Post Office will advance their closing hours to 4pm). Mobile post offices will be suspended from service.

Mail collection from posting boxes and mail delivery service (including that for Speedpost items) will remain normal. For buildings with COVID-19 confirmed cases within the past 14 days, Hongkong Post will maintain the service of mail delivery to the letter boxes in the lobbies for three times a week, yet door delivery service will remain suspended until the building concerned is removed from the list of buildings with confirmed cases within the past 14 days.

Hongkong Post will continue to adopt various measures on social distancing and infection control at all post offices, and provide frontline staff with protective gear such as face shields, protective goggles, masks, alcohol swabs, alcohol-based handrub and gloves.

Due to the adjustment of business hours of post offices, members of the public requiring counter services may expect longer waiting times. During this period, services of local, inbound and outbound mail will be subject to delay. Hongkong Post apologises for the inconvenience caused.

Hongkong Post will keep abreast of the situation and the latest announcement of the Government and make timely adjustments. For further enquiry, please call the Hongkong Post enquiry hotline at 2921 2222.

Issued at HKT 19:30

DH's Oral Maxillofacial Surgery and Dental Clinic of Pamela Youde Nethersole Eastern Hospital and Chai Wan Government Dental Clinic to undergo disinfection tomorrow

****

The Department of Health announced today (November 30) that its Oral Maxillofacial Surgery and Dental Clinic of Pamela Youde Nethersole Eastern Hospital (OMS&DC PYNEH) learned that a patient who tested positive for COVID-19 had earlier visited the premises for treatment. As the OMS&DC PYNEH and Chai Wan Government Dental Clinic (CWGDC) share a common waiting area, based on public health considerations, both clinics will undergo a thorough cleaning and disinfection tomorrow (December 1). Service appointments at the

OMS&DC will be suspended while the CWGDC will be closed. Affected clients will be contacted to reschedule their service appointments.

The client visited the OMS&DC on November 26 and had a mask on while waiting for treatment. The client subsequently tested positive for the COVID-19 infection on November 28. The staff attending were wearing masks with suitable protective equipment. At present, no staff members have developed symptoms, nor are confirmed cases at either clinic.

In view of the current epidemic situation, dental clinics have stepped up infection control measures, including temperature screening for all visitors before clinic entry and conducting a health declaration. Dental services have been strictly implementing various disease prevention measures during the epidemic, which include providing employees with masks and other protective equipment, and stepping up cleaning and sanitising measures of the clinics. All dental services' staff members are wearing masks at work and practising hand hygiene at all times. The DH is highly concerned about the COVID-19 situation and has reminded all staff again to maintain personal hygiene and be vigilant at all times.

Issued at HKT 20:00

FEHD reminds catering business operators and public again to continue complying with anti-epidemic regulations

****

In view of the COVID-19 epidemic situation, to minimise the risk of the spread of the virus, the Food and Environmental Hygiene Department (FEHD) today (November 30) reminded again catering business operators to strictly comply with the requirements and directions under the Prevention and Control of Disease (Requirements and Directions) (Business and Premises) Regulation (Cap. 599F), and the public to comply with the various restrictions in relation to group gatherings and mask-wearing under the anti-epidemic regulations and directions when patronising catering premises.

The FEHD also reminded persons responsible for carrying on catering businesses and scheduled premises in operation that, according to the directions issued by the Secretary for Food and Health, they must apply for a "LeaveHomeSafe" venue QR code from the Government website "LeaveHomeSafe" on or before December 2 (Wednesday), and display the QR code obtained at the entrance of the premises or at a conspicuous position within two working days upon receipt of the QR code.

An FEHD spokesman said, "To facilitate persons in charge of catering premises (including bars/pubs, night establishments/night clubs and karaoke establishments), places of public entertainment, private swimming pools and commercial bathhouses who have not yet applied for the 'LeaveHomeSafe' venue QR code, the FEHD and the Office of the Government Chief Information Officer have made special arrangements to simplify the application procedures and expedite the completion of the workflow. Applicants can enter the webpage 'Apply QR code for Catering and Scheduled Premises under Cap. 599F' of the 'LeaveHomeSafe' dedicated website (www.leavehomesafe.gov.hk/en/registration/599F/), fill in the licence number of the related FEHD licence and then verify the relevant information including the shop's name and address. If the information is correct, the 'LeaveHomeSafe' venue QR Code can then be downloaded and saved immediately. For premises which are not able to use the simplified procedures, applicants can follow the instructions on the webpage to submit their applications through the existing venue registration function."

The spokesman stressed that the FEHD will continue to step up inspections and take enforcement actions against offenders, to ensure that persons responsible for carrying on catering businesses and scheduled premises and the public strictly comply with relevant regulations so as to minimise the risk of transmission of COVID-19.

Issued at HKT 20:10

Alice Ho Miu Ling Nethersole Hospital announces a preliminary positive case of COVID-19

****

The following is issued on behalf of the Hospital Authority:

The spokesperson for the Alice Ho Miu Ling Nethersole Hospital made the following announcement today (November 30) regarding a preliminary positive case of COVID-19:

A 69-year-old male patient attended Accident & Emergency Department (A&E) yesterday (November 29) afternoon with fever and pneumonia symptoms. Since the patient had no contact history with COVID-19 confirmed cases, the healthcare staff conducted clinical examination and provided him with high-flow oxygen therapy in the A&E consultation room.

The patient was subsequently transferred to the isolation ward for further treatment and specimen was collected for COVID-19 test. In the early hours today, it was learnt that he had been preliminarily tested positive for COVID-19.

Upon knowing the patient's test result, the hospital Infection Control Unit conducted contact tracing for the healthcare workers and patients who had been in contact with the patient. Five patients who stayed in the same A&E fever cubicle with the patient concerned have been classified as close contacts. Their COVID-19 test results are negative and have been arranged for isolation treatment.

Meanwhile, nine A&E staff members who had not been wearing appropriate personal protective equipment (PPE) while in contact with the patient were also classified as close contacts. COVID-19 test were arranged for them, all results are negative and they have been arranged for quarantine. As a precautionary measure, the hospital has arranged another 16 A&E staff who were on duty on that day to conduct COVID-19 test. 15 of them are tested negative and the test result of the remaining staff is still pending.

The hospital has arranged thorough cleansing and disinfection in the A&E Department and will continue to closely monitor the health of our staff and patients and communicate with the Centre for Health Protection on the latest situation.

All healthcare workers are reminded to wear full PPE when performing high-risk medical procedures.

Issued at HKT 21:09

Specifications under Prevention and Control of Disease (Regulation of Cross-boundary Conveyances and Travellers) Regulation to be gazetted

****

In view of the global development and severity of the COVID-19 pandemic situation, the Government announced today (November 30) that it will gazette the specifications under the Prevention and Control of Disease (Regulation of Cross-boundary Conveyances and Travellers) Regulation (Cap. 599H) to include Romania as a specified place starting from December 7 to more effectively combat the epidemic.

A spokesman for the Food and Health Bureau said, "The global pandemic situation is becoming increasingly severe. The daily number of new cases increased from around 70 000 to 100 000 between late March and mid-May, and further increased to reach a new height of around 660 000 in mid-November. In view of the severe global pandemic situation, Hong Kong cannot afford to drop its guard on entry prevention and control measures."

Travellers who visited very high-risk places

The Government has earlier introduced Cap. 599H to impose testing and quarantine conditions on travellers coming to Hong Kong from very high-risk places to reduce the health risk they may bring to Hong Kong. The Secretary for Food and Health (SFH) has previously published in the Gazette specifications on the relevant measures applicable to 17 specified places (i.e. Bangladesh, Belgium, Ecuador, Ethiopia, France, Germany, India, Indonesia, Kazakhstan, Nepal, Pakistan, the Philippines, Russia, South Africa, Turkey, the United Kingdom and the United States of America) and adjusted the relevant conditions having regard to the circumstances on the ground since the implementation of the regulation.

Taking into account the latest public health risk assessment, and the changes and developments of the epidemic situation, the SFH will publish in the Gazette new specifications to maintain the conditions imposed and to include Romania as a specified place. The relevant specifications will come into effect on December 7 and remain until further notice.

According to the latest specifications, a traveller who, on the day on which the traveller boarded a civil aviation aircraft that arrives at, or is about to arrive at, Hong Kong (specified aircraft), or during the 14 days before that day, has stayed in one of the aforementioned specified places must provide the following documents:

(1) A test report in English or Chinese issued by a laboratory or healthcare institution bearing the name of the relevant traveller from the aforementioned specified places identical to that in his or her valid travel document to show that:

(a) the relevant traveller from the aforementioned specified places underwent a nucleic acid test for COVID-19, the sample for which was taken from the relevant traveller from the aforementioned specified places within 72 hours before the scheduled time of departure of the specified aircraft;

(b) the test conducted on the sample is a nucleic acid test for COVID-19; and

(c) the result of the test is that the relevant traveller from the aforementioned specified places was tested negative for COVID-19; and

(2) If the relevant report is not in English or Chinese or does not contain all of the above information, a written confirmation in English or Chinese issued by the laboratory or healthcare institution bearing the name of the relevant traveller from the aforementioned specified places identical to that in his or her valid travel document and setting out all of the above information. The said written confirmation should be presented together with the test report; and

(3) Documentary proof in English or Chinese to show that the laboratory or healthcare institution is ISO 15189 accredited or is recognised or approved by the relevant authority of the government of the place in which the laboratory or healthcare institution is located; and

(4) The relevant traveller from the aforementioned specified places has confirmation in English or Chinese of room reservation in a hotel in Hong Kong for not less than 14 nights starting on the day of the arrival in Hong Kong of the relevant traveller from the aforementioned specified places.

Travellers who visited any country outside China

The spokesman reminded with effect from November 13, 2020, a traveller who, on the day on which the traveller boarded a specified aircraft, or during the 14 days before that day, has stayed in a specified place outside China (excluding very high-risk areas specified otherwise), must provide confirmation in English or Chinese of room reservation in a hotel in Hong Kong for not less than 14 nights starting on the day of the arrival in Hong Kong of the relevant traveller from the rest of the world.

The operator of the specified aircraft should submit to the Department of Health (DH) before the specified aircraft arrives at Hong Kong a document in a form specified by the DH confirming that each relevant traveller from the rest of the world has, before being checked in for the flight to Hong Kong on the aircraft, produced for boarding on the aircraft the above document.

A person who is in transit in Hong Kong, a person exempted by the Chief Secretary for Administration from compulsory quarantine under section 4(1) of either the Compulsory Quarantine of Certain Persons Arriving at Hong Kong Regulation (Cap. 599C) or the Compulsory Quarantine of Persons Arriving at Hong Kong from Foreign Places Regulation (Cap. 599E), and a person who arrives at Hong Kong from Singapore and meets all conditions specified for Singapore as a Category 2 specified foreign place by the SFH under section 12(2) of Cap. 599E will not be affected.

Government continues to strengthen law enforcement

If any condition specified by the SFH is not met in relation to any relevant traveller on the conveyance, each of the operators of the conveyance commits an offence and is liable on conviction to the maximum penalty of a fine at level 5 ($50,000) and imprisonment for six months. If an operator fails to comply with a requirement to provide information, or knowingly or recklessly provides any information that is false or misleading in a material particular, he or she is liable on conviction to the maximum penalty of a fine at level 5 ($50,000) and imprisonment for six months.

As for travellers, if a traveller coming to Hong Kong fails to comply with a requirement to provide information, or knowingly or recklessly provides any information that is false or misleading in a material particular, he or she is liable on conviction to the maximum penalty of a fine at level 3 ($10,000) and imprisonment for six months.

Travellers to Hong Kong should note that they will be mandated to wait for their test results at a designated location after their deep throat saliva samples are collected for conducting testing for COVID-19 at the DH's Temporary Specimen Collection Centre pursuant to the Prevention and Control of Disease Regulation (Cap. 599A). If their test results are negative, they will be allowed to go to the hotel for which they made the reservation to continue the 14-day compulsory quarantine until completion. If their results are positive, the travellers will be transferred to hospital for isolation and treatment.

The Government will continue to monitor closely the situation including the developments of the epidemic situation both globally and locally and changes in the volume of cross-boundary passenger traffic, and will not hesitate to adopt more resolute and severe measures as and when necessary.

Issued at HKT 21:11

Transcript of remarks of press conference

****

The Chief Executive, Mrs Carrie Lam, held a press conference this afternoon (November 30). Also joining were the Secretary for Food and Health, Professor Sophia Chan; the Permanent Secretary for Food and Health (Health), Mr Thomas Chan; the Director of Health, Dr Constance Chan; and the Chief Executive of the Hospital Authority, Dr Tony Ko, Following is the transcript of remarks of the press conference.

Reporter: You've repeatedly said that infection control measures should be taken quickly, so why didn't the Government tighten these restrictions last week when the number of confirmed cases was clearly picking up? Secondly, you talked about the plan to increase the amount of fine for breaching some of the infection control measures. Why do you think there is a need to step up these penalties? Would you consider imposing a jail sentence for these offences? Thirdly, you also talked about setting up a hotline for people to report breaches of the social distancing measures. Do you think that it would be healthy for people to live in a society where people constantly monitor one another? Are you worried that people may abuse the system?

Chief Executive: Three questions. First of all, I have explained that this new wave of COVID-19 has hit Hong Kong very quickly, from around November 19 or 20, and every day we have been monitoring the situation. We have already announced measures that we have adopted in the past to deal with this pandemic. I wouldn't say that we have reacted too slowly. If you ask me, individual measures have been introduced in the same manner, or even in an accelerated manner than the previous wave, if you take individual measures. We are now closing almost everything except the restaurants because they are meeting the daily needs of the people. We are allowing a little bit of gym activities because people need this sort of thing to keep themselves healthy, whether it is physically or mentally. If I may just make a plea, it's very easy for an observer to say after the event that you should have done this earlier. If you are in the midst of the pandemic, you have to assess the situation and you have to introduce measures based on science and effectiveness, and of course the ability to undertake those measures.

The second thing about fine. Why do we need a fine? This is a very good question. If everybody is very concerned about the health of themselves, of Hong Kong people; if everybody wants to eradicate this wave as soon as possible, there is no need for any fines. People will self-behave, or self-discipline. Unfortunately, and maybe to a certain extent understandably, because of the fatigue associated with this prolonged period of pandemic - it's now almost one year - you have seen,- I have seen, reporters have taken a lot of photos and put on their front pages about

Hong Kong people ignoring the various regulations. They went out in groups, they did not wear their mask, they continued to enjoy themselves in parties. Even if party rooms were closed, they went to other private places to have parties. They danced in close contact. That is when we decided that perhaps the $2,000 fine at the moment does not serve the purpose of deterring people from this sort of activities, so we need to raise the fine. You can see in other places they also resort to fines. Fortunately, we have not seen some of the reactions that we have seen in some European cities, that is, people got so fed up that they went out to protest on human rights grounds, that they no longer accept the Government's restrictions on social distancing. I don't think Hong Kong will reach that stage. I still have confidence that the great majority of Hong Kong people are very sensible and very pragmatic. They want to help control this pandemic. But for some, you still need some instruments to deter them from doing this sort of behaviour.

A hotline is a hotline. The Government has all sorts of hotlines for members of the public to shoulder their civic responsibility to tell government departments that they suspect there are certain irregularities going on here and there. Then they report to us. Our enforcement colleagues will go there to investigate and to see whether there is indeed an irregularity that requires some actions to be taken. I hope people will not overreact. This is not sort of monitoring people and so on. People are jointly shouldering part of the responsibility, given the very serious pandemic situation that we are now facing. Thank you.

Secretary for Food and Health: Thank you, Chief Executive. I want to supplement in terms of the restrictions or tightening of social distancing measures. If you remember way back in September, we have already alerted the public that in winter there will be another wave coming, and that is something what we probably cannot avoid and is inevitable. So, we have been all along, together with the Department of Health and also the Hospital Authority, been preparing for something coming in winter. That's number one. Secondly, we talk about in November (when we) started (tightening the measures) even before the dancing groups have come into notice by the Department of Health. Since November 14 till now, this is already the fourth time that we are tightening the social distancing measures. We have (announced to) tighten the social distancing measures on November 14, 21 and 24. We are trying to be sophisticated and precise in terms of our social distancing measures. But, in terms of preparing for this wave, not only are we doing social distancing measures, we are also building our capacity, for example, in testing. That's why we are now rolling out different community testing centres, four (centres) in phase one, and then five (more centres). We will be rolling out further testing centres in the community, so that we can expand our testing. And also for border control measures, they are as important as restricting movement in the community because we want to prevent imported cases from bringing virus into the community. So, again, if you notice in the past few weeks, we have been issuing notices and we have been (adopting) different measures in tightening our border control measures. Thank you.

Reporter: Hi, Mrs Lam. Firstly, can I ask you about, you have asked for the tolerance of the general public to support the raft of measures that you've introduced today, and you've said that some of the measures are going back to the toughest period that we've seen before, in July for example, would you also offer the same amount of support – the maximum level of support to citizens who are following your policies, like closing down of premises etc? And perhaps give them the third round of Employment Support Scheme that people are facing with this policy? If not, what do you think the economic cost to them would be? Secondly, given some research has shown that the fourth wave of the epidemic has been caused by a new strain of virus being brought by travellers coming back from Nepal, who may have been quarantining at home, and also the fact that some dance studios were not actually covered in the original (Cap.599F) scheduled premises, do you feel you bear any responsibility for this oversight and for allowing this situation to happen, in other words, for the fourth wave that has come today? Thirdly, can I also ask you if it is still your intention to reopen borders with Mainland China in the New Year, given the latest situation? And given the latest situation, would you actually consider, for example, stopping Return2hk Scheme and stopping the flow of people from Mainland China and Macao without quarantine, in order to further curb the epidemic? Thank you.

Chief Executive: Thank you for the three questions. First question, I have actually answered. Since February this year, that is since the 2020-21 Budget and the three rounds of Anti-Epidemic Fund measures, the Government has already committed some $310 billion, that is over 10 per cent of our Gross Domestic Product. The Financial Secretary is projecting a deficit of over $300 billion this year. The public finance situation is equally very dire, as in the case of the pandemic situation. We fully understand the economic trauma experienced by some of the sectors, for example tourism, that's why I have offered in my 2020 Policy Address about $600 million to help the tourism sector, which has no business for over a year. It is not just COVID-19, they have not had businesses since the social unrest last year, so after a lot of soul-searching, we have identified this being the most hard-hit sector we will need to help. But at the moment, as I said, we are more focused on tackling the COVID-19 pandemic, we have no plans yet to do another round of relief measures which will incur quite significant public sector expenditure.

About the cause of the fourth wave or the cause of any outbreak in society, there are a lot of reasons, but I hope you understand that Hong Kong is not being singled out as a city that continuously face a wave after wave. Globally, I think we are still in the worst situation – "we" means the world except our country, Mainland China and Macao. The world is facing a worsening situation continuously. I think it has now been over 60 million cases and many cities in Europe have gone into complete city lockdown again, so your same question could be pointed to all those country government leaders. To be fair to Hong Kong, we are not doing bad at all. If you look at some of the statistics in terms of number of people confirmed per one million population, we are about 800; globally, that figure is about 8 000. Compared to the world, we are nine over 10 better if you put it that way. In terms of death, we are about 15 per one million population. If you look at the US, if you look at the UK and other countries, we are only a fraction of that. And on top of that, we manage through our strategy to allow the city to continue to operate. We never have a complete lockdown or "stay home" that creates a huge trauma on the economy and on individuals. I think as reporters you too should feel that we are not doing bad and you should promote that Hong Kong after all is not doing bad. Because we are such an open and free society, we cannot seal off the airport and the land borders for Hong Kong people not to come back. Now I got another wave of Hong Kong students who need to come back. Can I deny them from coming back? What will be the local reaction if they are not allowed to come back? All these are very practical issues that any government or any government leader has to seriously consider.

My message to you is Hong Kong is not doing bad. Please bear that in mind and try to tell exactly the Hong Kong story. But we can do better. I have said many times that in fighting an epidemic, there is no perfect solution. We need to continue to find the best solution to deal with the situation of the day. And now when we saw that the fourth wave was here and was likely to get worse - it's actually not as bad as late July yet when we have a peak of 148 cases a day - but with the anticipation of the worsening of situation, we should go back to the tight, the toughest measures that we have ever introduced. When you talk about the dance studios, everybody could rent a place in Hong Kong and start some dance tutorials. I am afraid we do not have a regulatory regime, but after this COVID-19, we may. I may ask for research and review on whether we should further regulate such activities happening in some of the premises. If you ask yourself, if there is one case of infection, either imported or local that has gone into community, if every member of community sticks to the rules of wearing a mask, no close contact, no social gathering and stays home as far as possible, we would not have seen this major cluster involving over 500 confirmed cases and more to come. So, do you want to blame the Hong Kong people as well? Let's face it. Now is not the time for argument. Now is not the time for blaming which party. This is a time for solidarity. This is a time for working together and make sure that Hong Kong will face the least trauma in this round of the pandemic.

On the final question, again, I have said on many occasions that we should build our strategy and measures on the basis of science. The Mainland of China and Macao are now almost free of cases, such a vast country has only a dozen of imported cases and episodic isolated cases here and there which they manage to stamp out in pretty short time. If you look at science, I have quoted you many figures previously. We have Cap. 599C which imposes quarantine orders on people from Mainland, Macao and Taiwan. We have a Cap. 599E imposing the same quarantine arrangement on people from overseas for nine to 10 months now. Over 300 000 quarantine orders have been issued for people coming in from Mainland China and Macao under Cap. 599C. Not a single confirmed case has been identified. This is very good scientific evidence that that place is very safe. When that place is very safe and we have thousands of Hong Kong people who have been stranded for months who want to come back to see a doctor to refill their drugs and to do some essential personal things, could I be that heartless to turn them away when the science is for them to come in? So, we have arranged for this scheme for them to come in but under certain precautions. They still have to get a negative COVID-19 test and we allow them to come in. My latest information is over 5 000 Hong Kong people have benefited from that measure, which means at least 5 000 families have addressed some of their problems because of the separation. For all of us sitting here as government officials, any decision we take is taken in the public interest for the people of Hong Kong. There is no question of suspecting that we were doing otherwise. Thank you very much.

Issued at HKT 22:06

CHP investigates 76 additional confirmed cases of COVID-19

****

The Centre for Health Protection (CHP) of the Department of Health announced that as of 0.00am, November 30, the CHP was investigating 76 additional confirmed cases of coronavirus disease 2019 (COVID-19), taking the number of cases to 6 315 in Hong Kong so far (comprising 6 314 confirmed cases and one probable case).

Among the newly reported cases announced, eight had a travel history during the incubation period.

A total of 780 cases have been recorded in the past 14 days (November 16 – 29), including 694 local cases of which 143 are from unknown sources.

The CHP's epidemiological investigations and relevant contact tracing on the confirmed cases are ongoing. For case details and contact tracing information, please see Annex One or the list of buildings with confirmed cases of COVID-19 in the past 14 days and the latest local situation of COVID-19 available on the website "COVID-19 Thematic Website" (www.coronavirus.gov.hk).

As a number of cases confirmed recently claimed that they had visited venues for dancing or singing, bars or gyms, and food premises, the CHP reminded those who had visited the specified venues (Annex Two) under the Prevention and Control of Disease (Compulsory Testing for Certain Persons) Regulation (Cap. 599J) to receive COVID-19 nucleic acid test according to the compulsory testing notice. The public are also urged to seek medical attention early if symptoms develop.

In view of the severe epidemic situation, the CHP called on members of the public to avoid going out, having social contact and dining out. They should put on a surgical mask and maintain stringent hand hygiene when they need to go out. The CHP strongly urged the elderly to stay home as far as possible and avoid going out. They should consider asking their family and friends to help with everyday tasks such as shopping for basic necessities.

In view of the latest epidemic developments in the Mainland, the previous arrangement to provide specimen collection containers to inbound travellers arriving via land boundary control points who have been to Shandong Province in the past 14 days will be cancelled from tomorrow (December 1). These travellers, if they are not exempted persons, are subject to compulsory quarantine for 14 days at a designated place (home or other accommodation) upon arrival in Hong Kong. For the arrangement of distributing specimen collection containers to inbound travellers who have been to Xinjiang, Shanghai, Tianjin and Inner Mongolia in the past 14 days arriving via land boundary control points, which has come into effect earlier, remains unchanged.

The spokesman said, "Given that the situation of COVID-19 infection remains severe and that there is a continuous increase in the number of cases reported around the world, members of the public are strongly urged to avoid all non-essential travel outside Hong Kong.

"The CHP also strongly urges the public to maintain at all times strict personal and environmental hygiene, which is key to personal protection against infection and prevention of the spread of the disease in the community. On a personal level, members of the public should wear a surgical mask when having respiratory symptoms, taking public transport or staying in crowded places. They should also perform hand hygiene frequently, especially before touching the mouth, nose or eyes.

"As for household environmental hygiene, members of the public are advised to maintain drainage pipes properly, regularly pour water into drain outlets (U-traps) and cover all floor drain outlets when they are not in use. After using the toilet, they should put the toilet lid down before flushing to avoid spreading germs."

Moreover, the Government has launched the website "COVID-19 Thematic Website" (www.coronavirus.gov.hk) for announcing the latest updates on various news on COVID-19 infection and health advice to help the public understand the latest updates. Members of the public may also gain access to information via the COVID-19 WhatsApp Helpline launched by the Office of the Government Chief Information Officer. Simply by saving 9617 1823 in their phone contacts or clicking the link wa.me/85296171823?text=hi, they will be able to obtain information on COVID-19 as well as the "StayHomeSafe" mobile app and wristband via WhatsApp.

Issued at HKT 23:20

www.ingramcontent.com/pod-product-compliance
Ingram Content Group UK Ltd.
Pitfield, Milton Keynes, MK11 3LW, UK
HW061707190726
53UKWH00008B/2445